Cooking for Halflings & Monsters: Volume 3

Celebrating Comfy, Cozy Foods from North America

Astrid Tuttle Winegar

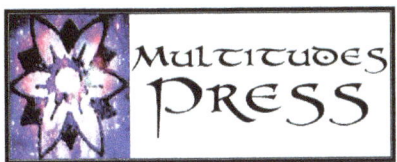

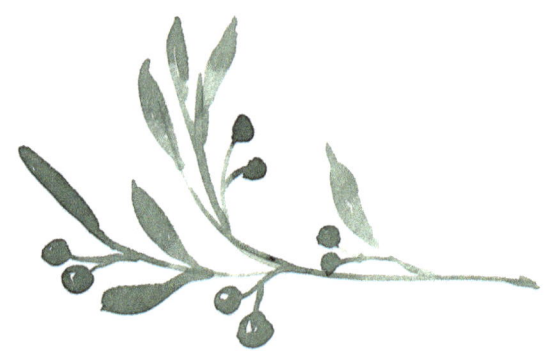

Cooking for Halflings & Monsters, Volume 3:
Celebrating Comfy, Cozy Foods from North America

Copyright © 2024 Astrid Tuttle Winegar

All rights reserved. No part of this book may be used or reproduced in any manner whatsoever, including internet usage, without written permission from the author, except in the case of brief quotations embedded in critical articles and reviews.

First edition © 2024
First printing

Paperback edition: 978-0-9994179-4-2
Ebook edition: 978-0-9994179-5-9

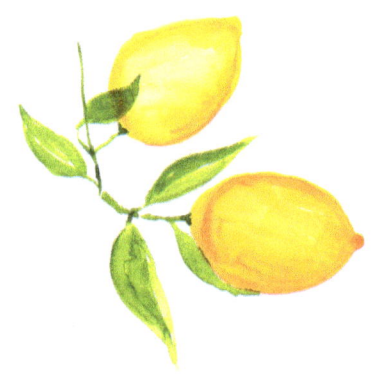

Printed in U.S.A.
Graphics © 2020 Opia Designs | Design Cuts
Graphics © 2024 Shutterstock
Photographs © 2024 Astrid Tuttle Winegar
Cover Design © 2024 Astrid Tuttle Winegar
Author Photo © 2024 Kate the Photographer

For more information, please see: astridwinegar.com.

DEDICATION

BEGIN: MARCH 10, 2020

(Approximately 3,900 Americans have died from COVID-19 as of this date, according to Johns Hopkins University.)

Though most of these recipes have been prepared in my kitchen for many years, I actually started typing them on my computer during the novel coronavirus (COVID-19) pandemic of 2020. New Mexico was one of the first states to institute a stay-at-home regimen, thanks to the quick thinking of our governor at the time. So, Americans (and others, of course) ended up with lots of time on their hands.

Not all of it involved Netflix (there was also plenty of Hulu, Disney+, Peacock, Max, and the inevitable viewing of older DVDs).

Not all of us wrote plays such as *King Lear* (which William Shakespeare supposedly accomplished during some plague quarantine or other...).

Not all of us were up to the challenge of restaging photos of famous works of art with items found in our attics and basements, toy chests and closets.

But many of us were grateful for the incredible sacrifices of healthcare professionals around the globe. They sacrificed their time and their health, and some of them sacrificed their lives, while fighting this vicious virus.

This cookbook is dedicated to those heroes. In your own search for heroes, look no further than your own community. They sacrificed for all of us.

END: MARCH 10, 2023

(Approximately 1,123,836 Americans have died from COVID-19 as of this date, according to Johns Hopkins University.)

TABLE OF CONTENTS

INTRODUCTION | I

    Garnishes & Photography | ii
        Nice New Mexican & Mexican Garnishes | ii
    Substitutions & Altitude | iv
    Vegetarian & Meat-Lovers Options and/or Substitutions | v
    Green Chile & Other Hot Stuff | v
    Seasoning, Salt, and Butter | vi
    Just one more thing… | vii
    My Biography | vii

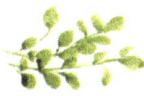

A FEW ESSENTIALS | XI

    Dry Seasoning Mixes | xi
    Magical, Mythical Garlic | xvii
    A Couple of Baking Essentials | xix
    Chile (NOT the country…) | xxiii
    Chile Pepper Protocols | xxiv
    Roasted Green Chile | xxv

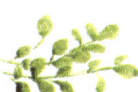

CHAPTER ONE—NEW YEAR'S EVE & DAY | 1

CHAPTER TWO—HALFLING HAPPY HOUR | 17

CHAPTER THREE—SUPER BOWL | 45

CHAPTER FOUR—COLD SALADS | 55

CHAPTER FIVE—VALENTINE'S DAY | 71

CHAPTER SIX—HOT SIDES | 83

CHAPTER SEVEN—CINCO DE MAYO | 99

CHAPTER EIGHT—LUNCHY STUFF | 111

CHAPTER NINE—THE FOURTH OF JULY | 137

CHAPTER TEN—MAIN EVENTS | 151

CHAPTER ELEVEN—THANKSGIVING | 181

CHAPTER TWELVE—PASTA | 213

CHAPTER THIRTEEN—BOB'S BIRTHDAY | 237

CHAPTER FOURTEEN—SUNDRY SWEETIES | 245

CHAPTER FIFTEEN—MONSTERS SCREAM FOR ICE CREAM! | 269

CONCLUSION | 289

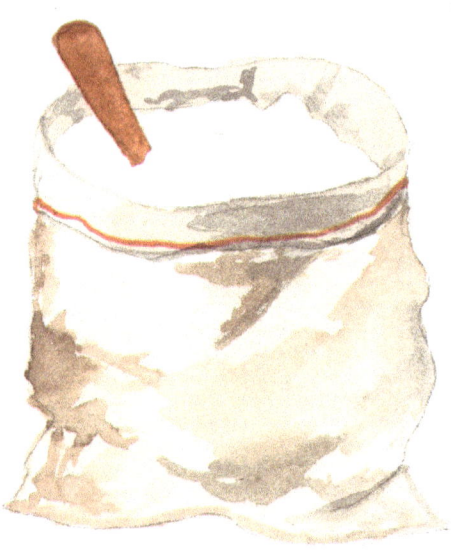

LIST OF KITCHEN UTENSILS | 291

    Cooking Utensils & Miscellaneous Items | 291
    Small & Large Appliances | 292
    Pots & Pans | 292
    Baking Essentials | 293

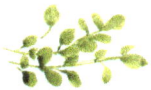

CONVERSION CHARTS | 295

    Dry Ingredients by Weight | 295
    Liquid Ingredients by Volume | 296
    Lengths & Widths | 297
    Temperatures | 297

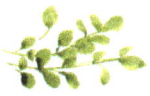

ACKNOWLEDGMENTS | 299

THE FELLOWSHIP OF THE RECIPE TESTERS | 301

WORKS CITED & SOURCED | 303

SHOPPING SOURCES | 307

INDEX | 309

AUTHOR'S BIOGRAPHY | 325

INTRODUCTION

A FEW YEARS ago, I wrote a cookbook that was influenced by the fictional land of Middle-earth. During the writing process, I used to joke about utilizing that fictional land for culinary inspiration, and then visiting other "fictional" lands, such as North America, Europe, and Asia. That idea always stuck with me, especially since I had ended up with three notebooks filled with recipes from each of these other regions. Fearing the cookbooks would become too large, I split off a majority of my soups, stews, chilis, and breads into a separate collection, which became my second cookbook.

Weird? Perhaps. An even weirder way of approaching my future cookbooks was when I envisioned dividing them into holiday sections, with subject sections in between. This concept loosely developed into a "holiday-year-in-the-life" kind of thing. Yes, it is a bit odd, but that is apparently who I am (definitely odd). I'm thinking you can handle it, dear reader.

So, Volume 3 in the Cooking for Halflings & Monsters series deals with North America, a land that has become even more fantastical than I ever could have imagined. Quite a lot of this cookbook will be based in the Southwest region of North America, which is where I reside—specifically, Albuquerque, New Mexico.

However, this is not at all a comprehensive examination of New Mexican or American cuisine, so please don't expect to see historical or specifically regional recipes. For example: I don't make tamales, because they require an awful lot of work and are better made with a collection of helpers in the kitchen. I don't have helpers, and I usually don't bother to make difficult foods if I can purchase a satisfactory product. It's one reason I don't like to make candy—it can be temperamental and frustrating, and the results often fail. I can easily go to a shop and buy it. I often do. Too often. It's the same with tamales—I can easily purchase some from stores or local restaurants, or I can go nuts and purchase some from enterprising neighbors. This cookbook is a collection of my own favorite stuff, which is heavily influenced by New Mexico but not in any sort of historical way. Maybe hysterical, but not historical.

Foolishly, I have made plans for future cookbooks. I say foolishly, because life often interferes with the best-laid plans. But I plan for Volume 4 to be based in Europe and Volume 5 to be based in Asia. Since I came to the writing career later in life, I'm afraid I won't have any time to explore the Southern Hemisphere. And that's the way the tamale crumbles (which it shouldn't do very much; a lovely tamale should be rather moist and tender, but I digress, and I am obviously feeling the urge to go out and get a tamale).

Introduction   i

Garnishes & Photography

MY SECOND COOKBOOK had tons of optional garnishing going on, but plenty of items within this volume do not require extra embellishments. Yet many recipes are based on New Mexican and Mexican cuisine, so I am going to reprint my extensive list of **NICE NEW MEXICAN & MEXICAN GARNISHES** for your convenience, in case you want some yummy suggestions to jazz up your enchiladas.

NICE NEW MEXICAN & MEXICAN GARNISHES

- ANY sort of onion, chopped or diced finely or coarsely
- Radishes, sliced thinly or chopped finely or coarsely
- Fresh cabbage, chopped or diced finely or shredded
- Avocado, sliced or diced; a scoop of guacamole can also serve as a garnish
- Any sort of lettuce or other greenery, torn or chopped coarsely or finely
- Tomatoes, chopped or diced coarsely
- Green or black olives; pitted, drained, sliced or whole (most any mild variety you like, though usually not Kalamatas, which are extra salty; use canned black ones, if those happen to be your favorites)
- Fresh jalapeños, sliced or chopped
- Sliced jalapeños, from a jar or can, drained; however spicy you can endure
- Other pickled chili peppers
- Any other assorted chopped vegetables you might like
- Mexican crema or crème fraîche
- Sour cream (I often use the light kind if it's available; I'm forever trying to save calories somewhere.)
- Cheeses such as cheddar, Monterey Jack, pepper jack; shredded
- Cheeses such as cotija, fresco, or panela; crumbled
- Fresh cilantro, minced or chopped coarsely
- Jicama, peeled and shredded; minced, diced, or chopped coarsely
- Lime wedges
- Hot sauce, whatever is your favorite variety
- Salsa—ANY variety you like, a tablespoon or two (or seven) over the top of whatever you like
- Red chile sauce and/or green chile sauce, same as above

- Fried eggs (These are occasionally served on top of a dish of enchiladas. You would fry an egg over medium and keep a runny yolk.)
- Tortilla chips, broken up (Fritos will also work... Oh, let's face it, any chip you like will work as a crunchy garnish)
- Thin strips of crispy corn tortillas

All my photography was taken outdoors, without flash, with a Samsung Galaxy A13 5G cellphone. All the foods, beverages, and garnishes were real and were consumed afterward. Apparently, food photography actually involves staging quite a lot of fake foods. But since I'm not a professional photographer creating magazine copy or commercials, I don't have the same concerns that pros do.

Because I'm not staging anything artificial, I've noticed that certain foods don't always photograph that well. The best example is a pan filled with enchiladas, which usually looks like a lake of cheese. After you dish a serving onto your plate, it generally doesn't show all the ingredients inside. I'll only supply a photo that represents the genuine food well. I was also concerned about the overall length of this cookbook and didn't want to waste page spreads on rather dull items such as dry mixes or cocktails.

All I am saying is that, unlike my first two cookbooks, I will not include a large, featured photo of each and every recipe. Some items will be left to your imagination and some items will be grouped together in what I hope are pleasing ways.

One more note, which also touches on the subject of conserving space here: I used to write recipe posts for a *Star Wars* website. These have all been designated to fit into my second cookbook, this one, and any future ones I get around to writing. I decided to just go ahead and embrace the original photography and story anecdotes that deal with the *Star Wars* universe. Instead of supplying two photographs and two anecdotes (and even two names!) for these recipe items (as I did in my second cookbook), I'm going all in and just using the photographic concepts and stories from the original staged photos. I also included the one and only *Star Trek* recipe I have ever developed (at least, as of this moment), because I wasn't really up to the task of boldly going into that culinary universe in depth. So, while there is no Cellular Peptide Cake with Mint Frosting, I do have a spicy, snazzy version of Hasperat in Chapter Eight.

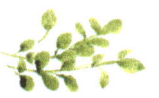

Introduction iii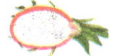

Substitutions & Altitude

THE INGREDIENTS UTILIZED within are fairly traditional. The only sugar substitutes I have tried are Truvia Cane Sugar Blend (which combines sugar, erythritol, and stevia leaf extract) and monk fruit (which is also combined with erythritol). If you are happy with the results of products such as Splenda, try them in the recipes. I have mixed erythritol with regular sugar (about 1:3) to cut back on calories and the results have produced good products.

If you are vegan, there are vegan substitutes available for many ingredients such as butter, mayonnaise, and cheese. If you are following a gluten-free diet, you can substitute almond flour or other products for recipes that require flour. I always use 1% milk and I generally try to use reduced-calorie dairy products. However, I never use fat-free products. If you prefer full-fat dairy products, you are free to use them; it shouldn't make too much difference in your results. Items such as oat milk and soy milk can substitute well for milk in many of the sweets recipes. As with all traditional recipes, however, if you substitute ingredients, you might have to make various modifications to each recipe. Sometimes, this could mean you might need to make relatively simple changes such as adding a bit more moisture to a cookie dough.

Your location might force you to make substitutions. For example, I have mentioned various cheeses within the cookbook that might not be available where you live. Mexican cheeses such as panela, fresco, blanca, cotija, etc., can easily be exchanged with items such as feta, mozzarella, paneer, etc., depending on the recipe. Internet searches can be helpful here.

Broth and stock are other items that you can substitute. Perhaps you only use a homemade product, and that is fine to use. I use both homemade and store-bought in a pinch. A quart of broth or stock can be whatever you like to use. A can of low-sodium broth is often convenient, but you can simply measure out a smidge over one and three-quarter cup's worth of your own broth to obtain the equivalent of a can.

I'm cooking at a mile-high altitude. This might affect your cooking and baking, but it might not. I've tried plenty of recipes that were most likely developed at sea level and have not needed to change anything. Nevertheless, you might need to consider things such as your overall cooking times (you might need a little more or a little less) and moisture (you might end up with too much or too little). I always strive to enlist recipe testers at different altitudes, and they have always let me know if there is a particular problem. So while cooking and baking can be fairly scientific, they can also be subject to the whims of weather and the individualistic whims of the cook, the baker, and the diner.

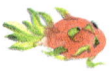

Vegetarian & Meat-Lovers Options and/or Substitutions

MY SECOND COOKBOOK was more conducive to offering many options to convert recipes to vegetarian or changing a vegetarian dish to one with meat. For this book, however, I thought it would be better to condense these options.

For many of the pasta dishes or hot vegetable sides that happen to be vegetarian, just add some leftover cooked meats, such as chicken or roast beef. Some of the cold salads might benefit from a bit of chilled cooked shrimp or chicken. Sometimes, dishes NEED bacon, so go for it.

If you would like to substitute ground turkey in all the recipes that might contain ground beef or pork, you certainly may. If you would like to go beyond meat by using your favorite vegetarian meat substitute, you definitely may. Your seasonings might need some adjustments, but that happens with many recipes, doesn't it?

While some of the recipes would be difficult to change (what would substitute for a filet mignon, I wonder…?), plenty of others are more flexible. I mainly didn't want to list every conceivable option with each recipe.

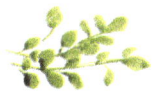

Green Chile & Other Hot Stuff

YES.

Oh, I mean to say that many recipes within have green or red chile as an ingredient. Since the internet now globally connects us, chile is available to all. Your best bets here are the jarred varieties, though canned chile is also completely acceptable and carried in many grocery stores. Thank goodness. Please see the chile recipes in the **Few Essentials** section for more information about preparing chile sauces. If you find yourself unable to purchase fresh chile peppers, please see the **Shopping Sources** section, which gives you a few website options beyond Amazon for your convenience.

Can't stand much spice? Choose the mild flavor and work your way up. Really can't stand any spice? Well… I guess you can omit it. Frowny face.

But don't worry—plenty of recipes contained within are not based on any spice at all. I really like to balance my own diet between mellow foods and spicy foods from day to day. Food is incredibly subjective, and we all have different tolerance levels for spice and other seasonings, such as salt and pepper. I even wonder if our tolerance levels vary from day to day, or according to our moods or hormone levels. But that's where you can experiment or place a jar of salsa, hot sauce, or Sriracha on the table. Sometimes diners need to add heat and that's fine.

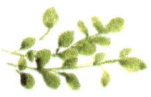

Seasoning, Salt, and Butter

I ALWAYS USE salted sweet cream butter in all my recipes, but unsalted butter might be fine. I try to be reasonable and moderate about salt, and I believe American doctors when they tell us to cut back on our salt consumption. If you need more salt, you may add it to your final seasoning. If you need to use a salt substitute, you are welcome to do so. I've included a few dry seasoning mixes in a later section (**A Few Essentials**) that contain less salt, so you might find nice options with some of those recipes.

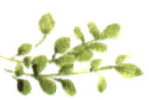

Just one more thing...

I DECIDED TO take a step into the modern world and supply you with preparation estimates. At first, I didn't want to clutter up the recipes with all this extra information, but then various people suggested that I include this type of feature. I'm going to model my estimates on my good old *Better Homes and Gardens* cookbook. This can be tricky stuff. I know sometimes I might take 15 minutes to do prep on a recipe, and another day, I might take 20 or 25 minutes because of fatigue or distractions of whatever kind. When determining these estimates I included assembling ingredients, and I've also erred on the side of more time rather than less.

Many recipes can have multiple operations going on at the same time, too, such as: "Start cooking your pasta. Meanwhile, chop up all your vegetables." I guess the most important features here are baking times, chilling times, marinating, standing, rising, cooling, etc. And, of course, what items need to be prepared in advance, such as boiling eggs or toasting nuts.

I'm going to hold the line when it comes to nutritional information, however. We really don't want that particular kind of clutter around here.

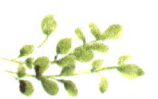

My Biography

IF THIS IS your first experience with my cookbooks, I should supply you with current biographical information. I was born in New York in 1962. In 1968, my family moved to the sunny state of New Mexico, and I've been here ever since. I have traveled abroad a couple of times, and I have participated in various adventures within the United States, but not recently. I'm a hobbity homebody—not like those weird hobbits who traipsed off to Mordor, just a Shire kind of hobbit.

I took up cooking and baking when I was around ten years old, as a hobby. In my teens I studied under a professional chef, and I later took baking courses at Albuquerque's community college. I've catered and supplied tons of food for various events. In my 20s and 30s, I was a professional dressmaker. I have a

bachelor's degree (2002) in English, with a minor in Latin. I have a master's degree (2008) in Comparative Literature and Cultural Studies. As a graduate student, I taught Latin for four years. During the college times of my life, I also managed to get married and have two daughters. So, my total time at the University of New Mexico was over 13 years; it started in 1980 and ended in 2008. I was busy.

When I was a freshman, I was going to minor in philosophy, but my minor ended up being in Latin. My philosophy dabbling started to extend to the kitchen, however, and I began to approach recipes with a sort of casual Platonic idealism—what would be the BEST version of a chocolate chip cookie? At least, the BEST, in my own humble opinion? So, that colors a lot of my recipe development.

Add to that an obsession with geeky/nerd culture (yes, mostly the works of J. R. R. Tolkien), and there you are. But I find that adhering rigidly to the realm of fantasy works can be stifling (plus, it can make you vulnerable to lawsuits, as I discovered with my first cookbook), so I released myself from those confines. I'm still cooking for halflings and monsters, however, in the sense of all my little darling halfling grandchildren (who act like monsters occasionally). You will find many kid-friendly recipes within, but this is definitely not a cookbook geared toward young children's skills, nor is it concerned with teaching basic skills in the kitchen. I would give this cookbook a rating of PG-13, bordering a bit on R, so tread carefully.

I'm sure if hobbits (halflings) were real, they would enjoy all the foods in my cookbooks—and yes, even the spicy dishes! Because it's all about comfy, cozy cooking, all the time. If you are looking for recipes that would be especially appealing to hobbity kinds of people, be sure to look for the various items that have been marked with a Halfling Alert, either in the title or in an anecdote.

ALLOW YOUR KITCHEN KRAKEN TO BREAK FREE, AND I HOPE YOU ENJOY THE RIDE!

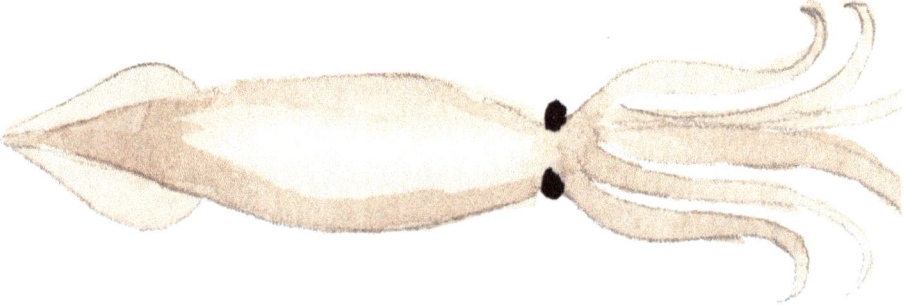

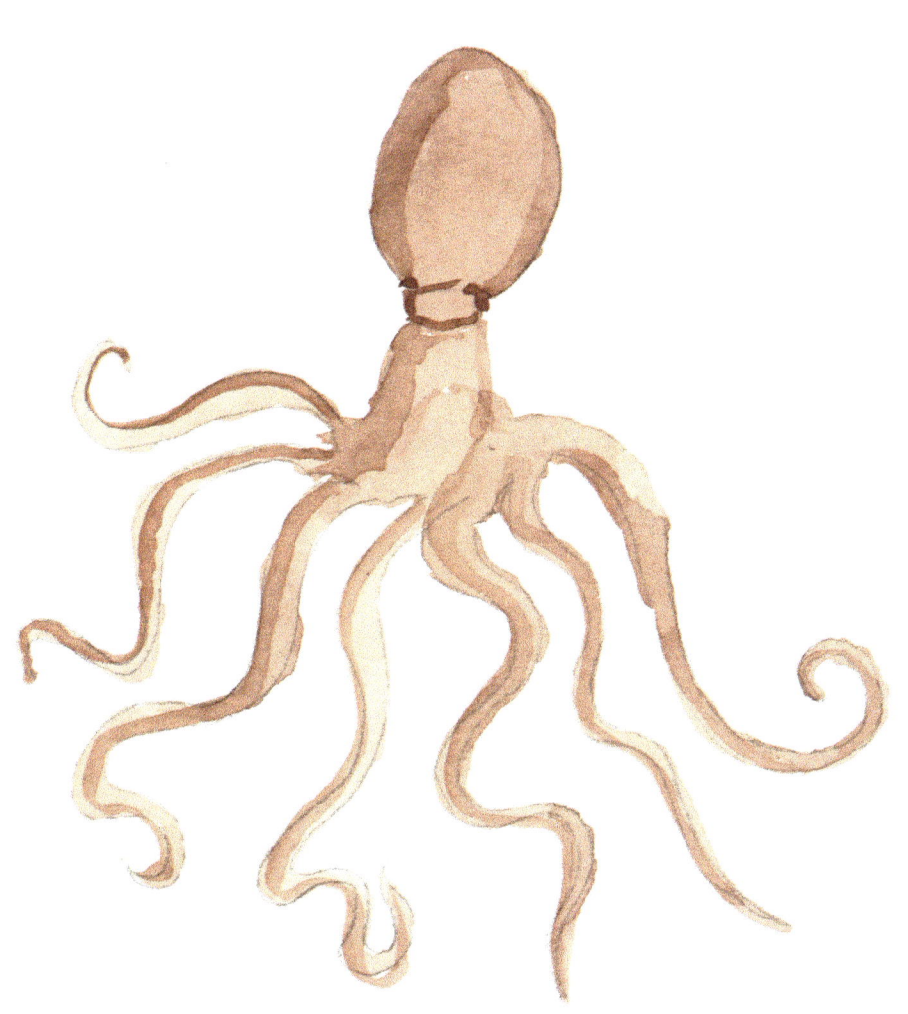

A Few Essentials

Dry Seasoning Mixes

BEFORE YOU DELVE into the chapters proper, you might want to check out these items first. I have included some dry seasoning mixes, preparations for red and green chile, and a few other basic items. While plenty of these items can be purchased easily, sometimes you really want the whole homemade experience.

Many of these mixes can be used interchangeably throughout this cookbook. I have written them as rather small portions. I've noticed that some cookbooks will require you to buy a particular mix, which inevitably comes in a two-ounce jar, or something like that. Then you use a teaspoon or two, and it sits in your cupboard for months. Years, even. By the time you get around to using that much seasoning, its flavor has probably faded. I just love hearing chefs and bloggers talk about replacing your herbs and spices every three to six months or so—who can afford to do that? Plus, isn't that unnecessarily contributing to the food waste crisis that is affecting our world? Anyway, I use mixes like these quite often. If I run out of something, I probably already have the basics on hand to whip up a new batch.

If you decide to swap seasonings, you might need to increase or decrease accordingly. Thus, if you wanted to substitute Mexican Mix for a recipe that calls for one teaspoon of Savory Seasoning, you might need to use one and a half teaspoons. You can judge it by the final taste test.

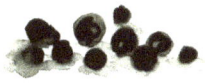

Savory Seasoning

START TO FINISH: ABOUT 8 MINUTES

This was invented for my first cookbook, *Cooking for Halflings & Monsters: 111 Comfy, Cozy Recipes for Fantasy-Loving Souls,* but I use it all the time in many other not-technically-hobbitish recipes. Though aren't all my recipes hobbitish? Probably. Anyway, here it is for your cooking convenience. You can grind this almost to a powder, but I like to leave some of the peppercorns nearly whole for more of an eye-opening experience.

2 tablespoons coarse sea salt
1 tablespoon whole peppercorns (all black or a mix of colors)
1 tablespoon dried parsley
1 tablespoon sugar
1 teaspoon onion powder
1 teaspoon garlic powder
½ teaspoon dried thyme
½ teaspoon dried marjoram
½ teaspoon rubbed sage
½ teaspoon crushed rosemary
½ teaspoon celery seed

COMBINE the salt and peppercorns in a blender or a small food processor. Pulse until the peppercorns are mostly broken; this will take about a minute. Add the remaining ingredients and pulse another 20 seconds or so. Keep in a tightly covered container in your pantry. Shake or stir before using. Makes about ⅓ cup and retains pungency for at least 3 months or more.

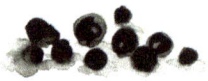

Easy Herbes de Provence

START TO FINISH: 5 MINUTES

Sometimes, it's nice to be able to whip up your own herby dry mix. You can use this fragrant mix almost everywhere! Use it on chicken, seafood, eggs, and vegetables. Maybe not on ice cream…

1 TEASPOON EACH, ALL IN DRIED FORM:
- parsley
- rubbed sage
- crushed rosemary
- thyme
- summer savory
- marjoram
- lavender (optional)

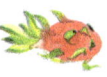

COMBINE all the ingredients in a small bowl. If you like, you may use a mortar and pestle if you want the herbs to be a finer consistency, or you can simply crush them a little with your fingers. Keep in an airtight container in your pantry. Makes about 2 tablespoons.

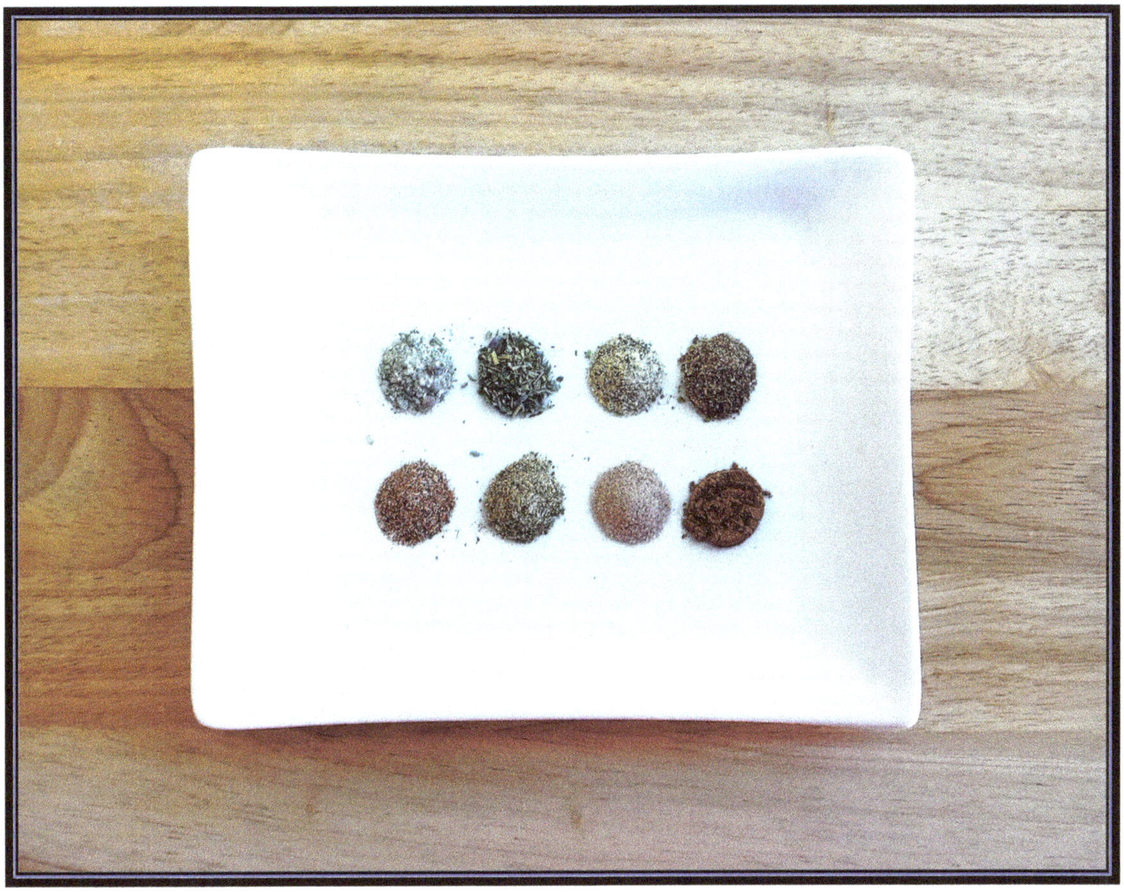

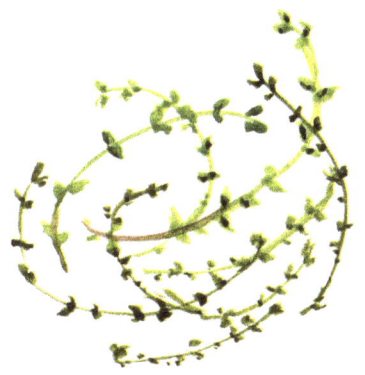

TOP ROW, LEFT TO RIGHT:
Savory Seasoning, page xi
Easy Herbes de Provence, page xii
Just the Basics, page xiv
Mexican Mix, page xiv

BOTTOM ROW, LEFT TO RIGHT:
Cajun Mix, page xv
New England Mix, page xv
Simple Cinnamon Sugar, page xvi
Pumpkin Pie Spice, page xvi

A Few Essentials xiii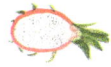

Just the Basics

START TO FINISH: 5 MINUTES

Perfect for pretty much anything. Yes, I'm vague about this, but you'll probably find many uses for this seasoning.

1 TEASPOON EACH: finely ground salt
finely ground black pepper (white pepper will also work)
onion powder
garlic powder

COMBINE all the ingredients in a small bowl. Keep in a tightly covered container in your pantry. Makes 4 teaspoons.

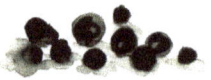

THE NEXT THREE RECIPES BUILD ON JUST THE BASICS.

Mexican Mix

START TO FINISH: 5 MINUTES

1 TEASPOON EACH: finely ground salt
finely ground black pepper (white pepper will also work)
onion powder
garlic powder
ground cumin
dried oregano
chili powder

COMBINE all the ingredients in a small bowl. Keep in a tightly covered container in your pantry. Makes a little over 2 tablespoons.

Cajun Mix

START TO FINISH: 5 MINUTES

1½ teaspoons smoked paprika
1½ teaspoons cayenne pepper
1 teaspoon finely ground salt
1 teaspoon finely ground black pepper
1 teaspoon onion powder
1 teaspoon garlic powder

COMBINE all the ingredients in a small bowl. Keep in a tightly covered container in your pantry. Makes a little over 2 tablespoons.

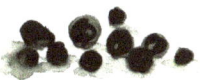

New England Mix

START TO FINISH: 5 MINUTES

2 teaspoons Old Bay Seasoning
1 teaspoon finely ground salt
1 teaspoon finely ground black pepper (white pepper will also work)
1 teaspoon onion powder
1 teaspoon garlic powder
1 teaspoon dried thyme, crushed with your fingers
1 teaspoon celery salt

COMBINE all the ingredients in a small bowl. Keep in a tightly covered container in your pantry. Makes almost 3 tablespoons.

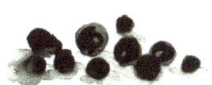

Simple Cinnamon Sugar

START TO FINISH: 5 MINUTES

For different flavor profiles, use one tablespoon of cinnamon and a tablespoon of some other spice, such as nutmeg (or any combination of other spices you might like: cardamom, cloves, allspice, mace, ginger, even five-spice powder).

1 cup sugar
2 tablespoons ground cinnamon

COMBINE all the ingredients in a medium bowl. Store in an airtight container in your pantry. Makes a little over 1 cup and keeps for a long time.

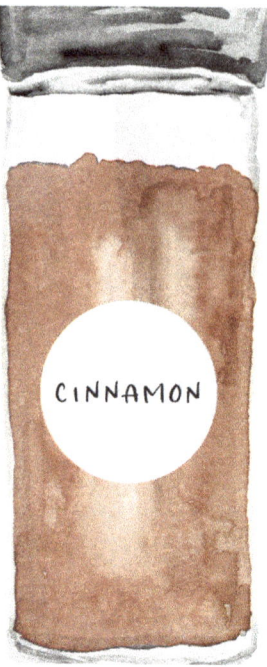

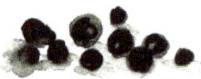

Pumpkin Pie Spice

START TO FINISH: 5 MINUTES

You know fall is in the air when the coffee shops start adding this to their beverages. Then everyone argues about whether they love it or hate it!

2 tablespoons ground cinnamon
2 teaspoons ground nutmeg
2 teaspoons ground ginger
1 teaspoon ground allspice
1 teaspoon ground cloves
1 teaspoon ground mace

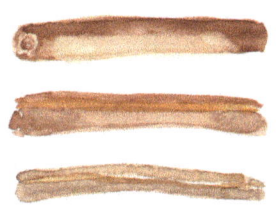

COMBINE all the ingredients in a small bowl. Store in an airtight container in your pantry. Makes a little over ¼ cup and keeps for a long time.

Magical, Mythical Garlic

GARLIC HAS BEEN around forever, so it's inevitable that it has developed all sorts of anecdotal information about its health benefits. The odor can be off-putting to some, so you either eat it with people you love or people you hate. After his expulsion from Eden, Satan supposedly placed his left foot on a garlic plant, which gave this modest herb a rather negative quality. But it also wards off vampires and can protect you from all sorts of other evil forces. I love garlic, as well as all the other members of the allium family: onions, chives, leeks, shallots, etc. Here are a couple of roasting treatments for one of my favorite flavors. You may use other types of oil if you like. Mix either recipe with a cup of mayonnaise and a pinch or three of extra salt, and you will end up with an instant aioli (purists would only use an olive oil-based mayo).

Regular Roast

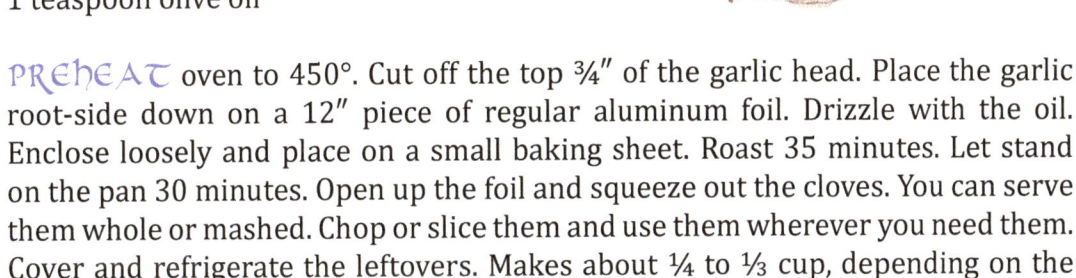

PREP: 5 MINUTES
ROAST: 35 MINUTES
STAND: 30 MINUTES
OVEN: 450°

A rather large head of regular garlic
1 teaspoon olive oil

PREHEAT oven to 450°. Cut off the top ¾" of the garlic head. Place the garlic root-side down on a 12" piece of regular aluminum foil. Drizzle with the oil. Enclose loosely and place on a small baking sheet. Roast 35 minutes. Let stand on the pan 30 minutes. Open up the foil and squeeze out the cloves. You can serve them whole or mashed. Chop or slice them and use them wherever you need them. Cover and refrigerate the leftovers. Makes about ¼ to ⅓ cup, depending on the size of the garlic.

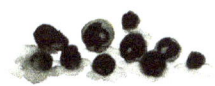

A Few Essentials xvii

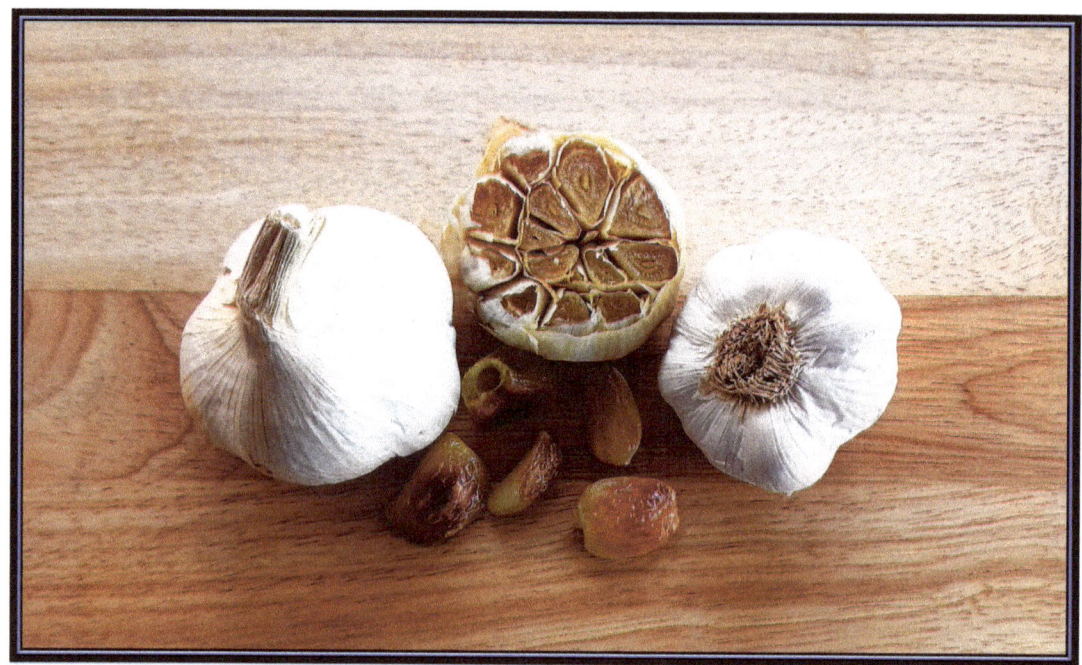

Elephant Roast

Prep: 5 minutes
Roast: 30 minutes
Stand: 30 minutes
Oven: 400°

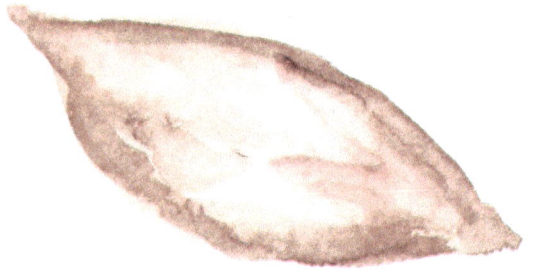

A large head of elephant garlic
1 tablespoon olive oil
¼ teaspoon salt

PREHEAT the oven to 400°. Peel all the cloves of the garlic and cut off any stems. Cut any really large cloves into about 1" chunks. Place on a 12" piece of regular aluminum foil. Drizzle the oil over all, then sprinkle with the salt. Enclose loosely and place on a small baking sheet. Roast 30 minutes. Let stand on the pan 30 minutes. Chop, slice, or mash the cloves and use them wherever you need them. Cover and refrigerate the leftovers. Makes about ½ cup, depending on the size of the garlic.

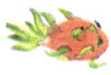

A Couple of Baking Essentials

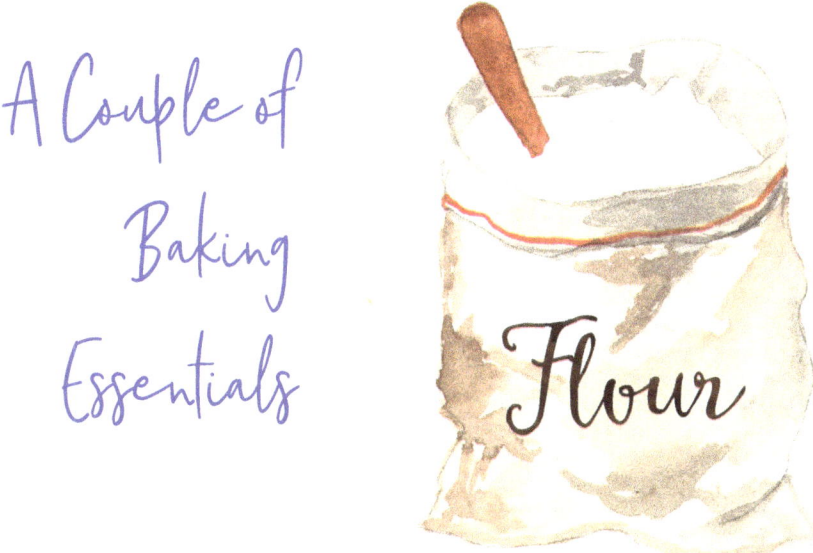

Halfling Alert Pie Crust

ACTIVE PREP: 20–25 MINUTES
CHILL: 1 HOUR

Named so because this is a generous amount of dough for your special pie or quiche creation. You will be able to fold over the edge for decorative fluting or crimping and you will also end up with scraps that can be cut into whimsical shapes for the top of your pie. These are essential to a halfling's happiness.

When it comes to shortening, you can go old school and use lard. Now, I know many people might object to that ingredient, but it is a traditional treatment in a pie crust. But you can certainly use other forms of shortening. Butter, margarine, or vegetable shortening will all work out well. You can even use combinations if you like; a good one is 2 ounces of lard and 1 ounce of butter (which is 2 tablespoons). Keep in mind that your choice of shortening might change the results of the product overall. Shortening should usually be rather cool or chilled before you cut or spoon it into smaller pieces.

Many people like to add some sort of acid to their pie crusts, such as vinegar. You can add white or cider vinegar, or lemon juice, or I have even heard of adding vodka. Supposedly, this inhibits gluten from forming and helps to produce a more tender crust. This is not really a scientific recommendation; it is more anecdotal. Every cook has his/her own little secrets when it comes to making something as deceptively simple as a basic pie crust. So many variables factor into your final product—altitude, flour hardness, the temperature of your shortening, how much you have mixed the dough, what kind of pan you use, exactly how hot your oven is, etc. No wonder we sometimes just buy a crust rather than mess around with making it from scratch.

I use a glass Pyrex pie dish, which measures 9½" in diameter. But perhaps you have a metal one or a pretty ceramic dish. This pie crust and your future pie creations will work in almost anything, but you might have to keep an eye on browning. This is easy to do with glass, but if you have an opaque style of dish, just pay attention to the visible crust and adjust your baking times accordingly.

½ cup water
A few ice cubes
1½ cups all-purpose flour
½ teaspoon salt
3 ounces chilled shortening, cut into ¼" bits or spooned out in small portions
1 teaspoon white vinegar (optional)

MEASURE water in a 1-cup glass measuring cup. Add ice and set aside.

IN a large bowl, combine the flour and salt. Cut in the shortening with a pastry blender until the mixture resembles coarse crumbs. Remove the ice from the water and measure ½ cup. Add vinegar (if you are using it) to the water and mix. Add the water mixture to the flour and combine until the dough is incorporated almost thoroughly. I use a wooden spoon at first; then, I use my floured hands to finish the mixing. If it seems too dry or too wet, adjust accordingly by adding a *smidge* more water or flour. Don't overwork the dough. Form the dough into a disk, place it on a lightly floured plate (I just use the pie dish in which I plan to bake the pie), and cover it with a cloth napkin or towel. Refrigerate 1 hour before using.

ON a floured surface and with a floured rolling pin, roll out the dough to a 13" circle and place it in a 9½" (glass) pie dish. Trim the pie crust to ½" beyond the edge of the dish, then fold the crust edges under nicely. Flute or crimp as desired. Save the scraps for decorations; cut these out with small cookie cutters. Proceed with your pie recipe and place the scrap decorations on top. Bake as directed. Makes a single pie crust.

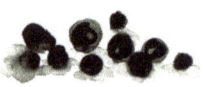

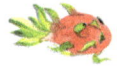 xx Celebrating Comfy, Cozy Foods from North America: CH&M, Volume 3

English Muffins

ACTIVE PREP: ABOUT 40 MINUTES
STAND: 25 MINUTES
RISE: ABOUT 1 HOUR (POSSIBLY MORE)
BAKE: 15 MINUTES PER BATCH
OVEN: 400°

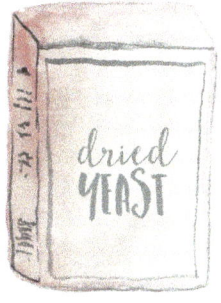 

Not English! Not a muffin! I was going to include these in my next (European) cookbook, but I discovered that what Americans think of as your basic English Muffin was actually invented in America. The inventor was English (he was Samuel Bath Thomas, of Thomas' English Muffins—talk about everlasting branding), but he created them in America. And they really resemble more of a crumpet, not what you think of as the soft, rather cakey and multi-flavored product you would bake in a muffin tin.

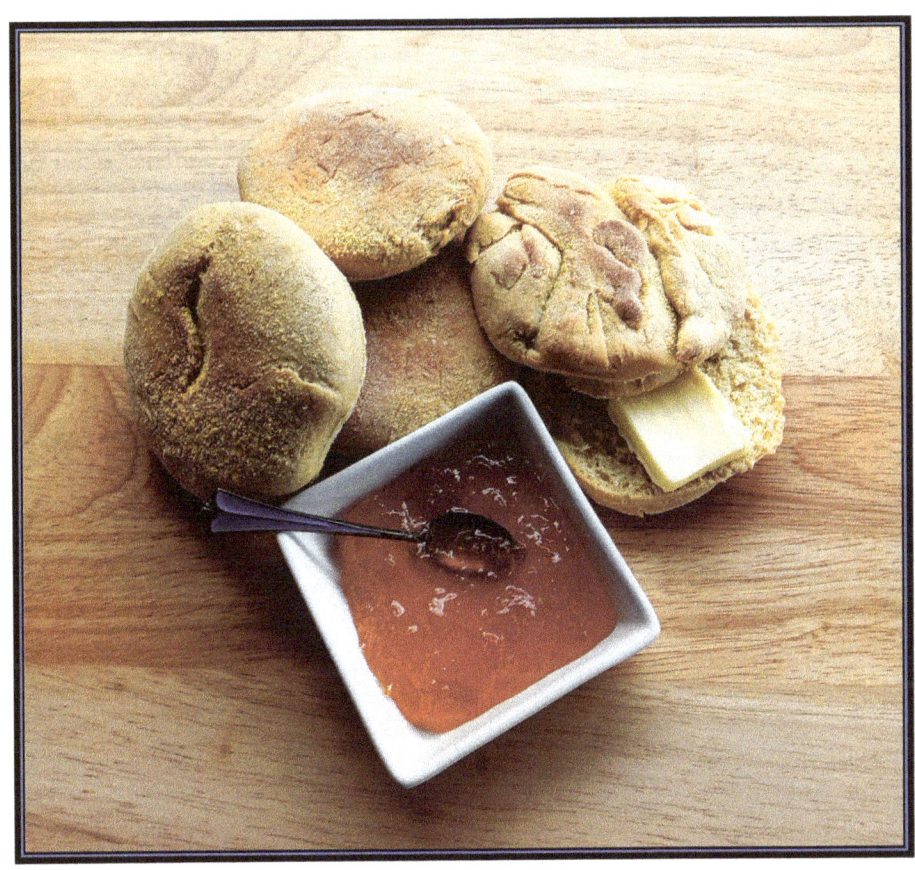

A Few Essentials
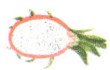

I started working on my own recipe to cut down on the amount of packaging that generally accompanies your basic English muffins. These freeze well and they are a good-tasting product. I also wanted to be able to bake them, instead of utilizing the more traditional method of cooking them on a griddle. This was mainly to save time and achieve more consistency. Griddles can be hard to regulate, especially when you are cooking a whole bunch of muffins. Nooks and crannies might occur, but they might not. If your tops and bottoms end up rather gnarly, don't worry about it; it only makes them taste better.

1 cup 1% milk
1 cup water
¼ cup salted butter
2 tablespoons sugar
1 tablespoon salt
3 tablespoons white vinegar
5½ cups all-purpose flour, divided
2 (¼-ounce) packets active dry yeast (4½ teaspoons)
1 tablespoon baking powder
1 tablespoon vegetable oil
¼ cup cornmeal

PLACE the milk, water, butter, sugar, salt, and vinegar in a 4-cup glass measuring cup. Microwave on HIGH for 2 minutes. Remove and let stand 15 minutes, then whisk well (the butter might not be completely melted, but don't worry about it).

PLACE 3 cups of flour, yeast, and baking powder in a very large mixing bowl, such as a stand mixer. Combine by hand with a paddle attachment or a wooden spoon. Whisk the milk mixture again, then add to the bowl. Mix on low speed 1 minute. Add the remaining flour and mix at the lowest speed 1 minute. Switch to a dough hook and mix at the lowest speed 6 minutes (you may also knead the dough by hand). Remove the dough from the bowl and place it on a cutting board. Place the oil in the bowl, then put the dough back in and turn it all over to grease the surface. Cover with a towel and let rise in a relatively warm draft-free place until it has doubled, about 1 hour (maybe longer, depending on various conditions).

PREHEAT the oven to 400°. Place the dough on a floured surface and press it down gently. Cover with a towel and let it rest 10 minutes. Place the cornmeal in a shallow bowl. Cut the dough in half, cover one half with the towel, and set aside. Roll out half of the dough to a scant ½" and cut 8 or 9 muffins with a 3½" round cutter. Reroll as needed. Press each side in the cornmeal and place on a large baking sheet. Bake on the center rack 10 minutes. Turn all of them over and bake another 5 minutes. Immediately place them on a cooling rack.

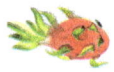

WHILE the first batch is baking, roll out the other half, cut them, then cover them with a towel until you are ready to bake them. Repeat the cornmeal application (any remaining cornmeal can be used in other baked goods). You can make a "mutant" muffin (maybe even 2; it'll depend on how thin your dough was) for your final one with all the end scraps. When cooler, you can cut them in half and toast them more, if desired, but when they are fresh, this is probably not necessary. Cover and keep them at room temperature or refrigerate them; they freeze well. Makes 16–18 (more or less, it depends on the dough).

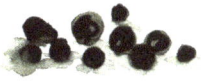

Chile (NOT the country...)

IN HIS SONG "Steam," Peter Gabriel's love interest might know his or her green from his or her red, but you might not (and he's probably not referring to chile, of course, but I always like to think he is). Here is a brief chile primer for you.

This information is exclusively about the New Mexican version of green chile; it is not about any of the hundreds of chile/chili/chilli peppers grown in many parts of the world. The first thing to know about your typical green chile is that it is one of the official state vegetables of New Mexico. The other is the pinto bean, and the two are often served together. What is a chile? Why is it sometimes green and sometimes red? Why is it mild, medium, or hot? What does Christmas mean? Not philosophically or culturally, but at a restaurant.

A young green chile resembles an elongated green bell pepper. New Mexican green chiles have been cultivated by Pueblo and Hispanic communities for hundreds of years, and they thrive in the climate, especially in the southern portions of the state. The best chiles come from Hatch, New Mexico. Sometimes, they are known as Anaheim peppers, a milder variety grown in California. Colorado has entered the chile-growing market, and NASA astronauts prepared "space tacos" from plants grown on the International Space Station in 2021. The heat of any chile pepper depends on various conditions, such as the particular pepper's genetic makeup, its ripeness, and the climate in which it has been grown. As you can imagine, chile crops can be successful or not, depending on many factors.

Usually, green chiles are roasted until very dark brown, almost black, spots appear on the skin. After a length of time for cooling, they are then peeled and usually chopped. Sometimes, they are left whole and stuffed with a variety of

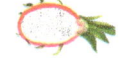

ingredients. They can be dried to become a powder, or they can be added to various sauces, either in roasted or dried form. Sometimes, they are used raw. Unadorned green chiles can be frozen for later use. They can be added to a surprising number of dishes. Green chile apple pie is sometimes featured in New Mexican restaurants. Some of our local Japanese restaurants serve green chile in sushi or deep-fried with a tempura batter.

A red chile is simply the more mature version of a green chile. The red chiles are dried and can be pulverized into powder. Others can be rehydrated, then usually used in a smoky, earthy sauce. Red chile sauce and roasted, chopped green chiles are often served to garnish the same dish; the two varieties work well together and complement many items. New Mexico is apparently the first state to have an official question: "Red or green?" Then you smile at your server and respond, "Christmas."

Chile Pepper Protocols

THESE APPLY TO all fresh chile/chili/chilli pepper preparations, including jalapeños and any other hot peppers one might use from all over the world. Any recipe with chile/chili/chilli peppers will be marked with the spicy hot little graphic you see below, so you can implement whatever handling protocols you feel are appropriate before you get started.

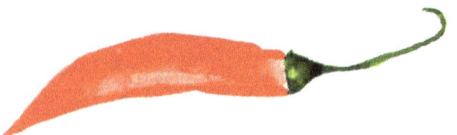

WARNING: Should you use thin latex (or other) disposable gloves to deal with chiles? If you have sensitive skin, this is probably wise. I let my hands go commando, because I can't really feel the skins well with gloves. Plus, I'm used to dealing with chiles, jalapeños, serranos, etc. all the time. Of course, then you have to wash your hands quite a few times and avoid touching sensitive areas, such as your eyes. I have had burned eyes before, but the burn passes eventually. You might rub some dairy product (such as milk) on irritated areas or pour some over your hands.

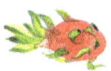

Should you wear a facial mask if your chiles are too pungent? Again, this depends on how sensitive you are to hot pepper fumes. Sometimes, I have been known to have coughing fits when I prepare chile. But onions can make me cry, too, and onion juice can irritate your eyes. Do I wear gloves to prepare onions? Nope.

Another small WARNING: If your chile pepper has black seeds within, you should discard that pepper. Green chile seeds are beige in color.

Roasted Green Chile

THE FIRST RECIPE makes about a cup of green chile and uses a broiler. The second version makes quite a lot more and roasts the chiles in the oven. I don't usually have to bother roasting my own green chile much at all since it's everywhere in my city, but in case you happen to see a few good-looking Hatch or Anaheim-type chiles at your market, you might want to try this. You can also set a few fresh green chiles either on a sheet of aluminum foil or directly on a grill rack and grill them until the skins blister. Then just follow the rest of the recipe for prepping them.

In August and September, chile starts appearing in New Mexican grocery stores. Chiles are generally packed in a fairly large box, and they can be roasted in a large roaster at the store where you have purchased them. The air becomes permeated with their singular scent. After roasting, you take them home and clean them up; peel them, chop them, then place them in conveniently sized containers or baggies in your freezer. They exude delicious juices and sometimes you will use this juice, but sometimes you might drain it off, depending on what you are making.

And even though I live in New Mexico, I usually just buy my chile already roasted and chopped, and packaged in 4-ounce plastic bags, from the freezer section at Costco, because it is more convenient and chile can be seasonal. You might find green chile in plastic containers in the freezer section. I have also purchased green chile in a glass jar. Usually jarred chiles have a smidge of salt or lime, which does not detract from the flavor of the pepper at all. Canned chile will do in a pinch, and they should be even more readily available to you. My grocery stores usually carry a four-ounce can and a seven-ounce can. That's rather annoying; why not just make it an eight-ounce can? If a recipe calls for eight ounces, don't skimp and buy the seven-ounce one; cave in and get two little cans. I know sometimes that is the only option available, and that is fine. All regional cookbooks have the same situation with regional ingredients, so you just have to make do with what you can get, right?

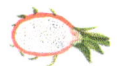

Just a Few Chiles

ACTIVE PREP: 13 MINUTES
BROIL: ABOUT 16 MINUTES
STAND: 40 MINUTES
BROILER: HIGH

About 1 pound of Hatch or Anaheim green chiles, preferably rather straight and approximately 6–8″ long

SET your oven rack to the level designated for broiling. Set the broiler to HIGH. Lay 2 feet of aluminum foil across a medium baking sheet. Let the foil hang over the long sides. Wash the chiles. Cut the stems down to about 1″. Pat them dry with a towel (which you will use later). Stagger the chiles, stem to end, on the foil. Broil 4 minutes. Turn them all a quarter turn; broil another 4 minutes. Repeat this process twice more, though you need to keep an eye on them. Move the chiles around on the pan if they start becoming too dark. You want them to be quite dark, but not burned. The skin will blister and peel. Curly or smaller peppers might not need as much time under the broiler; you can remove them and set them aside until all the chiles are done.

PLACE the pan on a rack. Fold both sides of the foil over the chiles, then lay the towel over all of them. Press down on all the chiles. Let stand around 40 minutes or so.

GENTLY pull out the stems. Peel off the blistered skin gently. Rinse them to help remove the seeds and seed membranes. A few stray seeds usually avoid removal, and that's okay. Cut the chiles into strips or dice. Cover and refrigerate or freeze. Makes about 1 cup.

A Big Bunch of Chiles

ACTIVE PREP: ABOUT 33 MINUTES
BAKE: ABOUT 35 MINUTES
STAND: 40 MINUTES
OVEN: 475°

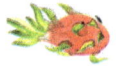

About 3 pounds of green chiles

PREHEAT the oven to 475°. Lay a piece of aluminum foil on a large baking sheet. Wash the chiles and pat them dry with a towel (you'll use the towel later). Cut the stems down to about 1″. Place all the chiles on the prepared pan and bake 15 minutes. Turn them all over and bake another 15–20 minutes. Judge if they need more roasting (see the previous recipe) and adjust the chiles accordingly; remove the ones that are done. Place the pan on a rack and lay another sheet of foil over all of them. Lay the towel on top and press down on the chiles. Let stand 40 minutes or so and proceed with peeling, cutting, and storage as described in the previous recipe. Makes around 3 cups.

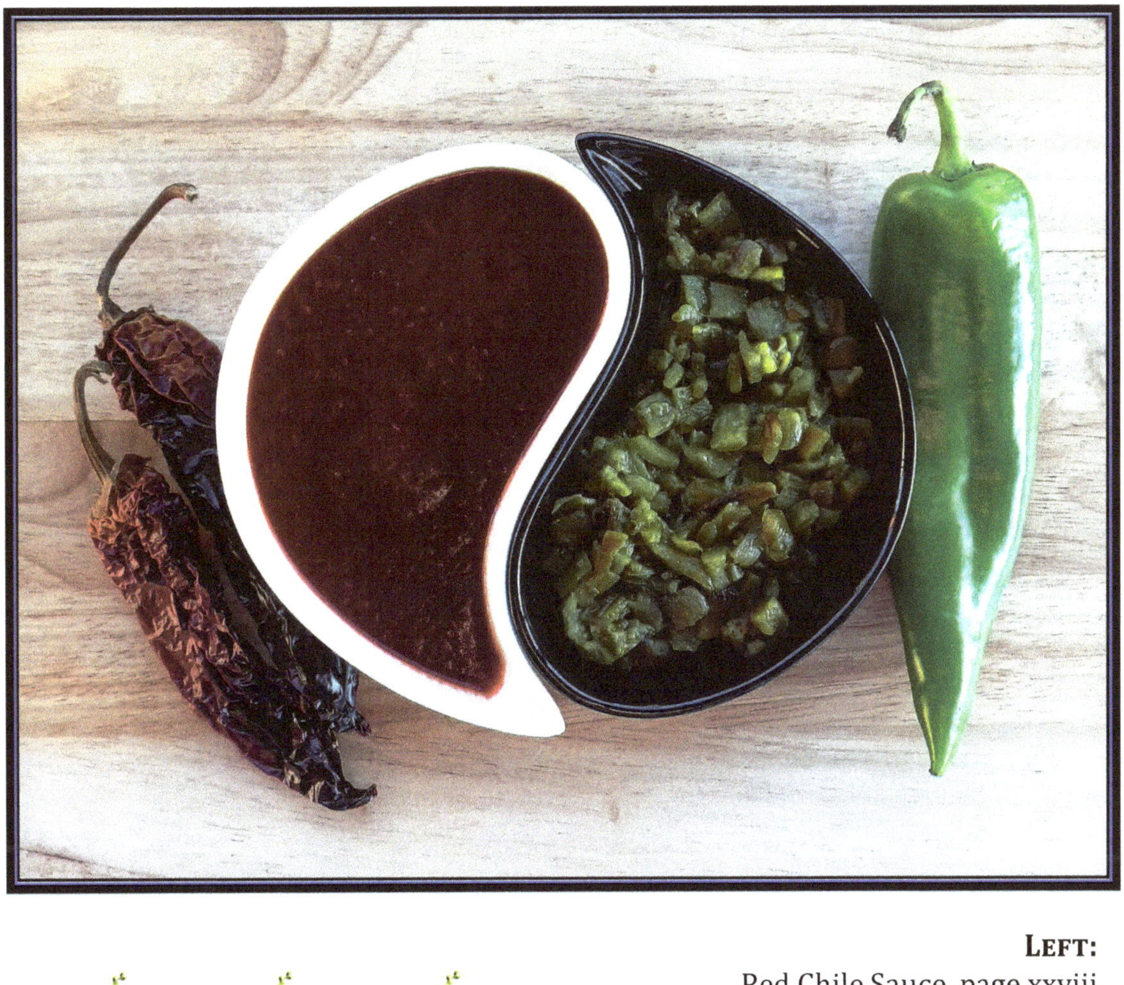

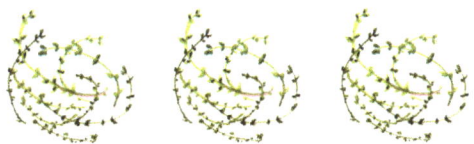

LEFT:
Red Chile Sauce, page xxviii

RIGHT:
Green Chiles, page xxvi

Red Chile Sauce

Prep: about 50 minutes
Stand: at least 75 minutes

Dried New Mexican red chiles (*capsicum annuum*) usually come in a plastic bag and they will keep in your pantry for a LONG time. But if you end up liking red chile, you'll end up using your peppers pretty fast. They are generally around five to six inches in length and a couple of inches wide at the top, though some of them end up rather curled and smaller. Sometimes, you'll see other names for basic red chile pods, such as *chile guajillo entero* or *chile pasilla ancho*. These will also work with this recipe. *Chile de árbol* are not appropriate for this recipe; they are way too small and way too spicy.

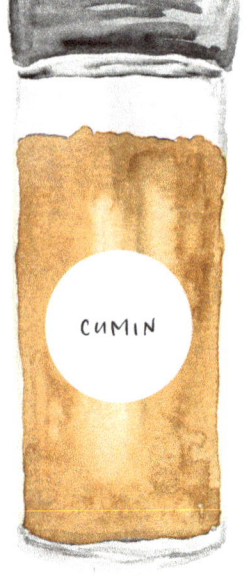

Remember to implement Chile Pepper Protocols if you find yourself to be extra-sensitive to chile, or at least wash your hands frequently afterward. But if you touch something sensitive on your body (usually it's your eyes), don't worry—this burn shall pass!

Spoon this sauce over mashed potatoes for a classic New Mexican side dish; combine a portion of this sauce with some cream and mix with cooked pasta (you could try something like a half cup of sauce, a cup of cream, and 8 to 12 ounces of pasta).

3 ounces dried New Mexican red chile pods
1 quart low-sodium chicken broth (vegetable broth is okay)
5–6 fairly large garlic cloves
2 tablespoons tomato paste
1 teaspoon dried oregano (2 tablespoons fresh, minced)
1 teaspoon ground cumin

PLACE the chiles in your kitchen sink. Fill the sink with very hot tap water to cover all and let them soak 15 minutes. Pull out the stems and discard. Break the pods apart and swish them in the water to remove as many of the seeds and membranes as you can. Place the pods in a 3-quart saucepan (don't worry about the few stray

seeds that will inevitably sneak into the pot). Add the broth and bring to a boil. Simmer on low heat, covered, 30 minutes. Stir a couple of times.

Add the remaining ingredients. Cover and let stand at least an hour (longer is okay). Pour into a 6-cup blender (if you have a smaller blender, you should do this in a couple of sections) and **BLEND THE ABSOLUTE SH*T OUT OF IT!!!** You shouldn't have to strain it if you blend it thoroughly enough. Pour it back into the saucepan and reheat over a gentle simmer. Cover and refrigerate the leftovers; you can freeze it, though it might get a little watery after thawing. Do not store this in plastic containers; it will stain them. Glass is best for storage. Makes 4 cups.

Perky Pico de Gallo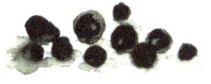

PREP: 20 MINUTES
CHILL: 1 HOUR

There are a gazillion types of salsas (*salsa* merely means *sauce*) available in your local grocery stores. While many are available in hermetically sealed jars for future consumption, other varieties are completely fresh and need to be consumed rather quickly. Here is a recipe for the latter, which is a good relish to put on all sorts of items, from omelets to grilled fish and chicken.

Pico de gallo literally means "beak of the rooster." This is supposedly because of the shape your thumb and index finger make when you want to pinch a bit of this relish. But it has come to mean something more like "fresh sauce" or "raw sauce." It's the perfect sauce to make with some freshly grown tomatoes from your garden. Since it is absolutely fresh, it won't necessarily keep very well for a long time, so I've designed this to be a rather small quantity.

An ingredient that is sometimes problematic is cilantro. This herb is often used in salsa, but many people don't care for it, and other people have a genetic predisposition that makes cilantro taste like soap. So, if you love cilantro, great. If you don't, leave it out. It'll still taste fine.

8 ounces Roma tomatoes (other varieties will also work)
¼ cup cilantro, coarsely chopped and loosely packed (optional)
2 rather large cloves of garlic
¼ cup red onion, finely chopped (white or yellow onions are also fine)
1 large jalapeño, cut off stem, remove seeds, and chop finely
1 teaspoon lime juice
¼ teaspoon salt
¼ teaspoon black pepper
¼ teaspoon ground cumin

CUT the tomatoes into quarters and slice off the stems. Place half of them in a small food processor. Add the cilantro and garlic. Process well. Scrape the sides and bottom of the bowl and process again. Place in a medium bowl and set aside.

CUT the remaining tomatoes into small chunks, about ½″ or so. Add these tomatoes and the remaining ingredients to the bowl and mix well. Season, if desired. Chill about an hour before serving. Cover and refrigerate the leftovers. Makes about 1½ cups.

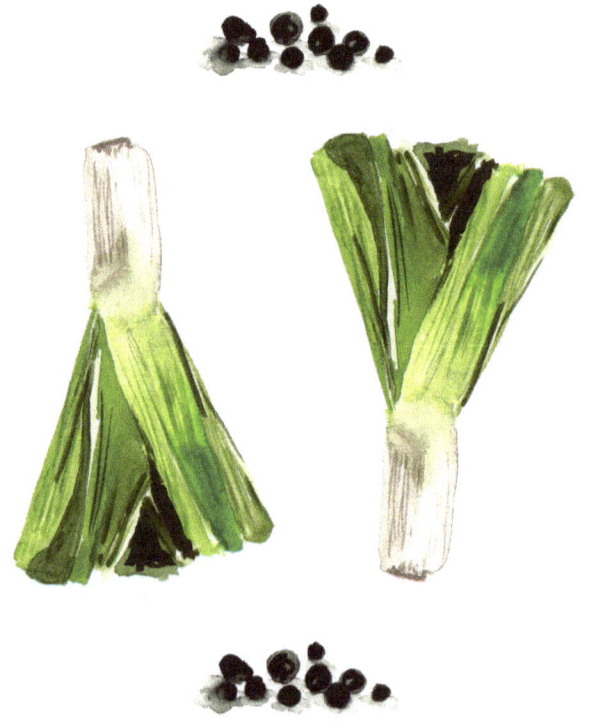

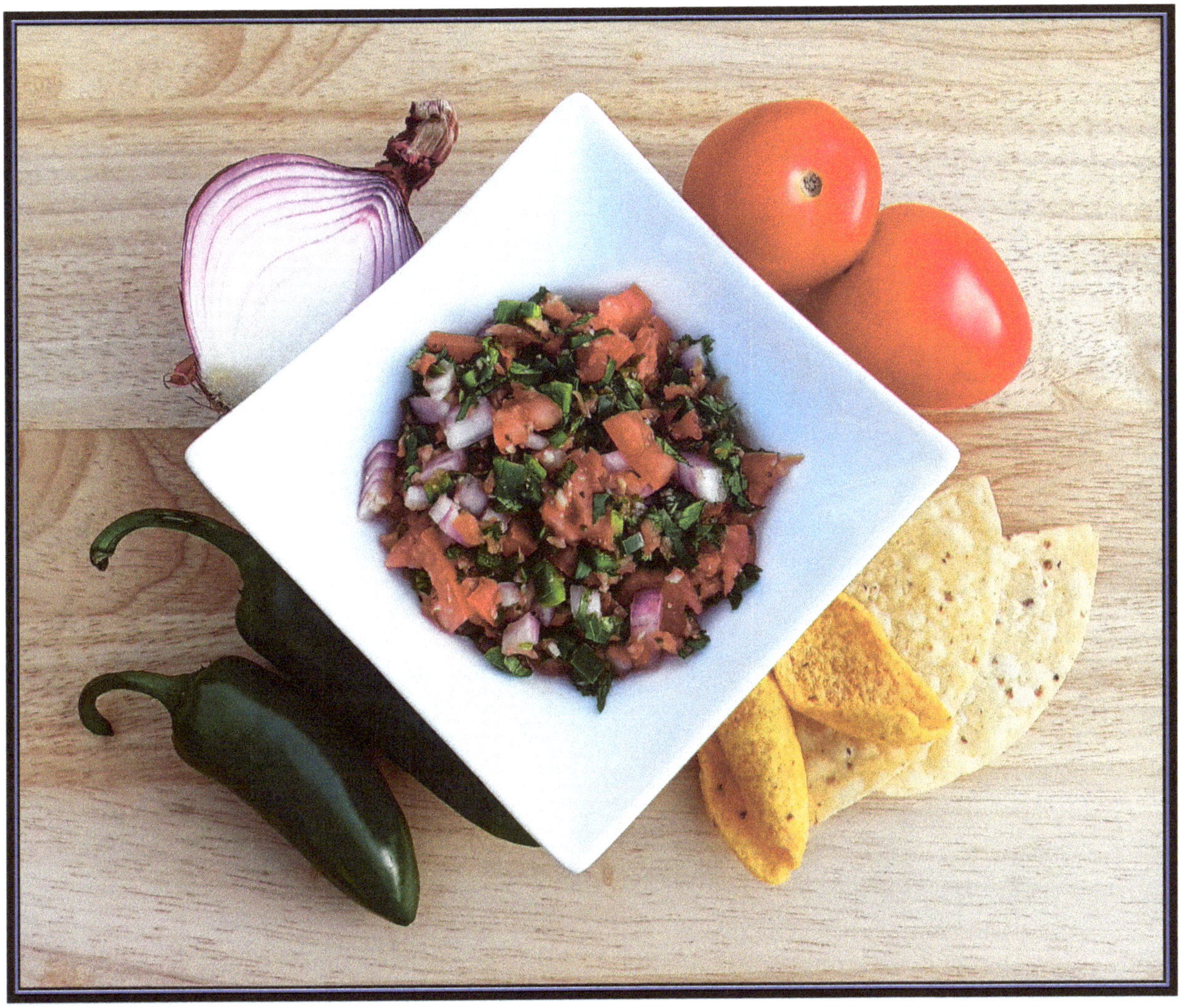

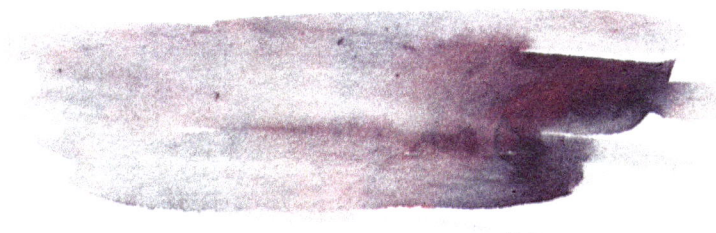

CHAPTER ONE

NEW YEAR'S EVE & DAY

EVE:

Mom's Spicy Meatballs

Green Chile Dip

Guacamole

Chile con Queso

R2-DChews

DAY:

NMNYBEP

NMNYBEP Soup

Pecan Pie

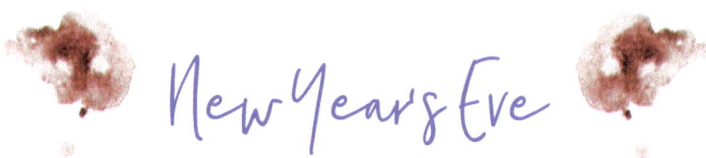
New Year's Eve

EVEN THOUGH HE'S been retired for a decade or so, my husband Bob is generally in bed by 9 p.m. and awake around 3 or 4 a.m. Back in the '90s, when our daughters were in elementary school, he decided to stay up until midnight on one particular New Year's Eve.

He never did *that* again.

We're not drinkers, partiers, or dancers. We are eaters, however, and most of the savory portions of this menu are usually served on New Year's Eve and Day. The dessert changes from year to year, but I'm including the R2-DChews as a nice accompaniment to all the chips; plus, they are made the night before you need them. Now, our household is generally down to two, but Mom's Spicy Meatballs are still a required item, no matter what else is served.

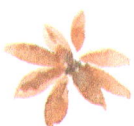

Mom's Spicy Meatballs

START TO FINISH: ABOUT 46 MINUTES

My mother never handed down many recipes at all. Why is that? I just don't know. Somehow, this one ended up in my repertoire. These are absolutely essential to our New Year's Eve celebration. They are only fun if you make them small! The recipe is easy to double and put in a chafing dish or fondue pot to keep warm at a party.

1 pound hot bulk pork sausage
1 large egg
⅓ cup seasoned breadcrumbs
¼ cup ketchup
¼ cup chili sauce (such as Heinz)
2 tablespoons packed light brown sugar
1 tablespoon soy sauce
1 tablespoon white vinegar

IN a medium bowl, combine the sausage, egg, and breadcrumbs with your hands. Roll into small balls (a scant ¾") and place on a dinner plate. Set aside.

IN a 2-quart saucepan, combine the remaining ingredients with a whisk. Bring barely to a boil on medium heat, then put on the lowest heat and cover.

COAT a large skillet with cooking spray and set on rather high heat. Fry all the meatballs. Shake the pan often until they are browned on all sides. Place in the saucepan and mix gently. Cook on the lowest setting 20 minutes, covered. Stir a couple of times, making sure all the meatballs are covered with sauce. Pour all into a chafing dish to keep warm, if desired. Cover and refrigerate the leftovers. Makes around 60–70 meatballs.

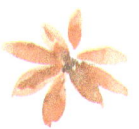

Green Chile Dip

PREP: 7 MINUTES
CHILL: AT LEAST 1 HOUR (OVERNIGHT IS FINE)

This dip is ubiquitous around New Mexico all year long and is delicious with pretty much anything you would consider dipping. You can make this the night before you plan to serve it, to let the flavors mingle.

2 full cups sour cream (light is okay)
1 teaspoon garlic powder
1 teaspoon onion powder
1 teaspoon jalapeño powder
1 teaspoon salt
8 ounces roasted and chopped green chile, well-drained

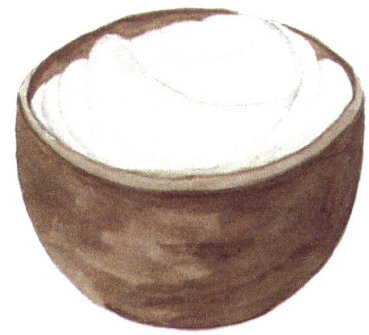

COMBINE the sour cream and the 4 seasonings in a large bowl. Whisk to combine well. Add the green chile and mix in. Season, if desired. Cover and refrigerate at least an hour or so before serving. Cover and refrigerate the leftovers. Makes about 3 cups.

Chapter One: New Year's Eve & Day 3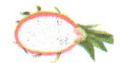

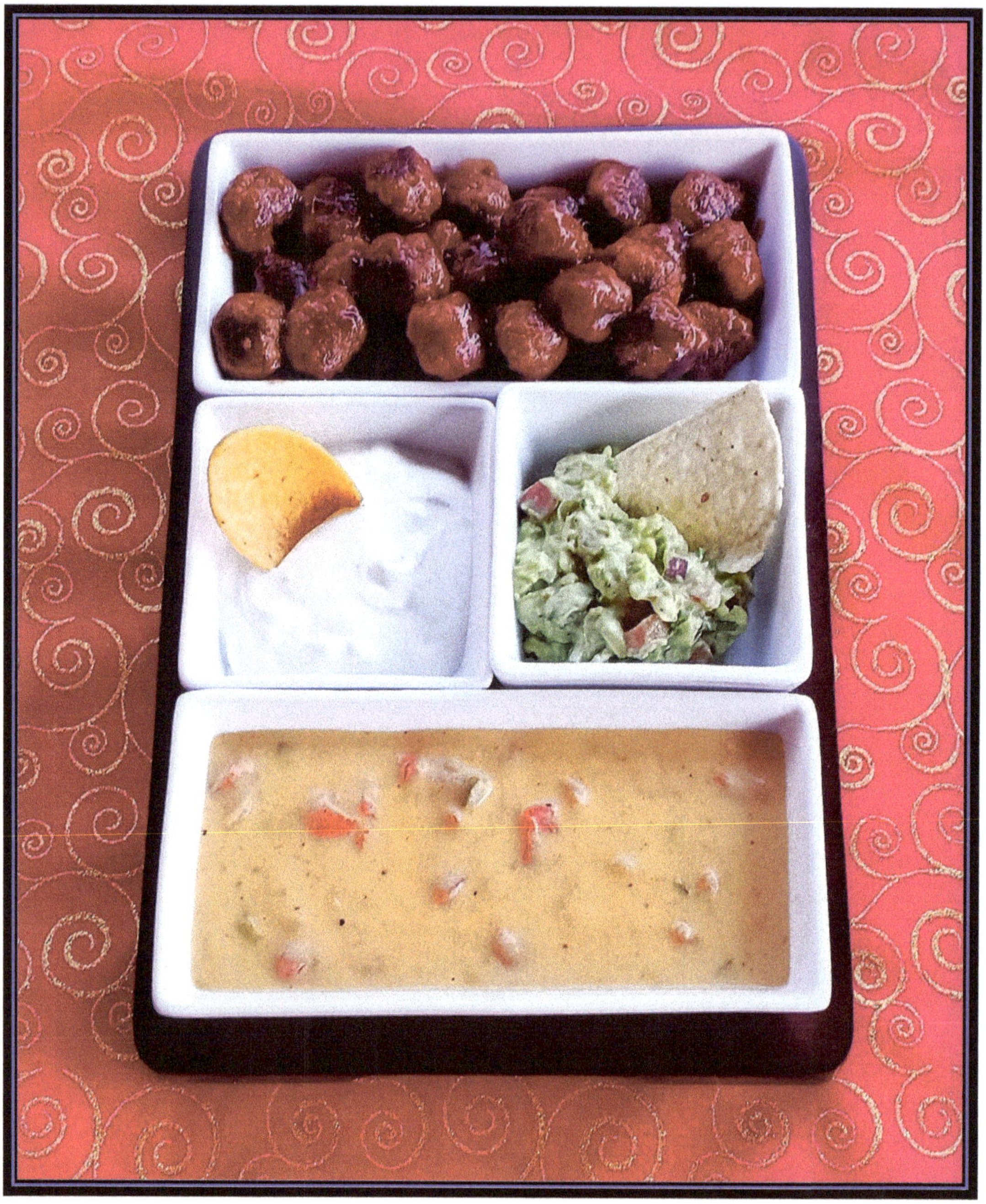

CLOCKWISE, FROM TOP:
Mom's Spicy Meatballs, page 2
Guacamole, page 5
Chile con Queso, page 6
Green Chile Dip, page 3

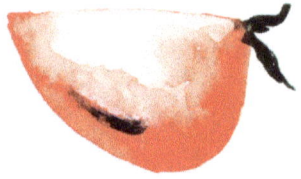

 Celebrating Comfy, Cozy Foods from North America: CH&M, Volume 3

Guacamole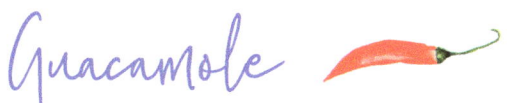

PREP: 18 MINUTES
CHILL: 1 HOUR

Avocados are one of those lovely vegetable-type fruits that can be hit or miss. When they are perfect, they can be sublime. Occasionally, however, you end up with brown spots and fibrous strings inside if you haven't picked the perfect day to use them. That can be disappointing. While avocado toast has become the trendy thing to eat as often as possible, there is really no substitute for chips and chunky guacamole (which can also be piled on toast).

1¼ pounds ripe avocados (not mushy)
8 ounces vine-ripened tomatoes, cut off stems, and cut into ½" chunks
½ cup red onion, finely chopped
4 teaspoons lime juice
1 teaspoon salt
1 teaspoon black pepper
1 teaspoon garlic powder
8 ounces roasted and chopped green chile, well-drained
½ cup cilantro, finely chopped and loosely packed (optional)

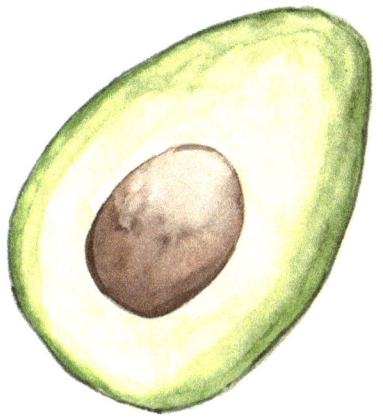

CUT the avocados in half and remove the pits (save them to store with any leftover guacamole; doing this *might* prevent your dip from turning brown). Remove the peel. Place half in a large bowl and mash with a fork. Cut the remaining avocado into small chunks and add to the bowl.

ADD the tomatoes and onion and mix well. Add the remaining ingredients and mix well. Season, if you like. Cover and refrigerate about an hour before serving. Guacamole doesn't keep too well; you might get an extra day or two out of it. Immersing the pits might help your guacamole last a little while longer. Freezing it can be problematic, but you might get lucky, and the texture won't change too much (it might get a bit watery). Makes about 4 cups.

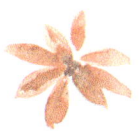

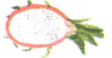

Chile con Queso

START TO FINISH: ABOUT 32 MINUTES

Chile with cheese makes for a killer hot dip. But you can also pour it over eggs, enchiladas, or meatloaf, or combine it with some cooked pasta.

4 ounces fresh jalapeños
2 tablespoons salted butter
½ cup onion, finely chopped
1 tablespoon minced garlic
1 teaspoon chili powder
½ teaspoon salt
½ teaspoon black pepper
½ teaspoon ground cumin
1 cup low-sodium chicken broth
1 cup half-and-half
10-ounce can diced tomatoes with green chiles, with juice (such as Ro*Tel)
8 ounces sharp cheddar cheese, shredded
8 ounces Velveeta cheese, shredded
3 tablespoons all-purpose flour

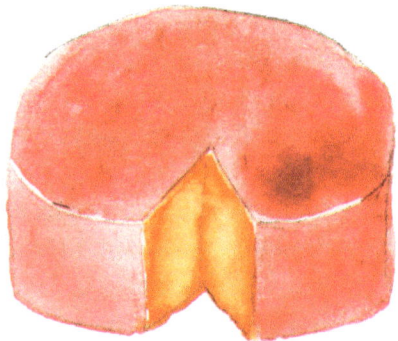

TO prepare the jalapeños, cut off the stems, cut in half vertically, then use a spoon to scrape out the seeds and membranes. Chop finely and set aside.

MELT the butter over rather high heat in a 3-quart saucepan. Add the onion, garlic, jalapeños, and the 4 seasonings and sauté about 4 minutes over moderate heat. Add the broth, half-and-half, and diced tomatoes with green chiles to the pot and bring to a boil. Reduce heat to medium and cook, uncovered, 5 minutes. Whisk a few times.

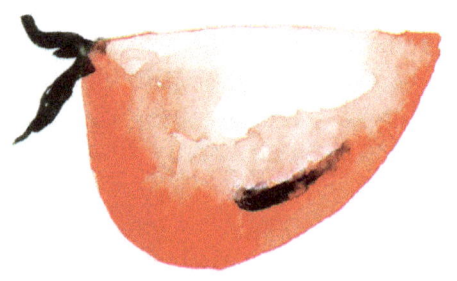

COMBINE the 2 cheeses and flour in a medium bowl. Turn heat to low and mix in the cheese mixture, a handful at a time. Cook on the lowest heat until the cheese is completely melted, about 10 minutes. Whisk a few times. Season, if desired. You can transfer this to a 2-quart fondue pot and keep on a low heat. Cover and refrigerate; reheat any leftovers slowly. Don't freeze. Makes 6 cups.

FOR A MEATY VERSION (*QUESO FUNDIDO*, WHICH MEANS "MOLTEN CHEESE"):

First fry up anywhere from 8 to 16 ounces of chorizo (or other ground sausage or meats, such as beef, pork, or poultry). Go with the whole pound if you want a substantial portion of meat. Break up the meat in a medium skillet and cook over rather high heat until all the pink is gone; drain and set aside. Add right at the end of cooking your queso.

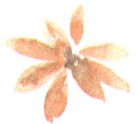

R2-DChews

IN ADVANCE: MELTING BUTTER AND LETTING IT COOL ABOUT 30 MINUTES
PREP: 20 MINUTES
BAKE: 48 MINUTES
COOL: 1 HOUR
CHILL: OVERNIGHT
OVEN: 350°

Here's my first *Star Wars* recipe in this cookbook. I'll just discuss each recipe from a *Star Wars* vantage point and include only one photo. If some important real-world details need to be mentioned, I'll bring them up as needed. Other flavors of preserves will also work in this recipe. **Prepare this the night before serving.**

I wouldn't be surprised at all if the feisty R2-D2 might have a small refrigerated compartment hidden somewhere in his body framework where he could store some goodies. If so, he might favor these delicious bars, which were designed with colors that are vaguely similar to his own outward appearance. I've always loved the insulting camaraderie between R2 and C-3PO; for every "beep boop chirp bleep bloop chirp," there is a "you nearsighted scrap pile" or "you overweight glob of grease." In the end, however, there is also, "You must repair him! Sir, if any of my circuits or gears will help, I'll gladly donate them." We should all have friends who are as loyal.

¼ cup salted butter, melted and cooled for 30 minutes or so
¾ cup sugar, divided
¼ cup all-purpose flour
½ teaspoon salt, divided
3 ounces graham crackers, broken into about 1″ pieces
1 pound light cream cheese (Neufchâtel), softened
2 large eggs
1 teaspoon vanilla extract
¼ cup 1% milk
1 cup blueberry preserves

THE NIGHT BEFORE SERVING: Preheat the oven to 350°. Coat an 8″ square baking dish with cooking spray or grease lightly; set aside. Place ¼ cup sugar, flour, ¼ teaspoon salt, and graham crackers in a large food processor and process well. Add the prepared butter and process until fully mixed. Press into the prepared pan evenly (don't bother washing the processor bowl or blade).

IN the processor bowl, combine the cream cheese, remaining sugar and salt, eggs, vanilla, and milk and process until fully mixed. Pour on top of the graham cracker crust. In a small bowl, stir the preserves well. Dollop all over the cheese mixture in tablespoon portions. Carefully swirl the batter with a butter knife without disturbing the crust. Bake 48 minutes. The center might still seem a bit moist, but it will firm up in the refrigerator. Place on a rack and cool 1 hour. Refrigerate overnight. Cut as desired. Cover and refrigerate the leftovers. Makes 16–20.

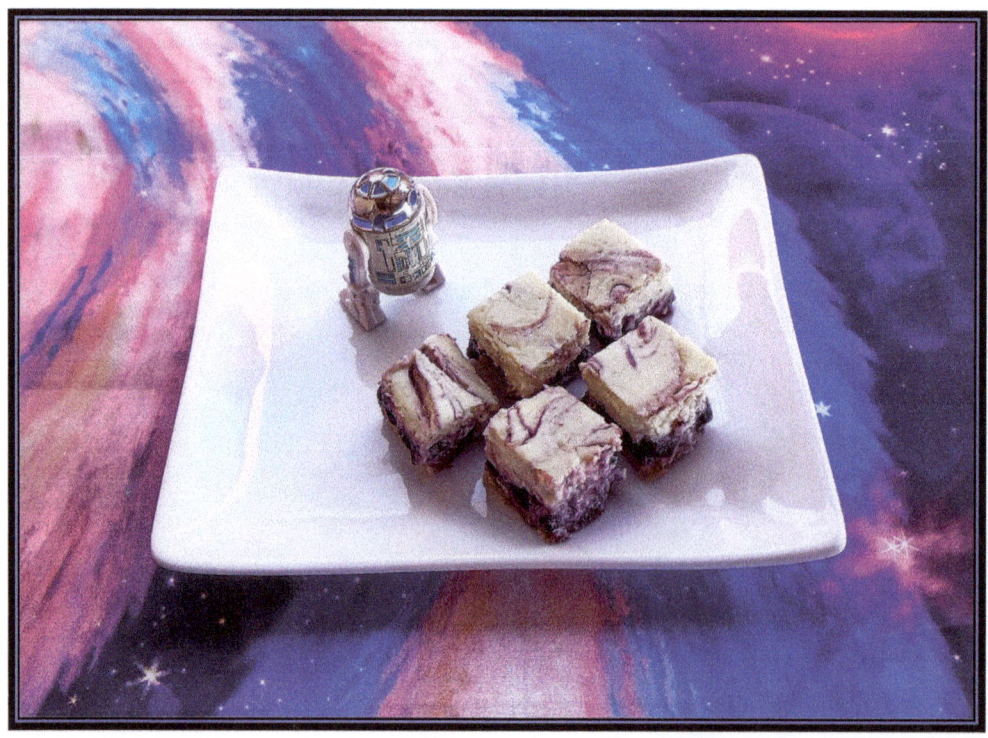

R2-D2 says: "Beep boop chirp. Bleep bloop chirp. Beep. Boop... Chirp?"

(Translation: "I got this recipe from the City's central computer. I know it's a stranger, but they really sounded good and easy to make. Maybe I should know better... but they do look delicious, don't they? Aw, come on, Threepio... sometimes you can be a real pain in my gearbox... well, BOOP to you, too!")

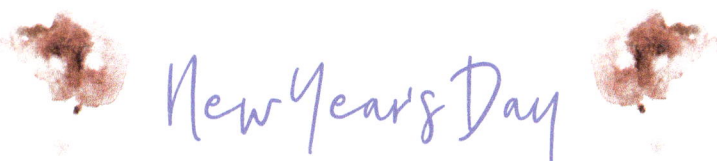

New Year's Day

I'VE NOTICED THAT you need to buy black-eyed peas much earlier than January, if you plan to cook some for New Year's luck. Though you never know any more about food availability—I was going to make these in August of 2023 and my neighborhood store didn't have a single package, so I substituted navy beans, and the dish was fine.

I'm not sure if I subscribe to food superstitions, but New Year's Day is the perfect time of year for a big pot of peas, anyway. Two of these recipes need to be started the day (or night) before, so if you need something to do while you are waiting for the New Year's ball to drop, here you go. To maximize your luck, the peas (which represent coins) should be accompanied by some cooked greens (which represent paper money) and cornbread (which represents gold). But a big green salad and some buttermilk biscuits will also make a nice supper. Apparently, nuts, in general, are lucky; they symbolize new life, so it's a good idea to start a new year with a pecan pie. Be sure to set aside three cups of peas to make the soup recipe below for a future meal.

NMNYBEP

ACTIVE PREP: ABOUT 20 MINUTES
STAND: OVERNIGHT, 10–11 HOURS
COOK: ABOUT 5 HOURS, MAYBE A BIT MORE

A.k.a. New Mexican New Year's Black-eyed Peas, this is a hearty meal to help you ring in the New Year. **Start this the night before you want to serve it.**

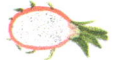

1 pound black-eyed peas
6 cups water
½ cup ketchup
⅓ cup chipotle peppers in adobo sauce, finely chopped
1 cup onion, coarsely chopped
2 tablespoons cornmeal
1 tablespoon minced garlic
½ teaspoon salt
½ teaspoon black pepper
½ teaspoon dried thyme (2-3 tablespoons fresh, finely minced)
2 packets (.2-ounce each) ham seasoning (such as Goya)
14.5-ounce can low-sodium chicken broth
1 pound smoked ham hocks (pork cut neck bones are also okay)

The night before serving: Combine the peas and water in a 5-quart slow cooker. Cover and let stand overnight.

About six hours before serving: Drain the peas; rinse and sort them now. Let them stand in the colander. Rinse out the slow cooker and dry it. Coat it with cooking spray or grease lightly. Whisk the ketchup, chipotle peppers, onion, cornmeal, garlic, the 4 seasonings, and the broth well in the cooker. Add the peas and mix in. Submerge the ham hocks in the peas. Cover and cook on HIGH 4 hours. Stir every hour or so.

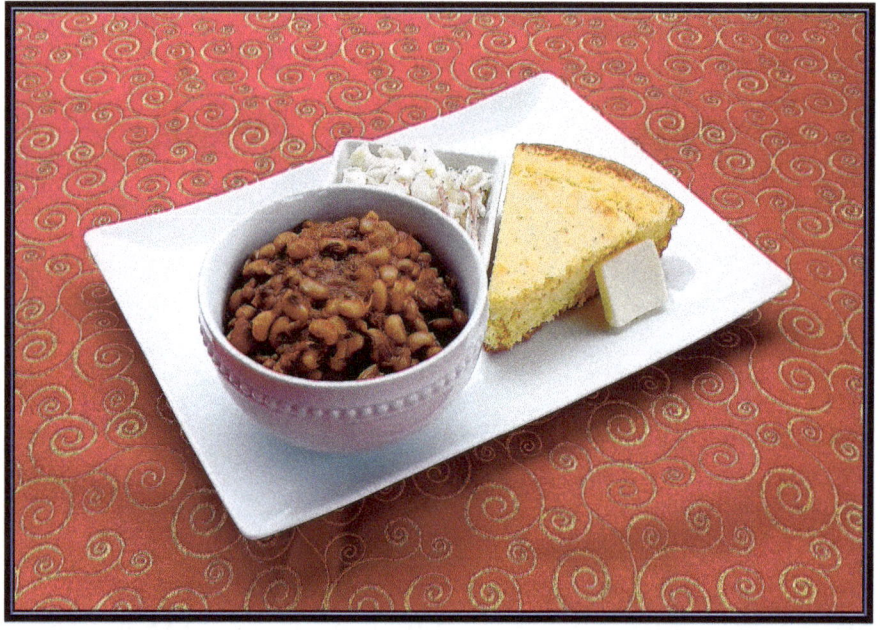

REMOVE the meat, brush off any stray peas back into the pot, and set the meat aside in a medium bowl. Cook the peas another hour or so on LOW, covered. When cooler, pick off any easy-to-access meat from the bones. Chop it coarsely and add it back to the pot. Cook the peas until they have reached the desired consistency and tenderness; stir a few times. The peas should be thicker and saucy but not dry. Season, but watch it! If the peas get done early, just let them stand, covered, until you need them. Reserve 3 cups for the following recipe, if desired. Cover and refrigerate the leftovers; they freeze well. Makes 6–8 servings.

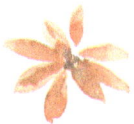

NMNYBEP Soup

START TO FINISH: ABOUT 55 MINUTES

If you have plenty of black-eyed peas left over from the previous recipe, take three cups of them and throw together this comfy, cozy, mildly spicy soup. Of course, any type of sturdy leftover beans will work here, either homemade or canned.

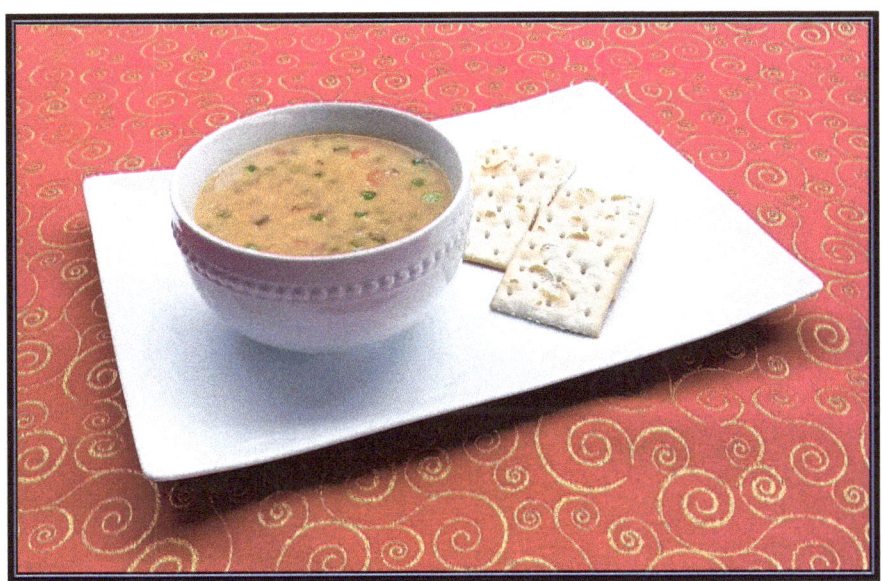

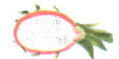

1 tablespoon olive oil
½ cup carrot, peeled and thinly sliced
½ cup scallions, thinly sliced
4 ounces ham, coarsely chopped
3 cups leftover NMNYBEP (page 9)
1 quart low-sodium chicken broth
8 ounces frozen lima beans (sliced okra or
   peas will also work)
¾ cup heavy cream
2 tablespoons all-purpose flour

COAT a 4-quart saucepan with cooking spray. Heat the oil on rather high, then sauté the carrot, scallions, and ham for 5 minutes over moderately high heat; stir frequently. Add the NMNYBEP and broth. Bring to a boil, then cook on medium heat 10 minutes, uncovered (a gentle boil). Stir a few times, scraping up any brown bits. Add the lima beans and cook another 15 minutes.

WHISK the cream and flour in a 2-cup glass measuring cup. Add about ¾ cup of the hot soup to this and mix well. Add this mixture to the pot. Bring to another boil, and cook on moderately high heat 3–4 minutes, uncovered, until it is thicker and the vegetables are tender. Season, if needed. Cover and refrigerate leftovers. Makes 4–6 servings.

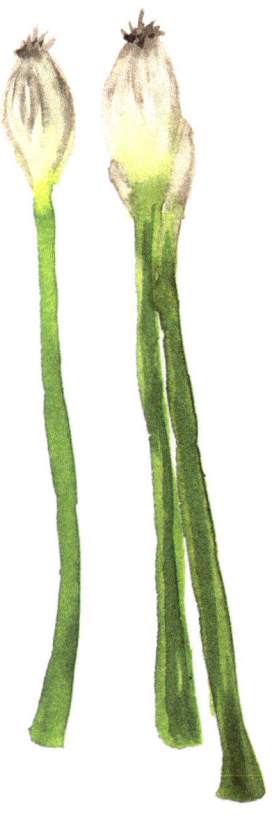

Pecan Pie

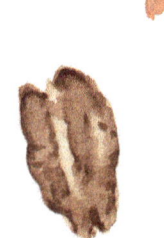
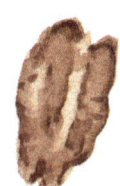

IN ADVANCE: PIE CRUST PREPARATION
IN ADVANCE: TOASTING NUTS AND COOLING
ACTIVE PREP: 20–25 MINUTES
BAKE: 1 HOUR
STAND: 30 MINUTES
COOL: 2 HOURS
CHILL: OVERNIGHT
OVEN: 350°

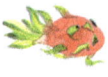

This almost ended up in my Thanksgiving chapter since it's a good make-in-advance option for that hectic holiday. **Prepare this the day before serving.**

A single pie crust (homemade is preferred; see page xix)
6 ounces pecan halves, lightly toasted and cooled in advance
½ cup salted butter
¾ cup light corn syrup
¾ cup sugar
1 tablespoon vanilla extract
2 large eggs
¼ teaspoon salt
½ cup old-fashioned oats
½ cup white chocolate chips

Garnish:

You can't go wrong with whipped cream or ice cream.

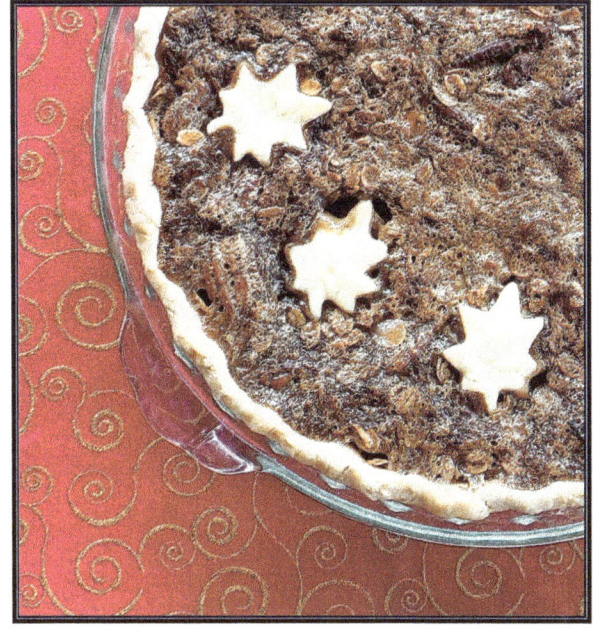

The Day Before Serving: Prepare your pie crust and pecans; set aside. Melt the butter in a 6-quart saucepan on medium heat. Turn heat to low and cook, undisturbed, anywhere from 10–12 minutes, until it becomes a lovely dark shade of brown (not burned). Let stand 30 minutes.

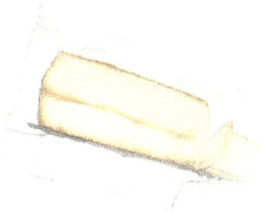

Meanwhile, preheat the oven to 350°. Finish your preparation for the crust and place it in a 9½" (glass) pie dish. Crimp or flute the edge generously (easier to do with a homemade crust). If using a homemade crust, you can cut small decorations out of the scraps if you like. Place the prepared pecans all over the crust. Set aside.

Add the corn syrup, sugar, vanilla, eggs, and salt to the browned butter and whisk well. Add the oats and chips and whisk well. Pour over the nuts evenly. Decorate, if desired. Bake 1 hour. Place on a rack and let it cool 2 hours. Refrigerate overnight. Bring to room temperature for about 3 hours before serving. To serve: slice and garnish as you like. Cover and chill long-term; bring to room temperature to serve again (though I have sometimes left a pecan pie on the counter and it's been fine, especially in cooler weather). Makes 8 servings.

HOW ABOUT A CHOCOLATE VERSION?

You just need to change three items.

After you have finished browning your butter, place 4 ounces of bittersweet (60–72% cacao) chocolate chips in the pot and let them stand for the 30 minutes. Whisk well, then proceed with adding the other ingredients. The second change is to use dark corn syrup instead of the light variety. The third change is to substitute dark brown sugar for the sugar. Everything else is the same. It ends up more like a brownie/pecan pie (as if that's a bad thing…).

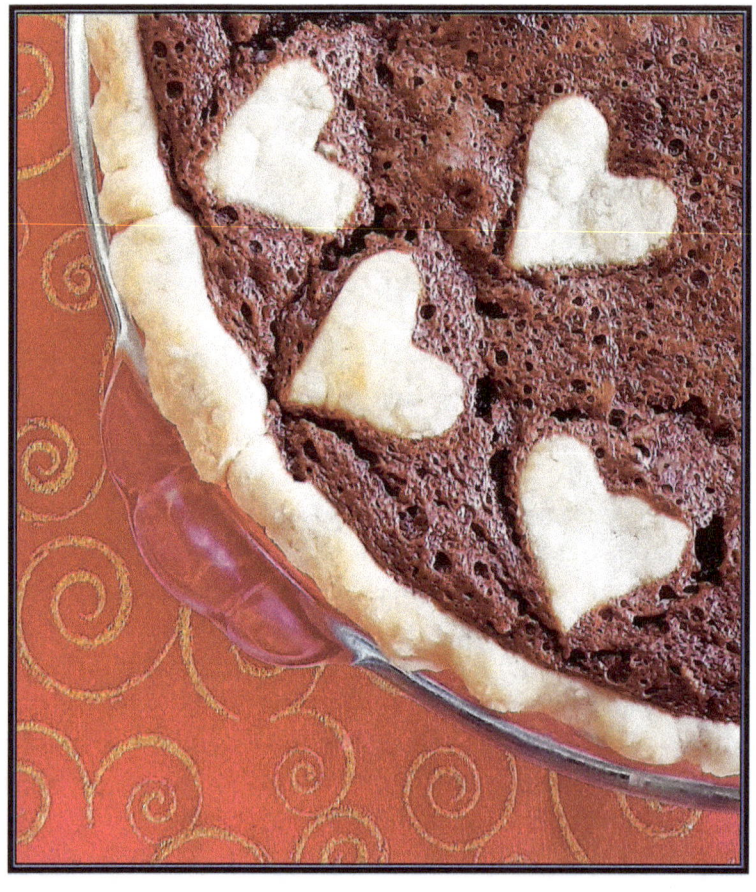

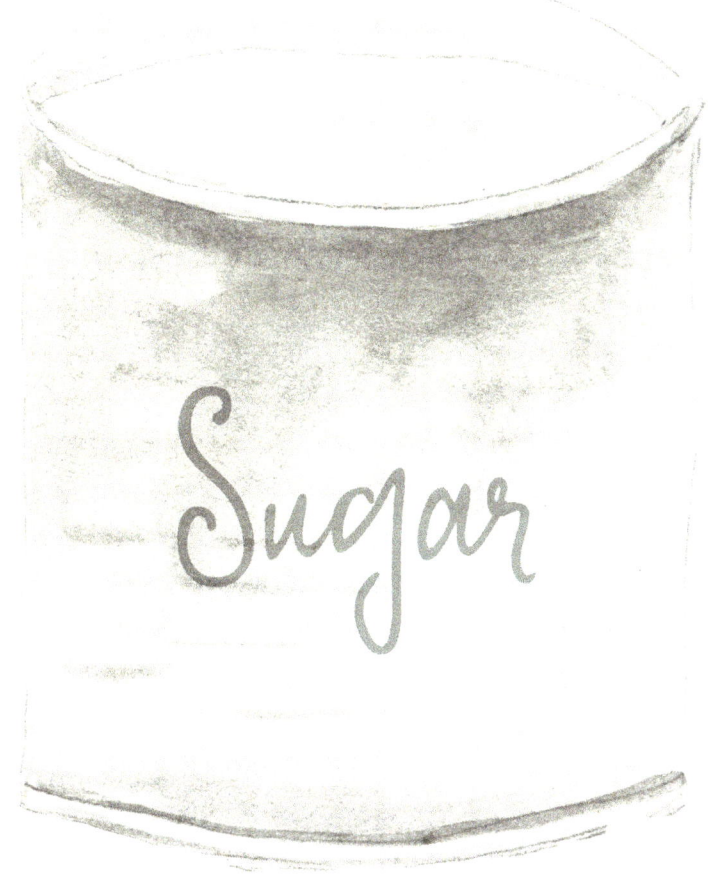

CHAPTER TWO

HALFLING HAPPY HOUR

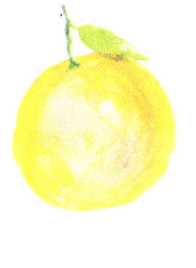
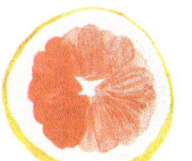

In which is included a plethora of perfectly cozy cocktails.

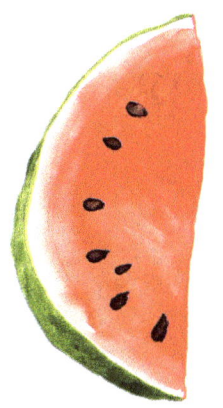

Pick your poison.

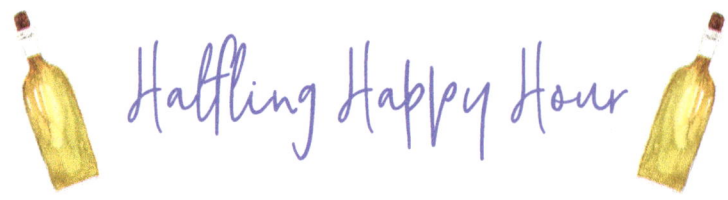

Halfling Happy Hour

THE COVID-19 QUARANTINE time led many of us to indulge in various pastimes more than usual. Shopping online. Sleeping. Crying. Making Zoom calls. Avoiding Zoom calls. Organizing bookshelves and closets. Doing puzzles. Deciding that you don't really care much about doing puzzles. Giving all your puzzles away to your neighbors by setting them out on your large front yard rocks and letting the Facebook group know they were free for the taking. Discovering that even when you have time for cleaning, this is not the pastime you usually choose. Cooking new foods for the novelty. Cooking old foods for the comfort. Baking. LOTS of baking. Then eating. LOTS of eating… Perhaps the number 19 could also refer to how many pounds some people put on during the pandemic.

When it came to baking, my immediate problem at the beginning of the quarantine was a lack of yeast and more unusual flours. I couldn't find yeast for a few months until I finally ordered some from King Arthur (the baking company, not the semi-historical figure). One of my biggest thrills during the quarantine was buying this special canister set from them: a hermetically sealed one-pound acrylic jar, one pound of active yeast, and a yeast measuring spoon. It actually measures out two and a quarter teaspoons! This is exactly what a packet of active dry yeast measures out to be. So, I finally had a stash of frozen yeast and a special spoon. Hurray! And isn't it pathetic how happy I was about this?

Many people tried more challenging baking projects, such as sourdough starters. I researched this for a few months before deciding that having a starter around seemed quite similar to getting a pet. You must feed it and keep track of what it is doing. I just wasn't up for the responsibility; plus, it felt like we would end up having too much bread around.

(Apparently, many people acquired new pets during the quarantine. I like to believe that these were all happy occasions and that all of these fur babies are still cherished members of their adoptive families.)

COVID-19 changed my whole grocery shopping routine to shopping every two weeks instead of weekly, with an occasional extra stop for fresh produce (I never did take much advantage of delivery or pickup services). I now make my own sandwich bread (using my Toasty Muffin Bread recipe from my second cookbook), which was a positive change and cut back significantly on our plastic bag usage.

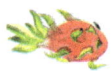

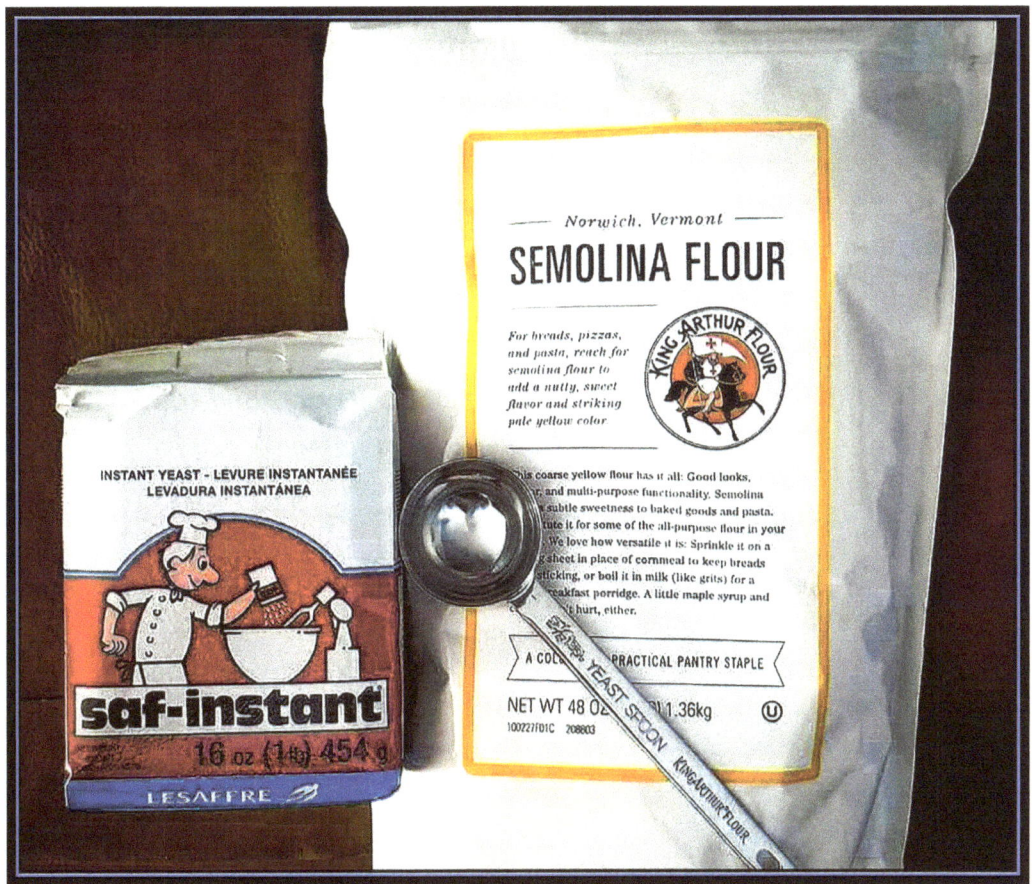

People worked on projects around the house. People watched tons of television. Movies. YouTube videos. People drank more than usual. Some of those people started to question whether this was a problem. Many people (mainly me, I suppose?) really started noticing that an inordinate number of characters in movies and television shows seem to drink absolute gallons of various alcohol products without ever appearing to suffer any sort of consequences, which probably doesn't set any sort of a good example for the viewers of said shows.

Did I drink too much during the COVID-19 quarantine of 2020–2021? Or just enough?

Yes. Yes, I did.

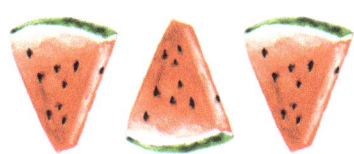

Chapter Two: Halfling Happy Hour

ANYWAY—I'm dividing these simple cocktails into three groups: Sours, Spritzies, and Sweets. OH MY!

Sours have a sour/bitter base, perhaps with a touch of spritz. Spritzies have more carbonation going on. Sweets tend to be fruitier and fun; you know, those yummy cocktails that are supposedly considered "girly drinks."

For almost a year in my early 20s, I was a bartender at a restaurant/lounge kind of place (not my favorite job). When you bartend, 98% of the time you will be serving beer, wine, or basic well drinks, such as gin and tonics. The other 2% of the time, you get to mix something fun and interesting. You meet some pleasant people. You meet some jerks. These people become bigger jerks once they start drinking. Here's my most annoying anecdote about my time bartending:

A man named "Misogynist Jerk" was a rather regular customer. He took a disliking to me immediately. And I to him, though I tried (and generally succeeded for the most part) to hide my distaste. After a few visits, he came in with a couple of friends, one male and one female. He expected them to match his alcohol consumption.

The woman subtly shook her head "no" to me. I stupidly asked her what she would like instead. "MJ" was offended and complained to my manager. This was rather upsetting, but, for the moment I was still employed.

A week or so later, he popped in again.

He said, "You still working here?"

And, in one of those fortuitous moments when one is actually blessed with the perfect words to make the perfect comeback PLUS the courage to articulate those words, I said, with a perfectly arched eyebrow: "You still coming here?"

He stopped bothering me after that.

I was fired for other reasons a few months later. Then the whole restaurant/bar went under because various members of the management were taking bottles of booze home every single day and generally spending much of their profits on cocaine...

BUT ANYWAY. Oh, the experiences of our young adulthood are not always pleasant, are they?

My television viewing and recipe creations sometimes coincided here. I hope you will enjoy—within reason! Some of these cocktails are stronger than others, so time your imbibing accordingly. All recipes (except for the final one, on page 43) serve ONE.

Everything is simple to make. All these ingredients should be easily and readily available from well-stocked liquor stores. I will occasionally list good substitutes in parentheses next to various ingredients. I am also well aware that sometimes people want the experience of whipping up a cocktail but might desire not to imbibe in alcohol. Non-alcoholic options are definitely available online and even in various liquor stores. However, I was so overwhelmed by how many products qualified as non-alcoholic (NA) that it was not possible for me to purchase enough to recommend options for you. Of the products I did try, I would say the results were mixed. And mixed is probably the best way to prepare NA distillations; served straight, some of them are merely fancy water. Not that that is inherently a bad thing. NA beers are now plentiful, however, with many flavor options, many of which are quite good.

Suffice it to say that if you are striving to live your best #soberlife, you can probably achieve this status now more than ever. Your liver will thank you.

Here are a few basics:

Tools of the trade, as required in this particular cookbook:

Stocking a bar is relatively easy and inexpensive. You need a cocktail shaker, preferably with a strainer attached to the top. You need some sort of a measuring container (that is, a jigger) whereby you can measure out at least one ounce, with smaller increments etched somewhere. Jiggers come in many different styles. A 1-cup glass measuring cup probably already exists in your kitchen for larger amounts. A blender comes in handy.

I like using a metal straw for stirring and sipping. This can be used for years and never needs to be discarded or recycled since you can wash it repeatedly. The following items make up your essential barware:

- A coupe or martini glass, 5–8 ounces
- A lowball glass (a.k.a. rocks or old-fashioned), 6–10 ounces
- A highball glass (a.k.a. rocks or Collins), 10–14 ounces
- A pint glass, 16 ounces

You might also add a margarita glass and a copper mug to this list, though margaritas and mules will certainly fit in the above glasses. If you are interested in garnishing your cocktails, you might invest in a fancy cocktail pick. Everything else you might need is probably already stocked in your kitchen.

MEASUREMENTS

JUST A LITTLE CHART FOR CONVERSIONS IF YOU DON'T HAPPEN TO HAVE A JIGGER:

¼ ounce = ½ tablespoon
½ ounce = 1 tablespoon
¾ ounce = 1½ tablespoons
1 ounce = 2 tablespoons
1½ ounces = 3 tablespoons
2 ounces = 4 tablespoons = ¼ cup

Rich Simple Syrup

PREP: ABOUT 7 MINUTES
COOL: ABOUT 1 HOUR

A large number of cocktails require a simple syrup as an essential ingredient. You can easily whip up an inexpensive syrup at home and avoid using plastic bottles filled with non-essential ingredients. A preservative-free syrup such as this can develop mold if stored in the refrigerator for too long (meaning six months or so), so make only half a recipe if you think you might not use this in a timely manner. I've got vanilla in this to give it a richer flavor, but you can omit it if you want. Simple syrup can also be used in other beverages, such as cold coffee or tea; the sugar is already dissolved, so you won't have granules floating around in your drink.

For all the cocktails included in the cookbook, you could substitute orgeat (which is pronounced ôr-zhā or ôr-zhat) syrup if you might prefer a subtle almond flavoring in your drinks. You can easily turn this syrup into an orgeat by adding 1 teaspoon of almond extract. You might also consider having honey syrup around as an option for your cocktails. For this, you would use equal parts water and honey and follow the directions below.

1 cup water
1¼ cups sugar (granulated, brown, raw; you can experiment
    and even use combinations)
½ teaspoon vanilla extract (other extracts are fine, though
    this is an optional ingredient)

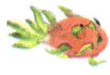

COMBINE all the ingredients with a whisk in a 1-quart saucepan and bring to a gentle boil. Reduce heat to a simmer and whisk a few times until the sugar dissolves completely, about 2 minutes or so. Let it cool, then place in a tightly covered 2-cup container and refrigerate. Makes about 1½ cups (maybe a bit more). Store covered in the refrigerator.

> **SKIP A TRIP:**
>
> Meaning, skip a trip to the local coffee franchise, and whip up a yummy cold beverage at home for a fraction of the cost. In a large highball or a pint glass, combine 8 ounces of chilled, previously brewed coffee, 1-2-3 tablespoons half-and-half, and anywhere from 1-2-3 tablespoons of Rich Simple Syrup, depending on how creamy and sweet you like your iced coffee. Add some ice. Try not to drink it all in one gulp. Better yet—find a really large glass, double this, and make it a grande.

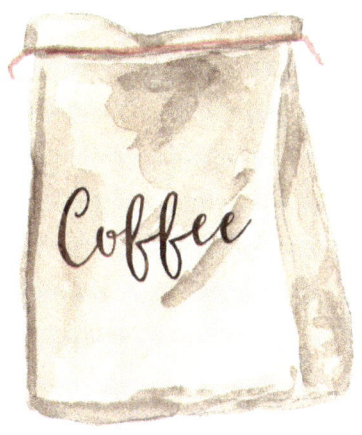

Chapter Two: Halfling Happy Hour   23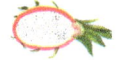

Sours

Though a couple are called "spritzies," they are here because the primary ingredient is sour.

Aperol Spritzie

START TO FINISH: 5 MINUTES

Aperol is an *amaro,* which means "bitter" in Italian. Quite a few varieties of *amari* are available; probably the most well-known is Campari (owned by the same company). The gorgeously orange Aperol is a bit sweeter and contains less alcohol than Campari, so they can be rather interchangeable in a pinch.

You can make many types of refreshing cocktails simply with prosecco mixed with various clear liqueurs or liquors. You usually wouldn't mix creamy types with prosecco, however.

2 ounces Aperol
3 ounces chilled prosecco
Ice

PLACE Aperol and prosecco in a highball glass. Add ice. Makes 1 serving.

Negroni Spritzie

START TO FINISH: 5 MINUTES

During the early days of the pandemic, the actor Stanley Tucci filmed a video of himself making a Negroni. This is a classic Italian cocktail that I find to be murderously strong. So I came up with a tamer version, which is more of an Americano. It might not be up to Tucci's standards, but that's too bad.

1 ounce gin
1 ounce Campari (Aperol will also be okay, and prettier)
1 ounce sweet red vermouth
1 ounce simple syrup
½ ounce lime juice
6–8 drops orange bitters
A few ice cubes
4 ounces chilled club soda
Fresh ice

GARNISH: an orange twist

COMBINE the gin, Campari, vermouth, simple syrup, lime juice, bitters, and a few ice cubes in a cocktail shaker. Shake for 20–30 seconds, then strain into a highball or pint glass. Add the club soda and a few fresh ice cubes. Garnish, if you like. Makes 1 serving.

The Cavett

START TO FINISH: 5 MINUTES

One night, Dick Cavett guest starred on *The Late Show with Stephen Colbert*, and they enjoyed a cocktail together. It's a refreshing summery drink. Aperol will also work here, or any other *amari* you might prefer.

2 ounces Campari
6 ounces chilled orange juice
Ice

GARNISH: an orange slice

COMBINE the Campari and juice in a highball or pint glass. Add ice. Garnish, if desired. Makes 1 serving.

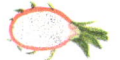

SPRITZIES

These are on the sweeter side, with carbonation.

The Colbert

START TO FINISH: 5 MINUTES

On another night, Stephen Colbert had a drink with the actor Sam Heughan (from the series *Outlander*), who brought along a bottle of his own whisky brand, the Sassenach. Colbert proceeded to pour some Fresca in his glass and Heughan seemed rather annoyed. I figured I'd give this a try and here is a recipe. It works with any whisky/whiskey you like, though I haven't gotten around to trying the Sassenach yet. Maybe I will add it to my wish list.

    Well, is it whisky or whiskey? Generally, if your bottle comes from Scotland, Canada, India, or Japan, it will be spelled whisky (plural: whiskies). If it comes from Ireland or the United States, it will be spelled whiskey (plural: whiskeys). Generally. The spellings for this spirit can be inconsistent. Does it matter that much? Probably not; everyone will know what you mean, no matter how you spell it. Can you substitute your favorite scotch, rye, or bourbon here? Of course you can!

    I WATCH TOO MUCH *LATE SHOW*! Substitute a good quality tequila for the whiskey and you have made a drink called a "Fresquila." On *The Late Show with Stephen Colbert,* Andy Cohen suggested this one, but his show companion Anderson Cooper grimaced at his first sip, then proceeded to get quick-silly-drunk off a shot of plain tequila. Colbert said it made him feel like it was 1977 and he should be smoking a Virginia Slim. Oddly enough, when I used to smoke, my chosen brand was Virginia Slims 120s. Those cigarettes are so long, it was like holding on to a skinny pool cue. I gave up that habit when I got pregnant in 1988. I don't miss it.

    During January 2023, Tom Hanks was on, and he and Colbert shared what I'm going to call The Hanks, which looked something like 6 ounces of Diet Coke mixed with about 2–3 ounces of champagne over ice. I'm not keen on Coke, so I didn't try this. THEN... Hugh Jackman was on, and he and Colbert had an espresso martini, which looked YUM, but by now I can't keep track of all these cocktails, so I give up! Then the writer's/actor's strike was going on for a while, and I started watching *Mad Men* again to vicariously experience all the tobacco and alcohol I was (mostly) not using in real life.

    And another Dry January bit the dust...

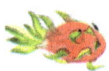

2 ounces whiskey (whisky)
6–8 ounces chilled Fresca (any flavor)
Ice

COMBINE the whiskey and Fresca in a highball or pint glass. Add ice. Makes 1 serving.

Jackie D's Nancy Drew

START TO FINISH: 5 MINUTES

In one of my top five favorite sitcoms, *30 Rock,* the ultra-masculine Jack Donaghy orders a "white rum with diet ginger ale and a splash of lime," whereby his ultra-feminist girlfriend C.C. (who impresses him by ordering a whiskey straight up) claims he must be a sorority girl for ordering such a ridiculous thing. Jack says if a man orders this cocktail, it's called a Hardy Boy. Hmm. Regardless of gender politics, here's my tropical spin on it.

2 ounces coconut rum
½ ounce lime juice (key lime juice would make it extra
     tart, if you like)
6–8 ounces chilled ginger ale (diet or regular)
Ice

GARNISH: a wedge or slice of lime

COMBINE the rum, lime, and ginger ale in a highball or pint glass. Add ice.
Garnish, if desired.
Makes 1 serving.

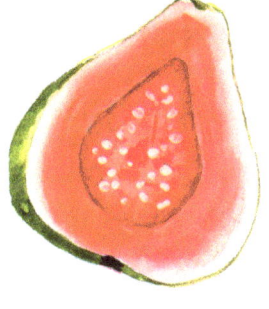
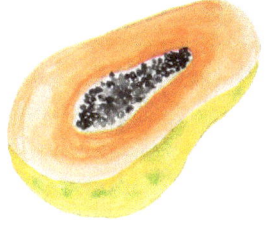

Chapter Two: Halfling Happy Hour 27

Kickin' Moscow Mule

START TO FINISH: 6 MINUTES

A typical Moscow mule is made with vodka, lime, and ginger beer served in a copper mug. Is the mug necessary? Not at all (strangely, copper mugs were banned in Iowa back in 2017). Then, of course, bartenders have created all sorts of variations on the mule theme. You can simply substitute tequila, gin, whiskey, or rum for the vodka. You can use any flavor of vodka you like. You can muddle up some soft, fresh fruit, such as raspberries, and mix them in.

2 ounces vanilla vodka
½ ounce lime juice
½ teaspoon crushed ginger
4 drops bitters
⅛ teaspoon hot sauce (optional)
6–8 ounces chilled ginger beer
Ice

GARNISH: a lime wedge or slice and/or a sprig of fresh mint

COMBINE the vodka, lime juice, ginger, bitters, and hot sauce well in a copper mug (a highball or pint glass will also be fine). Add the ginger beer and ice. Garnish, if desired. Makes 1 serving.

Sloe Your Roll Fizz

START TO FINISH: 6 MINUTES

Sloe Gin Fizzes were invented in America in the early 20th century but fell out of fashion in the '60s and '70s. Try mixing a couple ounces of sloe gin with three ounces of prosecco for a change. Generally, a fizz is served straight up, but you can serve some fresh rocks with your cocktail if you like (be sure to use a highball or pint glass for this treatment).

1½ ounces sloe gin
1 ounce gin
1 ounce simple syrup
½ ounce lemon juice
A few ice cubes
4 ounces chilled club soda

COMBINE the sloe gin, gin, simple syrup, lemon juice, and ice in a cocktail shaker. Shake for 20–30 seconds, then strain into a lowball (one that can hold at least 8 ounces) or highball glass. Add the club soda. Makes 1 serving.

Tickin' Time Bomb

START TO FINISH: 5 MINUTES

Here's another cocktail that has many variations, but I'm sticking with this one because I ended up with a bottle of spiced dark rum with a kraken on the label. A coconut rum will also work well here.

2 ounces spiced dark rum
1 ounce Kahlua
4 ounces chilled cola
Ice

COMBINE the rum, Kahlua, and cola in a highball or pint glass. Add ice. Makes 1 serving.

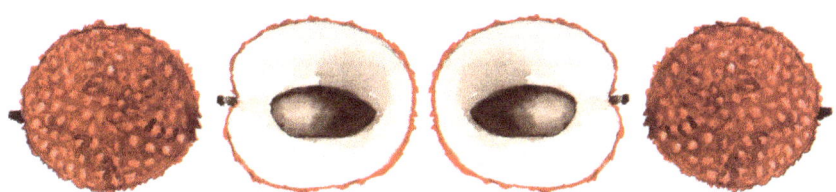

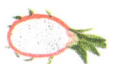

Ooooo-ti-ni!

START TO FINISH: 6 MINUTES

As you can see, this is another one of my *Star Wars* recipes. Besides the amaretto, other good alcohol choices are clear, fruity ones such as St-Germain or Cointreau. Or try your favorite whiskey or bourbon. Make it non-alcoholic by substituting orange juice for the amaretto (BTW, *amaretto* means "a little bitter," an Italian word derived from *amaro*).

> After a long, hard week scavenging droids, your average Jawa likes nothing better than to kick back over the weekend and enjoy a refreshing alcoholic beverage. Water becomes so tiresome. Tatooine becomes so tiresome. It is, after all, the planet that is farthest from the bright center of the universe, to paraphrase Luke Skywalker.
>
> As shown, an old-school Jawa is about to imbibe; he's got his parasol to shield him from the relentless heat, and he's about to relax. But along comes some newfangled creature who can't even keep his head from bobbling around who wants to move in on his treat. The full conversation goes like this: "Omu'sata. Yanna kuzu peekay; togo togu! Tandi kwa! A beton nya mombay m'bwa!" This translates to: "Shut up. This is not for sale; hands off! Give it back! This is mine, all mine!"

2 ounces amaretto
1 ounce lemon juice
1 ounce simple syrup (use orgeat syrup for extra almond flavor)
½ ounce lime juice
6 drops bitters
A few ice cubes
4 ounces chilled club soda
Fresh ice

GARNISH:

Items such as maraschino cherries or various citrus wedges, twists, or slices will work.

COMBINE the amaretto, lemon juice, simple syrup, lime juice, bitters, and a few ice cubes in a cocktail shaker. Shake 20–30 seconds, then strain into a highball or pint glass. Add the soda and some fresh ice. Garnish, if you like. Makes 1 serving.

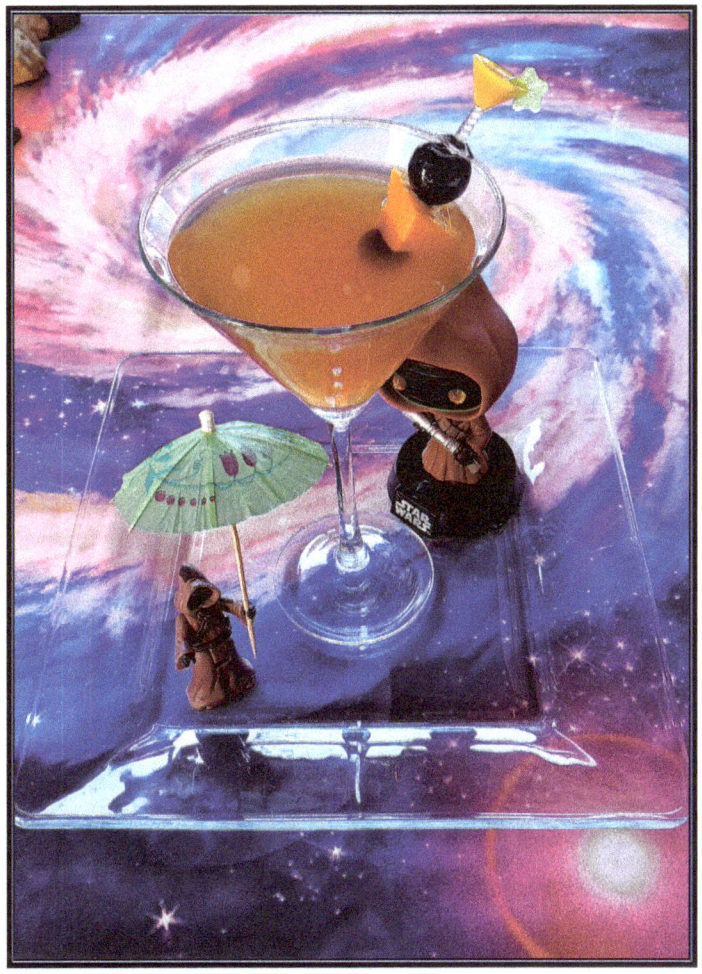

OLD-SCHOOL JAWA SAYS: "A BETON NYA MOMBAY M'BWA!"

(Translation: "This is mine, all mine!")

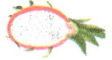

Sweets

Just a bunch of "girly drinks."

Chocolate Chip Cookie

START TO FINISH: 5 MINUTES

For the next three cocktails, you can use any other sort of Irish-creamy type of liqueur, rum creams, or other whiskey/bourbon creams. Try Amarula for a different flavor profile.

2 ounces Irish cream liqueur (such as Bailey's)
1 ounce clear crème de cacao
1 ounce Frangelico (or amaretto)
A few ice cubes

GARNISH: chocolate shavings

COMBINE the ingredients in a cocktail shaker. Shake for 20–30 seconds, then strain into a coupe. Garnish, if desired. Makes 1 serving.

Lemon Cake

START TO FINISH: 5 MINUTES

Limoncello (an Italian liqueur based on lemon, sugar, and usually vodka) should be enjoyed quite cold, yet sipped slowly. This seems like a contradiction, but you could freeze your glass and keep your limoncello in the freezer for an extra chill. I usually don't bother; shaking it over ice is enough for me. Limoncello is refreshing on its own, but it is also a nice mixer with club soda or prosecco.

2 ounces rum cream liqueur (such as Rumchata)
2 ounces limoncello (homemade or your favorite brand)
A few ice cubes

Garnish: a lemon twist

COMBINE the ingredients in a cocktail shaker. Shake for 20–30 seconds, then strain into a coupe. Garnish, if desired. Makes 1 serving.

> **Need to Make Your Own Limoncello?**
>
> Your liquor store might stock a few lovely limoncellos, but if you have some time and patience, you could concoct your own. Pour a 750 ml. bottle of plain vodka (80 or 100 proof) into a 4-cup container (rinse and save the bottle for later!). Add a cup of lemon zest (you'll need about 8 good-sized lemons for this; be sure to juice these lemons for other uses). Cover tightly and let it stand on your counter for 3–4 weeks or so.
>
> When you get tired of waiting, pour your lemon-flavored vodka into a 6-cup container using a fine mesh strainer. Add a refrigerated batch of the Rich Simple Syrup recipe on page 22 and stir well. Using a funnel, carefully pour most of it back into the original vodka bottle (the extra can just be poured into a smaller container). Refrigerate or freeze. Makes about 4½ cups (though this recipe is easy to cut in half, using 1½ cups of vodka, 4 lemons, and ¾ cup of simple syrup).

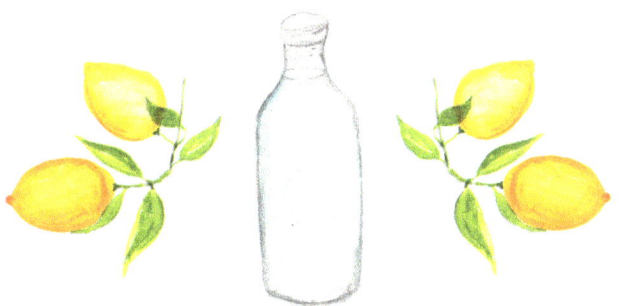

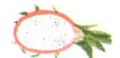

Cinnamon Bun

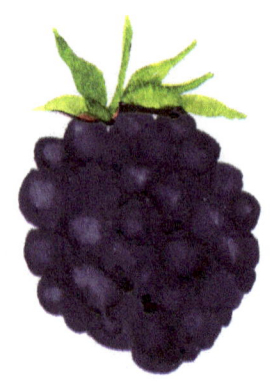

START TO FINISH: 5 MINUTES

This is a yummy little dessert cocktail.

2 ounces rum cream liqueur (such as Rumchata)
2 ounces Kahlua
A few ice cubes

GARNISH: a sprinkling of cinnamon sugar

COMBINE the ingredients in a cocktail shaker. Shake for 20–30 seconds, then strain into a coupe. Garnish, if desired. Makes 1 serving.

Screaming Orgasm

START TO FINISH: 5 MINUTES

For a nice finish (after a meal, I mean!!!), try this dreamy dessert cocktail.

1 ounce vodka
1 ounce Kahlua
1 ounce amaretto (or Frangelico)
1 ounce Irish cream liqueur (such as Bailey's)
1 ounce half-and-half
A few ice cubes

GARNISH:

    A good orgasm requires none.

COMBINE the ingredients in a cocktail shaker. Shake for 20–30 seconds, then strain into a coupe, or pour over some fresh rocks in a low- or highball glass. Makes 1 serving.

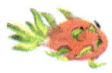

Carrie's Crazy Cosmo

START TO FINISH: 5 MINUTES

Speaking of screaming orgasms, remember all the gals in *Sex and the City*? In their 30s, drinking cosmos, wearing stilettos, and bedding everyone? The clothes. The city. The friendship. The rabbit.

Flash forward 20 years. Samantha is gone, Carrie needs hip surgery, Charlotte is still Charlotte but more so, and Miranda drunk-Amazon-orders *Quit Like a Woman*. And just like that—Miranda was done drinking.

Well, that was easy, wasn't it?

2 ounces vanilla vodka
2 ounces cranberry raspberry juice
½ ounce Cointreau
½ ounce lime juice
½ ounce simple syrup
A few ice cubes

GARNISH: lime or orange twists

COMBINE all the ingredients in a cocktail shaker. Shake 20–30 seconds, then strain into a coupe. Garnish, if desired. Makes 1 serving.

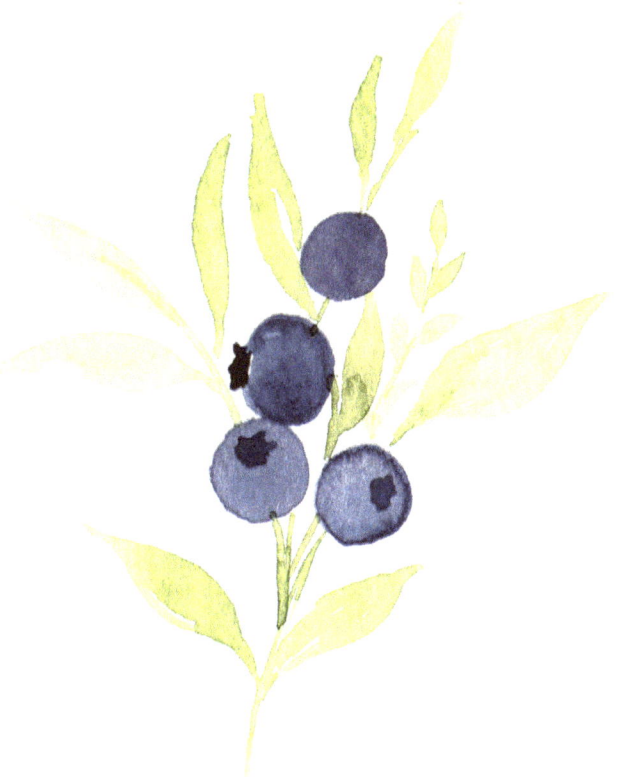

Fruity Martuity

START TO FINISH: 5 MINUTES

Feel free to substitute Grand Marnier or any other orange-flavored liqueur for the Cointreau here and in the previous recipe.

3 ounces unsweetened pineapple juice
1½ ounces vanilla vodka
1½ ounces Cointreau
A few ice cubes

GARNISH: a wedge of fresh pineapple

COMBINE all the ingredients in a cocktail shaker. Shake for 20–30 seconds, then strain into a coupe or a lowball. Garnish, as desired. Makes 1 serving.

Manhattan Madness

START TO FINISH: 5 MINUTES

The typical Manhattan (invented in the eponymous city way back in the 1870s) is made with rye, sweet vermouth, bitters, and cherries. But don't skimp on your cherries—get some luxurious ones, not the cheap kind you would put on a (child's) ice cream sundae. You can use whiskey or bourbon or scotch in this cocktail. A highly flavored liquor is usually not used here (meaning, don't waste your Crown Royal Vanilla here, or your Skrewball or Fireball types). Of course, there are all sorts of variations on this cocktail. I like to keep it fairly basic, but of good quality.

One lovely variation is to substitute amaretto instead of vermouth for an Italian version of this cocktail. Call that version Milan Madness. Substitute Benedictine and call that one Marseille Madness.

2 ounces (rye) whiskey
1 ounce sweet red vermouth
2–3 drops (orange) bitters
1 teaspoon premium quality maraschino cherry juice
A few ice cubes

MANDATORY GARNISH: a few luxury maraschino cherries

COMBINE all the ingredients in a cocktail shaker. Mix them for about 30 seconds with a cocktail stirrer or a metal straw. Strain into a coupe. You must garnish this cocktail. Makes 1 serving.

Old-Fogey-Fashioned

START TO FINISH: ABOUT 8 MINUTES

This classic whiskey cocktail also became well established in America in the 1800s. Its exact origins are a bit muddled, just like the typical sugar cube, bitters, and bit of water that traditionally start the cocktail. You can use any sort of bourbon, rye, or whiskey for this drink. I like to use these large brown sugar cubes I discovered in my pantry (though they really seem more suitable for English tea) and some orange bitters. You may substitute ½ ounce simple syrup for the sugar and water, if you prefer. You might also add half an ounce of clear liqueurs to jazz it up a bit (amaretto is a nice choice, or orange-flavored ones).

A sugar cube (white or brown, or use 1 teaspoon of sugar)
3 dashes orange bitters
½ ounce water
Ice
2 ounces whiskey

GARNISH: a generous orange twist and a maraschino cherry

PLACE the sugar in a rocks glass. Add the bitters and water and set aside for a few minutes. You can muddle this with a spoon or metal straw. Add a few ice cubes. Pour in the whiskey and stir. Garnish, if you like. Makes 1 serving.

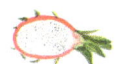

J.D.'s Awesome Appletini

START TO FINISH: 5 MINUTES

Though sometimes ridiculed for his drinking choices on the sitcom *Scrubs,* J.D. sticks with his appletinis: "They make me feel fancy."

1½ ounces apple vodka
1 ounce apple schnapps
½ ounce Calvados
½ ounce lemon juice
½ ounce simple syrup
A few ice cubes

GARNISH:

A paper-thin slice of green apple could be attached to the side of your glass.

COMBINE all the ingredients in a cocktail shaker. Shake 20–30 seconds, then strain into a coupe. Garnish, if desired. Makes 1 serving.

The More Mature Scherbatsky

START TO FINISH: 6 MINUTES

On the show *How I Met Your Mother,* Marshall and Robin discuss the Minnesota Tidal Wave, which is apparently the girliest of all girly drinks. At their usual watering hole (which is the second home for these characters), Marshall gets his wife, Lily, to order it for him. Lily casually and incompletely lists the ingredients: "Five tablespoons of sugar, a whisper of vanilla vodka, and you're done." Too embarrassed to be ordering such a drink for himself, Marshall coughs out the words "maraschino cherries" behind his hand, which apparently means a "handful on top." The bartender says you must have meant to order a Robin Scherbatsky. She orders so many, he says, that they added it to the menu. A swirly plastic straw completes the cocktail.

I figured this needed a more grown-up treatment. If you do an internet search for this mythical cocktail, you will actually find the words "whisper" and "splash" and "handful" when you read a recipe list. But those words are open to many interpretations. You will also find the five tablespoons of sugar. Yes, five. I've come up with a version that still qualifies as a dessert, but probably won't put you into a diabetic coma. You also won't need a hurricane glass, just a lowball. And you can skip the swirly plastic straw; those things are too hard to clean…

This drink is—wait for it—**LEGENDARY**.

1 ounce peach schnapps
1 ounce strawberry crème liqueur (I used Bailey's)
1 ounce cranberry raspberry juice
½ ounce coconut rum
½ ounce vanilla vodka
½ ounce simple syrup
A few ice cubes

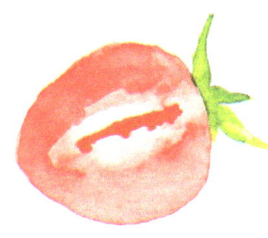

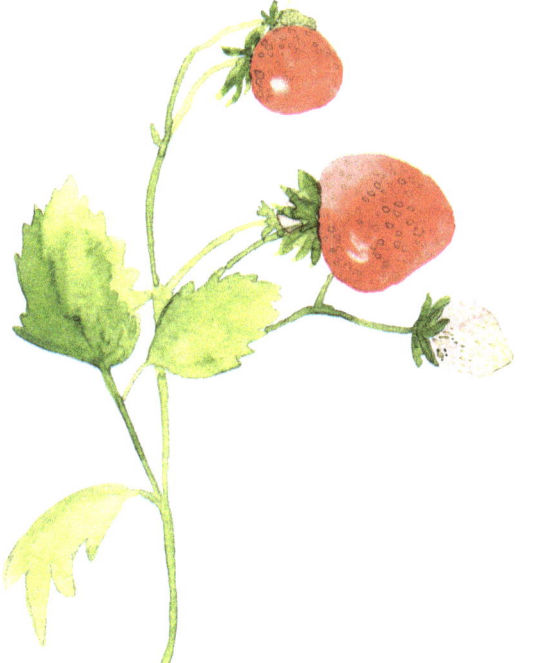

MANDATORY GARNISH:

You must use a few luxury maraschino cherries, because you are a grown-up now. I use 6 cherries, which might seem like a lot, but is certainly not a whole handful. I'm not sure how many cherries would constitute a handful, maybe 20? That's too many.

COMBINE all the ingredients in a cocktail shaker. Shake 20–30 seconds, then strain into a lowball glass. You are obligated to garnish this cocktail. Makes 1 serving.

Chapter Two: Halfling Happy Hour   39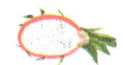

The Black-eyed Susan

START TO FINISH: 6 MINUTES

Black-eyed Susans are the state flower of Maryland. This refreshing cocktail has quite a few variations, though vodka and orange juice are two essential ingredients, regardless of whatever else you end up using. Even Maryland's Preakness Stakes has its own official recipe, though they use a standard sour mix, which I have never used since my bartending days. You can certainly drink it straight up, but serving it over some crushed ice is traditional.

2 ounces chilled orange juice
2 ounces chilled unsweetened pineapple juice
1 ounce vodka
1 ounce peach schnapps
½ ounce Cointreau
½ ounce white rum
½ ounce lime juice
A few ice cubes
Crushed ice

GARNISH: fruity items, such as maraschino cherries, orange slices, pineapple wedges

PLACE the first 8 ingredients in a cocktail shaker. Shake for 20–30 seconds, then strain into a highball or pint glass. Add some crushed ice. Garnish, if you like. Makes 1 serving.

Marvelous Margarita

PREP: 5 MINUTES
GARNISH PREP: 5 MINUTES

Apparently, American states are known for various beverages (such as milk), but they don't officially list alcoholic cocktails. If they did, however, a margarita would have to be the official New Mexico cocktail. I like them to be served in rather traditional ways, either straight up or on the rocks. But you can get frozen varieties with all sorts of additions, from coconut to strawberries, or avocado to mint.

In a nutshell, a margarita consists of tequila, orange liqueur, sugar, and lime. That's it. Below, I'll give you two versions that work out well. There are perhaps hundreds of tequila varieties and dozens of orange liqueur varieties, so you can experiment. Use a blue Curaçao to give your margarita a lovely blue tint.

You don't have to garnish the rim of your glass, but if you would like to do this, you would spread a tablespoon or so of coarse salt on a small plate. Rub a wedge of lime around the rim of your glass. Lightly dip your glass into the salt. Set it aside while you make your cocktail (you can use this salt for cooking afterward). At some restaurants, I've seen frozen blue margaritas pass by coated with almost half an inch of toasted coconut around the edge of the glass. That's overkill to me, but you have to drink what makes you happy, right? To accomplish this task, you would need to place toasted coconut (a half cup or so) in a shallow bowl and spread something sticky (like honey) around the rim of your glass.

SILVER

1½ ounces silver tequila
1 ounce lime juice
½ ounce Cointreau
½ ounce simple syrup
A few ice cubes

GOLD

1½ ounces gold tequila
1 ounce lime juice
½ ounce Grand Marnier
½ ounce simple syrup
A few ice cubes

GARNISH FOR BOTH VERSIONS:

Salt the rim of your (coupe) glass, as described above.

If you plan to garnish your drink, do that first. Combine the ingredients in a cocktail shaker. Shake 20–30 seconds, then strain into a coupe. Makes 1 serving.

Chapter Two: Halfling Happy Hour   41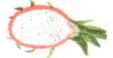

Just Another Tequila Sunrise

START TO FINISH: 5 MINUTES

Any kind of tequila will work here, though you can cruise the internet to read about all the expert opinions on which tequila should go where. Use what you like!

A few ice cubes
2 ounces tequila
4 ounces chilled orange juice
½ ounce grenadine syrup

GARNISH: orange slice and a couple of maraschino cherries on a pick

PLACE ice in a highball or pint glass. Add the tequila and orange juice and stir a bit. Pour the grenadine syrup slowly down one side of the glass to achieve a red glow at the bottom of the glass. Garnish, if you like. Makes 1 serving.

Hot Tamale

START TO FINISH: 5 MINUTES

This can be presented as a layered drink; if you happen to be an expert at that kind of pour, you drink it as a shot. I prefer this cold cocktail version, which is easy to mix up in your shaker. Adjust the hot sauce accordingly.

1½ ounces Kahlua
1½ ounces gold tequila
¼ teaspoon hot sauce (more or less to taste)
A few ice cubes

COMBINE all the ingredients in a cocktail shaker. Shake 20–30 seconds, then strain into a coupe. Makes 1 serving.

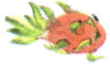

The Watergate

START TO FINISH: 7 MINUTES

I was going to title this one Trickie Dickie's Secret Deep Throat Delight, but that's quite a mouthful in more ways than one; plus, now you know why this isn't a cookbook for little children, if you haven't figured that out already.

Please skip over to Chapter Four and read the introductory paragraphs to the first recipe, the Post-Watergate Chicken Salad (page 56), to see why I invented this decadent ice cream concoction. This will serve two or three people, but if you need to store it for whatever reason, it will keep in the freezer for a while. Let it stand on your counter for 10–15 minutes before serving again (or you can place it in your fridge for an hour or so); stir it up and enjoy the brain freeze.

1 full pint pistachio ice cream, softened a bit
3 ounces whipped cream vodka (or marshmallow flavor)
3 ounces amaretto
2 ounces chilled unsweetened pineapple juice
10 drops Peychaud's bitters
2 drops of green food coloring (optional)

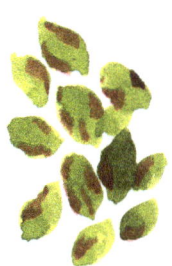

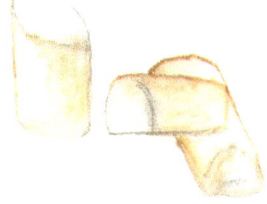

GARNISH:

If you are ambitious and like marshmallows, you could toast a plump one and place it on a long stick, along with a chunk of fresh or even dried pineapple, and a maraschino cherry or two.

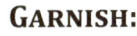 the ice cream into a blender. Add the remaining ingredients and blend on low speed, then increase to high speed and blend thoroughly for a minute or so, until the ice cream has been well combined. Pour into 2 or 3 lowball or highball glasses. Serve immediately, or you can set them in the freezer for a while. Garnish, if desired. Any leftovers can be kept covered and frozen for future use. Makes 2–3 servings.

CHAPTER THREE

SUPER BOWL

Ultimate Nachos

Tomatillo Salsa

It's My Pie, Nacho Pie

Fudge Bomb Brownies

Super Bowl

THIS IS A giant, highly anticipated, and almost sacred holiday for many Americans. It is such an important holiday that some people end up needing to take the following Monday off from work. I mainly pay attention to some of the commercials and the halftime show. Bob is still waiting for his favorite team, the Minnesota Vikings, to win. Lately, they haven't even made it to the playoffs. Oh, well. I mentioned this in my first cookbook, which was written quite a few years ago. I wonder if I will mention this again in another few years. Probably…

My New Year's Eve menu would also be a great Super Bowl buffet, or if you expect many people, you might consider preparing both chapters. Or get your guests to do part of it and make it a potluck, especially if you know someone who specializes in preparing chicken wings.

Ultimate Nachos

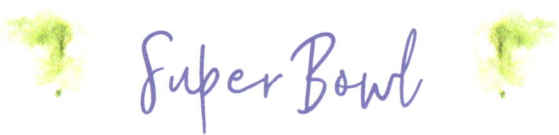

PREP: ABOUT 35 MINUTES
BAKE: 15 MINUTES
STAND: 2 MINUTES
OVEN: 425°

I suppose you can make nachos by simply sprinkling some grated cheese all over some tortilla chips and running them through a cycle on the microwave, but why not make a substantial meal out of them? Customize the spice level here by using either sliced tamed or hot jalapeños. You might be surprised, but I usually use the tamed ones. If you end up with leftover nachos, fret not! See the pie recipe on page 50 for a way to repurpose them.

What does nacho mean? It's the nickname for the man who invented them, Ignacio Anaya. Ignacio means "fiery one" (nacha would be the feminine version for the name Ignacia). This particular dish originated back in 1940, when he invented this beloved combination on the fly. He was the maître d'hôtel of the Victory Club in Piedras Negras, Mexico, which is situated right near the Texan border. Some American women came in after the kitchen was closed, and Ignacio improvised. He cut some corn tortillas into triangles, melted colby jack cheese all over them, topped them with pickled jalapeño slices, and voilà! He named them Nacho's Special.

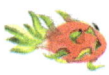

1 pound ground beef sirloin
1 cup onion, coarsely chopped
1 tablespoon chili powder
½ teaspoon salt
½ teaspoon black pepper
15.5-ounce can pinto beans, drained and rinsed
12 ounces tortilla chips (such as Tostitos)
1½ cups mild olives, pitted, drained, and sliced (green or black)
16-ounce jar sliced jalapeños, drained (tamed or hot)
15-ounce jar chile con queso (or use 2 cups from the recipe on page 6)
4 ounces fiesta blend cheese, finely shredded (sharp cheddar or
     colby jack are okay)

GARNISH:

> If desired, take a look at the **NICE NEW MEXICAN & MEXICAN GARNISHES** list and cut up some fresh vegetables to serve on top of this concoction. Your best bet is to make a garnish buffet and let your guests dress up their nachos by themselves.

COAT a 3-quart deep skillet with cooking spray. Place the beef, onion, and the 3 seasonings in the pan and sauté on a rather high heat, breaking up the meat. Fry until the pink is gone and it is almost dry. Mix in the beans, season if necessary, then let it stand.

PREHEAT the oven to 425°. Liberally coat a large sheet pan (18″ by 13″) with cooking spray. Layer evenly:

> Half of the tortilla chips
> Half of the prepared meat mixture
> Half of the olives
> Half of the jalapeños
> 1 cup of the chile con queso, drizzled all over
>   (warm up in the microwave if it is too thick)

REPEAT the layering with the remaining ingredients listed above. Sprinkle the shredded cheese evenly over all of them. Bake 15 minutes. Let stand a couple of minutes before serving. Garnish, if desired. Cover and refrigerate the leftovers. Nachos should be reheated in a warm oven; a microwave might make them chewy and/or soggy. Makes 6 servings, maybe more or less.

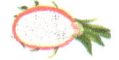

Tomatillo Salsa

ACTIVE PREP: 15 MINUTES
ROAST: 20 MINUTES
STAND: 30 MINUTES
CHILL: 1 HOUR
OVEN: 400°

Although tomatillo means "little tomato" in Spanish, they are not actually tomatoes. This fun little fruity vegetable can be a bit tart when raw, but this recipe roasts them for a while to produce a delicious green salsa. Besides serving with chips, pour this over chicken or fish, top an omelet, or serve anywhere you would serve a regular tomato salsa.

1 pound tomatillos
2 poblano peppers, about 6" long
2 serrano peppers, about 3" long
4 large garlic cloves, peeled
1 teaspoon salt, divided
2 tablespoons vegetable oil
1 pound avocados (ripe, but not mushy)

PREHEAT the oven to 400°. Coat an 8" square glass baking dish with cooking spray. Remove the husks from the tomatillos. Wash them, cut into quarters, cut off the stems, then place them in the prepared pan. Cut the poblanos in half lengthwise. Remove the stems, seeds, and membranes. Cut them into 1" chunks; add to the pan. Cut the stems off the serranos, then cut the peppers into thirds; add them and the garlic to the pan. Sprinkle with ½ teaspoon salt evenly. Pour oil all over and mix well. Roast 20 minutes. Mix halfway through cooking, then after cooking. Let stand in the pan about 30 minutes. Blend completely (you can prepare this the night before you need it; cover and refrigerate).

PEEL and pit the avocados. Mash half of them with the remaining salt in a medium bowl. Add the tomatillo puree and mix in well. Cut the remaining avocados into small bits and mix in. Season, if needed. Cover and refrigerate 1 hour before serving. Makes about 4 cups.

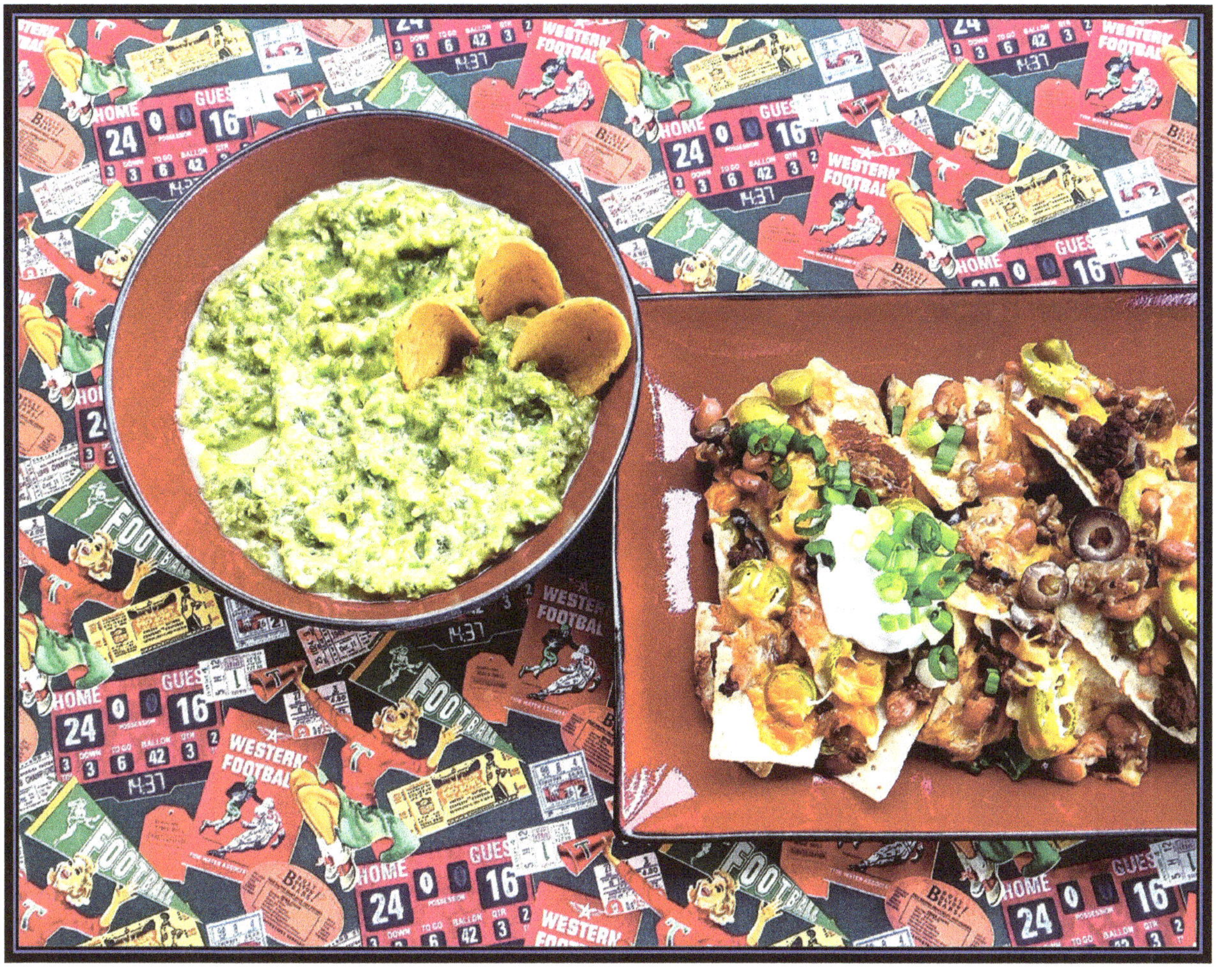

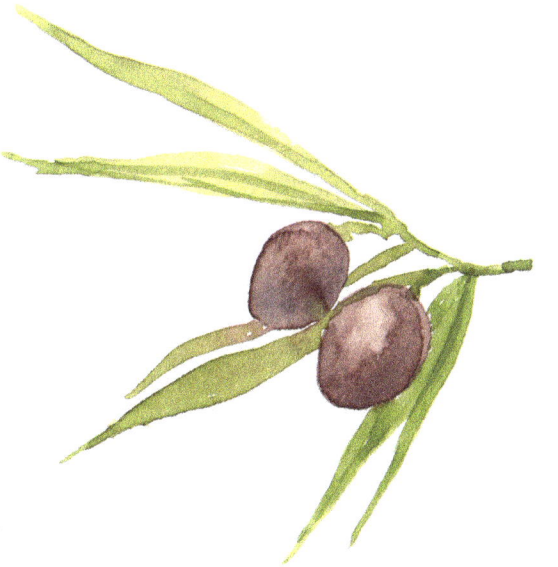

Left:
Tomatillo Salsa, page 48

Right:
Ultimate Nachos, page 46

It's My Pie, Nacho Pie

PREP: 10 MINUTES
BAKE: ABOUT 50 MINUTES
STAND: ABOUT 10 MINUTES
OVEN: 375°

Let's say you have ended up with a pile of leftover nachos, either from some you prepared at home, or maybe you brought some home from a restaurant. Nachos don't always lend themselves to a reheat (the microwave will make them soggy, and the oven might make them dry out if you're not careful). Here's a recipe that can utilize those leftovers in a tasty way. Serve with a green salad on the side.

1 pound cold leftover nachos (any variety)
1 cup 1% milk
4 large eggs
1 teaspoon chili powder
½ teaspoon salt
½ teaspoon black pepper
½ teaspoon garlic powder
4 ounces roasted and chopped green chile,
    with juice
2 ounces sharp cheddar cheese, finely shredded
    (fiesta blend is also fine)

GARNISH:

Tomatillo Salsa (page 48) is excellent poured over this pie, but you could also dress this up with some fresh **NEW MEXICAN & MEXICAN GARNISHES** from the list at the beginning of the cookbook.

PREHEAT the oven to 375°. Coat an 8" square baking dish with cooking spray or grease lightly. Break up the nachos and place in the pan relatively evenly. Place the milk, eggs, the 4 seasonings, and the green chile in a large bowl and whisk well. Pour over all the nachos. Press the chips down a bit with a spatula. Sprinkle the shredded cheese all over. Bake 46–50 minutes, until the center is firm. Let stand 5–10 minutes before cutting. Garnish, if desired. Cover and refrigerate the leftovers. Makes 4–6 servings.

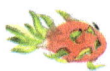

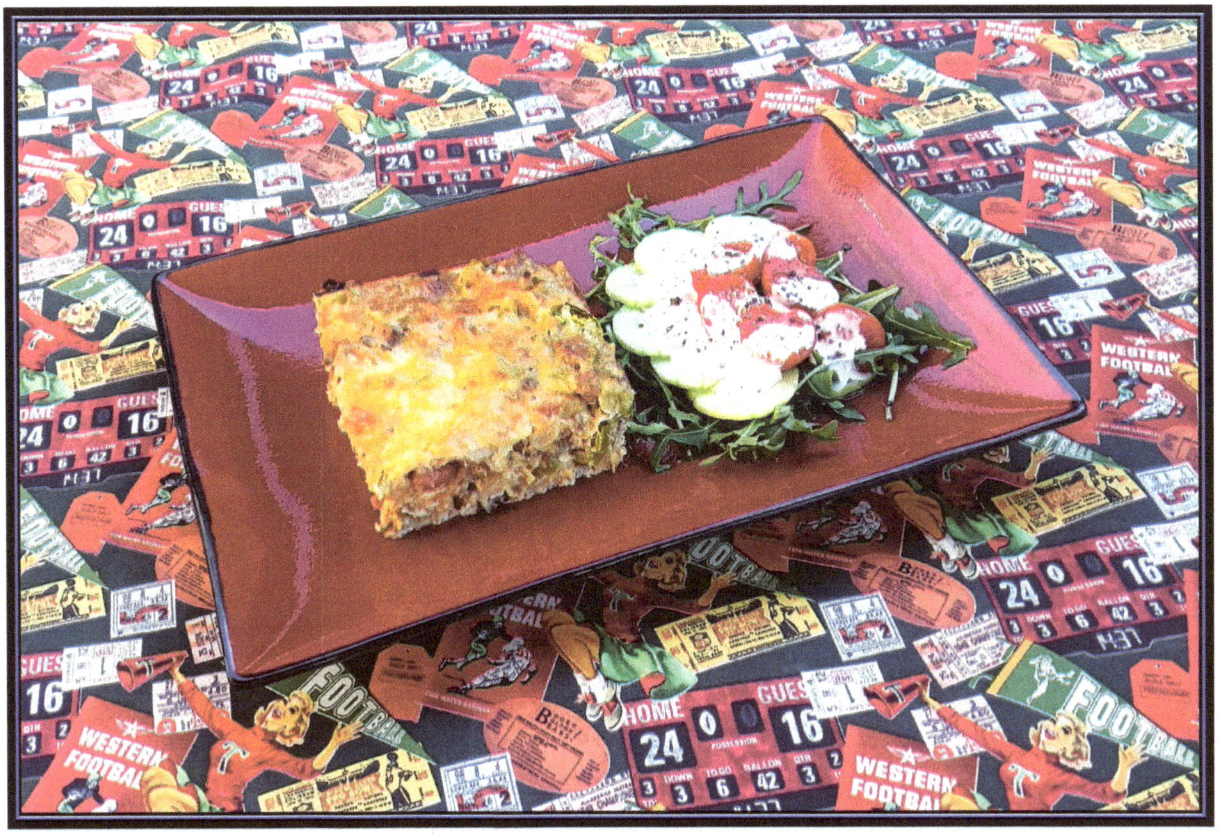

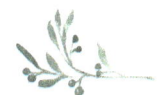

Chapter Three: Super Bowl 51

Fudge Bomb Brownies

IN ADVANCE: TOASTING NUTS, COOLING, AND CHOPPING
PREP: 15 MINUTES
BAKE: 38 MINUTES
COOL: 2 HOURS
OVEN 350°

What's better than some decadent chocolatey goodness to round out your game day? If you were really ambitious, you could cut these in advance, squirt a bit of whipped cream or premade frosting on the top, and decorate each with a tiny sugar football (if you can find some already made up around the end of January). Make them mocha by adding anywhere from 1–2 tablespoons of instant espresso powder to the butter mixture.

6 ounces pecans, lightly toasted, cooled, and chopped coarsely in advance
4 ounces unsweetened chocolate, broken into smaller squares
¾ cup salted butter
1 cup sugar
1 cup packed light brown sugar
2 tablespoons 1% milk
1 tablespoon vanilla extract
3 large eggs, room temperature
1 cup all-purpose flour
¼ cup unsweetened cocoa powder
1 teaspoon salt
½ teaspoon baking powder
3 ounces white chocolate chips

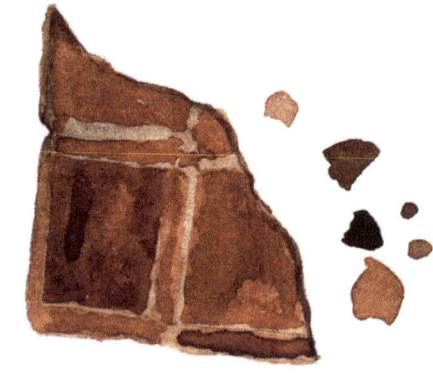

PREHEAT the oven to 350°. Coat an 11" by 7" baking dish with cooking spray or grease lightly; set aside.

PLACE the unsweetened chocolate and butter in a very large glass bowl. Microwave on HIGH in 20-second intervals until melted. Whisk to mix well. Whisk the sugar, brown sugar, milk, and vanilla into the butter mixture. Whisk the eggs in well. Add the flour, cocoa powder, salt, and baking powder and mix in well. Add the prepared pecans and white chocolate chips and mix well. Spread in the prepared pan. Bake 38 minutes. Place on a rack and cool 2 hours before cutting. Cover and keep at room temperature. Makes 18–24, or less, if you like giant brownies.

FAN
WESTERN FOOTBALL
FOOTBALL
HOME
24
0
16
POSSESSION
DOWN
TO GO
BALLON
QTR
3
3
6
42
3
14:37

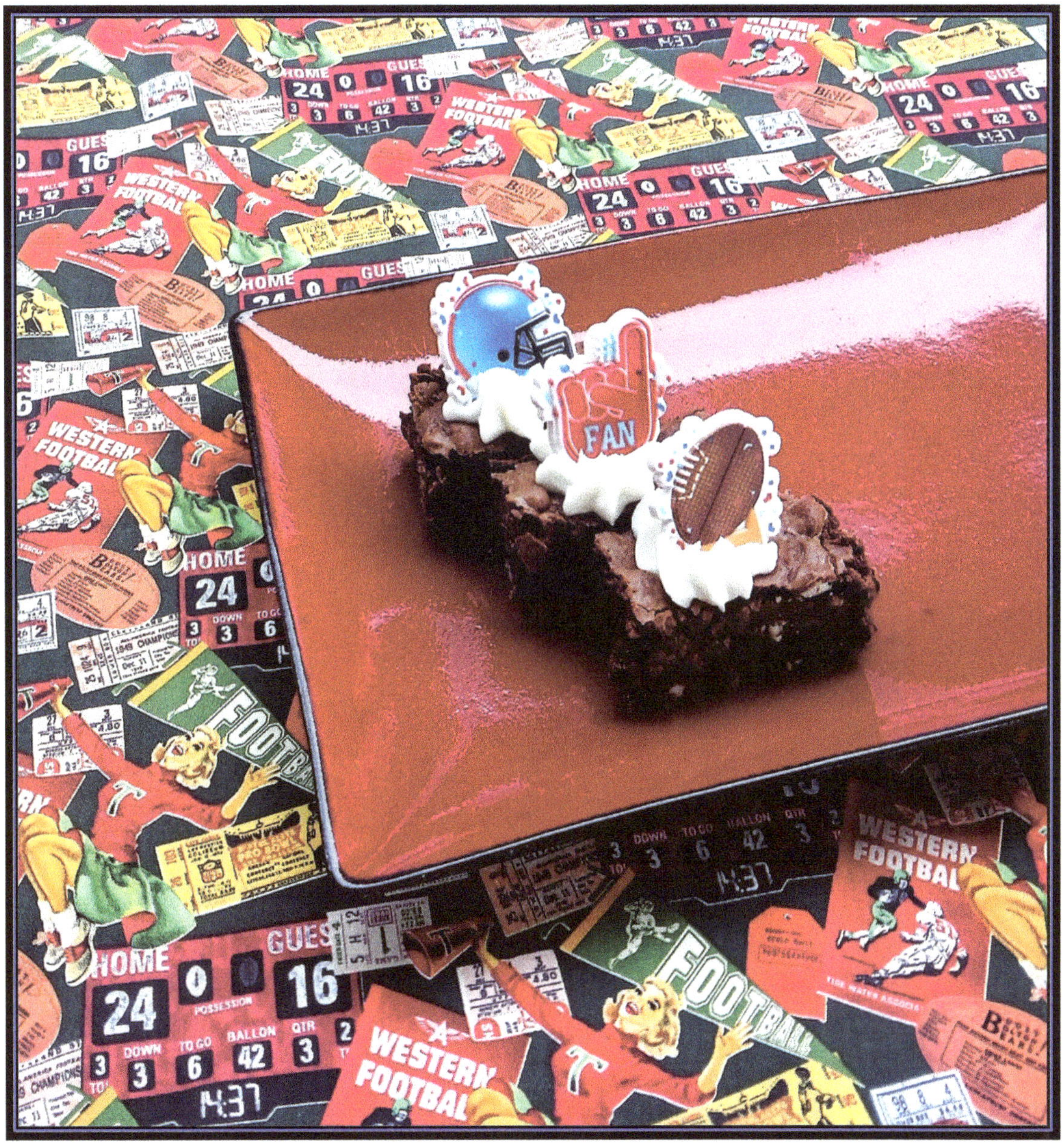

Chapter Four

Cold Salads

Post-Watergate Chicken Salad

Black Bean Salad

You Can't Name Everything After Bob Potato Salad

Three Bean Salad

Bacon Mac Salad

Super Savory Salad

All Hail the Caesar Salad

Naked Ambrosia

Cold Salads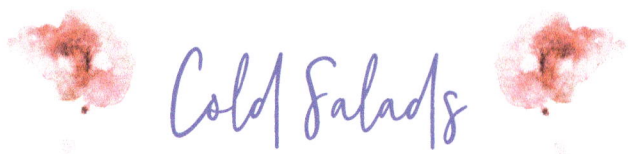

I HAVEN'T ASSIGNED these particular salads to fancy holiday chapters, but you can certainly interchange them with other recipes, if you like.

Post-Watergate Chicken Salad

START TO FINISH: ABOUT 20 MINUTES

A few years ago, I occasionally played this bizarre role-playing/trivia game on my phone called *Quiz RPG: World of Mystic Wiz.* You roamed around medieval/fantasy settings and collected spirits, all of which were beautifully drawn. You encountered enemies/bosses and had to answer trivia questions to proceed. Yes, I know that sounds pretty goofy, but it was good for taking your mind off your other exasperating game called *Candy Crush* (which I deleted long ago).

One night, I was playing *Quiz RPG* and I got this question: "Which of these nuts is usually in a 'Watergate Salad?'" The possible answers were: walnuts, peanuts, pistachios, or Brazil nuts. I had no idea what a Watergate Salad was, but I figured it was an American invention so I went with peanuts. This was the wrong answer; apparently, pistachios were the correct nuts. I demolished the boss in the game; then, I did some research on this mysterious item.

It's amazing how often American cuisine attaches the word "salad" to various obviously unhealthy items. Perhaps this stems from potlucks; you know, you get stuck bringing a "salad," but you really want to bring something that guests will enjoy, not just a bunch of greenery, which you know you are going to end up taking home. Nobody eats much of the vegetable trays with ranch dressing or the fruit trays. Perhaps if just one ingredient were a fruit or a vegetable, it could then qualify as a salad. Even if your fruit is merely a maraschino cherry, it would count as a salad. With this logic, you could concoct pretty much anything and then assign your new recipe to the salad section of the menu.

The Watergate Salad's origins are hard to pinpoint. Apparently, it is not definite that it was invented by a chef at the eponymous hotel, nor can we pin down whether it originated in the Midwest or the Deep South. Perhaps Kraft Foods invented it merely to market their pistachio pudding mix. But the name was attached to it in the mid-'70s and most likely is related, however obscurely, to the

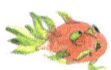

political scandal that took place at the time. It is also known as "green stuff," or "pistachio fluff." Most cooks who write about it love it—it is a great dish to bring to a potluck or serve on a holiday. It definitely falls into the "Seventies Food Trends" category, but before you go all snobby/foodie and relegate all old-fashioned foods to the discard bin, remember that every decade has food trends that fall out of favor eventually (gelatinous hot dog salads should definitely remain in the discard bin, however). What will be ridiculed as the trends of the early 21st century? I'm thinking it'll be kale…

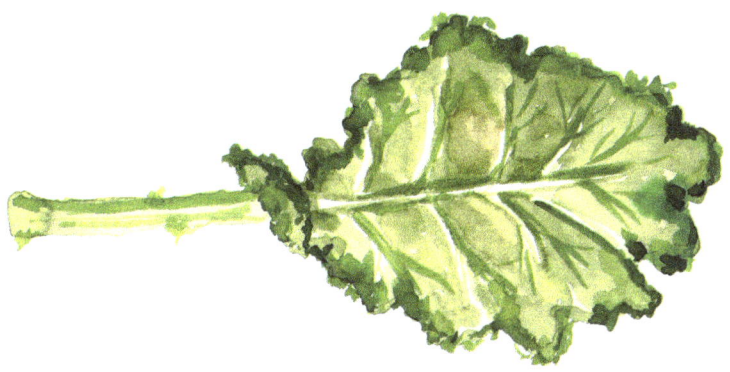

The salad is generally composed of these particular ingredients: Cool Whip, miniature marshmallows, pecans, pistachio pudding, and canned crushed pineapple in juice. There are many variations on this theme. You could add (or substitute) items, such as sliced almonds, maraschino cherries, fruit cocktail, chunky pineapple, sour cream, etc.

My automatic response to this salad was "BLECH," mainly because I really don't like marshmallows (just the actual candy's texture; I'm okay with marshmallow creme mixed into recipes, such as what you would put in a Rice Krispies Treat), but I was intrigued by the combination of flavors. Bob would probably love it, except for the canned pineapple. At first, I came up with the concept of an alcoholic beverage, which I was going to call something like "Deep Throat Delight." But then I had trouble finding pistachio liqueur locally and I was reluctant to order it through the mail; I hated the idea of receiving a broken bottle of booze. It's probably expensive stuff, too. You can check out Chapter Two (page 43) to see what I did with that idea.

My other thought was a main dish/salad, so I came up with this. This is lovely served over a bed of delicate greens, or crackers, or as a sandwich. For the dried pineapple, you may use the sweetened or unsweetened variety; either will work. Would this work at a potluck? Maybe. Bring along some crackers and see.

Chapter Four: Cold Salads   57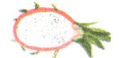

1 tablespoon salted butter
1½ teaspoons sugar, divided
¼ teaspoon cayenne pepper (use ½ teaspoon for a bigger kick)
1 ounce pecan halves, coarsely chopped
1 ounce dry roasted and salted pistachios, coarsely chopped
¼ cup sour cream (light is okay)
¼ cup mayonnaise
2 tablespoons unsweetened pineapple juice
1 teaspoon lemon juice
½ teaspoon salt
½ teaspoon white pepper
8 ounces cooked chicken, coarsely chopped
3 ounces dried pineapple, coarsely chopped (preferably unsweetened)
½ cup scallions, thinly sliced

In a small skillet, melt the butter over rather high heat. Add 1 teaspoon sugar and the cayenne. Add the nuts and sauté 1 minute, stirring frequently. Set aside.

In a large bowl, combine the remaining sugar, sour cream, mayonnaise, the 2 juices, and the 2 seasonings with a whisk until smooth. Add the chicken, pineapple, scallions, and nuts (break them up gently with a spatula, if necessary) and combine well. Cover and refrigerate the leftovers. Makes about 2¾ cups.

Black Bean Salad

START TO FINISH: ABOUT 15 MINUTES

Hearty and full of fiber, this is a fine fit as a Southwestern side dish.

15-ounce can black beans
1 tablespoon vegetable oil
1 tablespoon lime juice
1 tablespoon amber agave syrup (molasses or dark corn syrup will also work)
½ teaspoon salt
½ teaspoon black pepper
½ teaspoon dried oregano (2 tablespoons fresh, minced)

½ teaspoon cayenne pepper
1 large jalapeño
8 ounces Roma tomatoes
3 ounces feta cheese, crumbled coarsely (cotija will also work)

DRAIN and rinse the beans. Shake off the excess water and let stand in the strainer until they are fairly dry. Whisk the oil, lime juice, agave, and the 4 seasonings well in a medium bowl; set aside.

CUT the stem off the jalapeño, cut in half vertically, then scrape out the seeds and membranes with a spoon. Cut into ¼" pieces. Add the beans and jalapeño to the bowl. Cut the tomatoes into ½" chunks and place in the strainer. Shake off any excess liquid, then add them to the bowl. Add the cheese and mix well. Season, if desired. Refrigerate for an hour. Mix, then serve with a slotted spoon. Cover and refrigerate the leftovers. Makes about 4 cups.

You Can't Name Everything After Bob Potato Salad

IN ADVANCE: HARD BOILING EGGS AND CHILLING (APPROXIMATELY 2 HOURS)
IN ADVANCE: COOKING POTATOES AND COOLING (APPROXIMATELY 1 HOUR)
PREP: 20 MINUTES
CHILL: 1 HOUR

I've always disliked potato salads that are full of mushy potatoes and not much else. So, this is a chunky version filled with various goodies. No raisins, however. Raisins in potato salad were a strange addition people kept arguing about around the time I was writing this cookbook. Not that I'm against dried fruit in certain cold salads, but raisins and potatoes do not seem at all compatible. But you never know.

And in case you were wondering, yes, this is Bob's favorite potato salad.

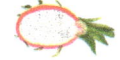

2 large eggs, hard-boiled and chilled in advance
1¾ teaspoons salt, divided
2 quarts water
1½ pounds baby Dutch yellow potatoes
½ cup mayonnaise
½ cup sour cream (light is okay)
2 tablespoons Dijon mustard
2 tablespoons white wine vinegar
2 tablespoons sweet pickle juice
½ teaspoon Savory Seasoning (page xi)
½ teaspoon white pepper
½ cup celery, finely chopped
½ cup sweet gherkins, finely chopped
½ cup scallions, ¼" slices
½ cup radishes, thinly sliced

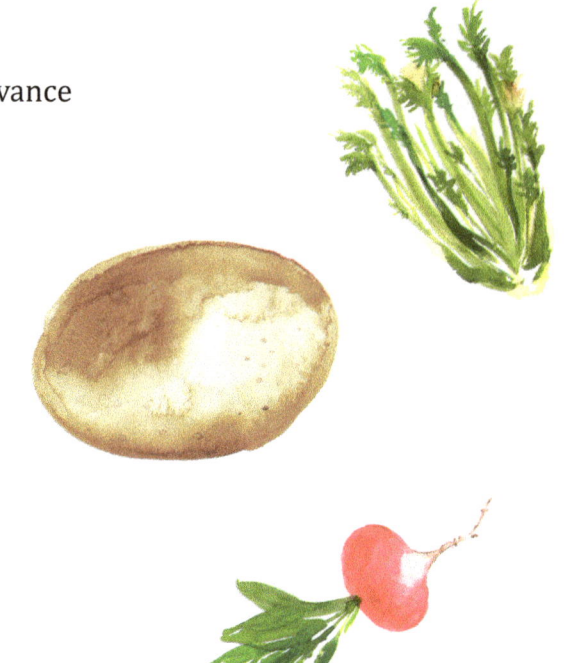

Garnish: a sprinkling of parsley and/or paprika

COMBINE 1 teaspoon salt, water, and potatoes in a 4-quart saucepan. Bring to a boil, then cook on rather high heat, uncovered, anywhere from 10–15 minutes, until all the potatoes are sharp-knife tender. Bigger ones might need a few more minutes. Drain and set aside. When cooler, cut into ¾" chunks and set aside (don't peel).

WHISK the mayonnaise, sour cream, mustard, vinegar, pickle juice, ¾ teaspoon salt, Savory Seasoning, and pepper well in a large bowl. Add the celery, gherkins, scallions, and radishes and mix in. Peel the cooled eggs, rinse them off, then chop coarsely. Add the prepared eggs and potatoes to the dressing and mix gently. Season, if necessary. Place in a 2-quart dish, cover, and refrigerate 1 hour before serving. Cover and refrigerate the leftovers. Makes 6–8 servings.

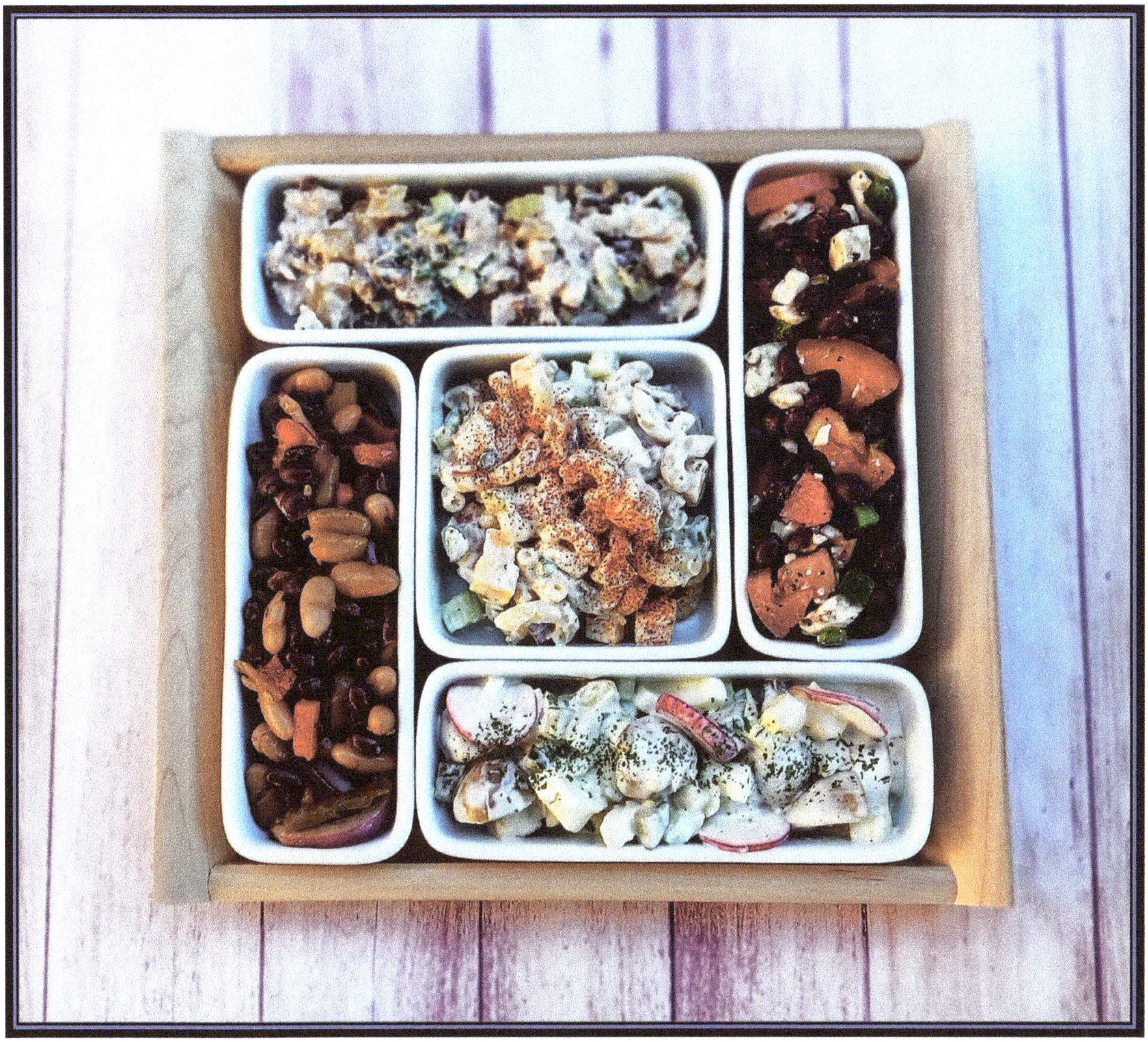

Clockwise, from top left:
Post-Watergate Chicken Salad, page 56
Black Bean Salad, page 58
You Can't Name Everything After Bob Potato Salad, page 59
Three Bean Salad, page 62

Center:
Bacon Mac Salad, page 63

Chapter Four: Cold Salads   61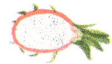

Three Bean Salad

START TO FINISH: ABOUT 15 MINUTES
CHILL: 1 HOUR

This salad is full of fiber and less sweet than your typical jarred varieties. This is my specific recipe with specific choices, but you can definitely change the beans, or the color of the pepper or the onion. How about Italian green beans, pinto beans, garbanzo beans, and some sweet Vidalia onion with a yellow bell pepper? That'll work, too.

14.5-ounce can whole green beans
15-ounce can black beans
15.5-ounce can cannellini beans
1 good-sized red bell pepper; remove core and chop coarsely
1 cup red onion, cut into ¼" slivers
⅓ cup balsamic vinegar (dark or golden)
⅓ cup vegetable oil
2 tablespoons sugar
¾ teaspoon salt
¾ teaspoon black pepper
¾ teaspoon celery seed
¾ teaspoon crushed red pepper flakes

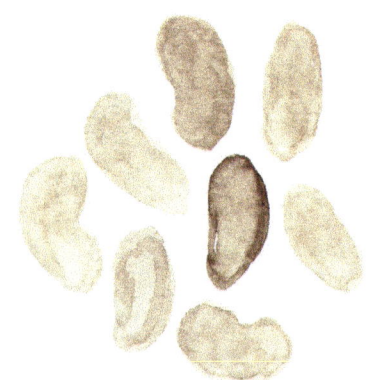

DRAIN the green beans and place them in a large bowl. Drain and rinse the other beans. Place them in the bowl, along with the bell pepper and onion; set aside.

COMBINE the remaining ingredients well in a shaker jar. Combine with the vegetables and mix well. Season, if desired. Place in a 2-quart container, cover, and refrigerate about 1 hour before serving. Stir a couple of times. Stir before serving with a slotted spoon. Cover and refrigerate the leftovers. Makes about 7 cups.

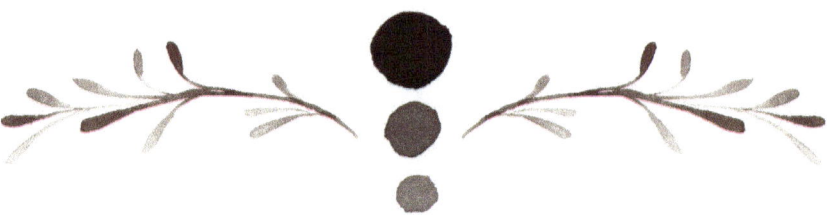

Bacon Mac Salad

START TO FINISH: ABOUT 35 MINUTES
CHILL: 30–60 MINUTES

Here's a macaroni salad that's substantial enough to be a main course, if you like.

8 ounces elbow macaroni (or other small pasta)
2 ounces precooked bacon
½ cup mayonnaise
2 tablespoons sour cream (light is okay)
2 tablespoons sweet pickle relish
3 tablespoons half-and-half
1 tablespoon Dijon mustard
¾ teaspoon salt
¾ teaspoon black pepper
¾ teaspoon Savory Seasoning (page xi)
¾ cup celery, finely chopped
¾ cup scallions, thinly sliced
4 ounces sharp cheddar cheese, cut into small cubes

GARNISH: a sprinkling of smoked paprika

COOK pasta as directed on the package in a 4-quart saucepan. Drain; rinse with cold water and let stand in the colander. Reuse the pot. In a large skillet, fry the bacon until it is crispy/chewy. Lay on paper towels to blot the fat. Set aside.

MEANWHILE, place the mayonnaise, sour cream, relish, half-and-half, mustard, and the 3 seasonings in the pot. Whisk well. Add the pasta, celery, scallions, and cheese and combine. Crumble or chop the bacon and add. Mix well, season, then place in a 2-quart container. Cover and refrigerate 30–60 minutes. Garnish, if desired. Cover and refrigerate leftovers; when serving again, add a smidge of milk if the pasta absorbs too much liquid. Makes 6–8 servings.

Super Savory Salad

IN ADVANCE: HARD BOILING EGGS AND CHILLING (APPROXIMATELY 2 HOURS)
START TO FINISH: ABOUT 30 MINUTES

Bob and I have a "Chef Salad" every two weeks or so and he is a ranch dressing fanatic. Southwestify the dressing below by adding a half cup of roasted, chopped, and well-drained green chile. For a dip, simply reduce the buttermilk to one-third of a cup and chill for an hour before serving (this makes about 1¼ cups). Of course, you can change the salad ingredients below with various items depending on what's around the grocery store or your garden.

Ranch-type dressings and seasonings are quintessentially American. The original was invented in 1949 by Nebraska native Steve Henson. He was a plumbing contractor who moved to Alaska and invented the dressing to keep his employees happy. A few years later, he moved to California, bought a ranch, and named it Hidden Valley. Henson was a peripatetic kind of guy, later moving to Colorado and back to Nebraska during his life. Eventually, he ended up packaging a dry mix, which was a great success. Competitors soon came up with their own recipes. Lawsuits proliferated. In the end, ranch dressing and ranch flavoring are about as ubiquitous as apple pie in America.

A nice variation for the eggs would be avocado. Two average ripe avocados could be sliced or diced and served instead of the eggs. Or... why not both?

4 chilled hard-boiled eggs; peeled, rinsed, and sliced in advance
4 ounces fresh baby spinach (other types of lettuce will be fine,
    torn into bite-sized pieces)
1 cup celery
1 cup carrot, peeled
1 cup cucumber, peeled or not
    (or partially peeled)
24 cherry or grape tomatoes
8 ounces thinly sliced roast beef,
    coarsely chopped or julienned
4 ounces sharp cheddar cheese, shredded

GARNISH: ½ cup dry roasted sunflower seeds

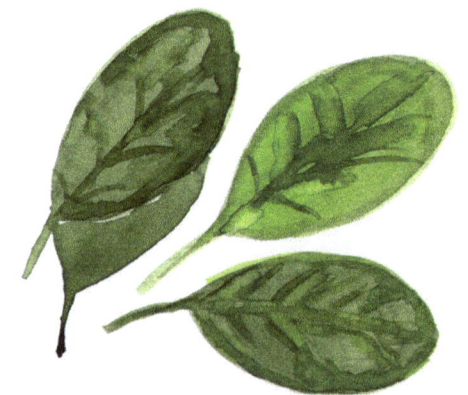

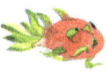

Savory Seasoning Ranch Dressing

¾ cup fresh buttermilk
½ cup mayonnaise
½ cup sour cream (or crème fraiche; light sour cream is okay)
2 teaspoons sugar
1 teaspoon Savory Seasoning (page xi)
1 teaspoon dry mustard
½ teaspoon garlic salt
½ teaspoon onion salt
¼ teaspoon cayenne pepper

DIVIDE the spinach between 4 dinner plates. Slice, dice, or chop the celery, carrot, and cucumber as desired and arrange on top of the spinach. Place 6 tomatoes around the edge of each plate. Divide and arrange the meat, cheese, and eggs as you like.

WHISK all the dressing ingredients well in a medium bowl or a 4-cup glass measuring cup. Season, if necessary. Dress each salad as desired, then top each with sunflower seeds. Cover and refrigerate any leftover dressing. Makes 4 servings. The dressing makes about 1¾ cups.

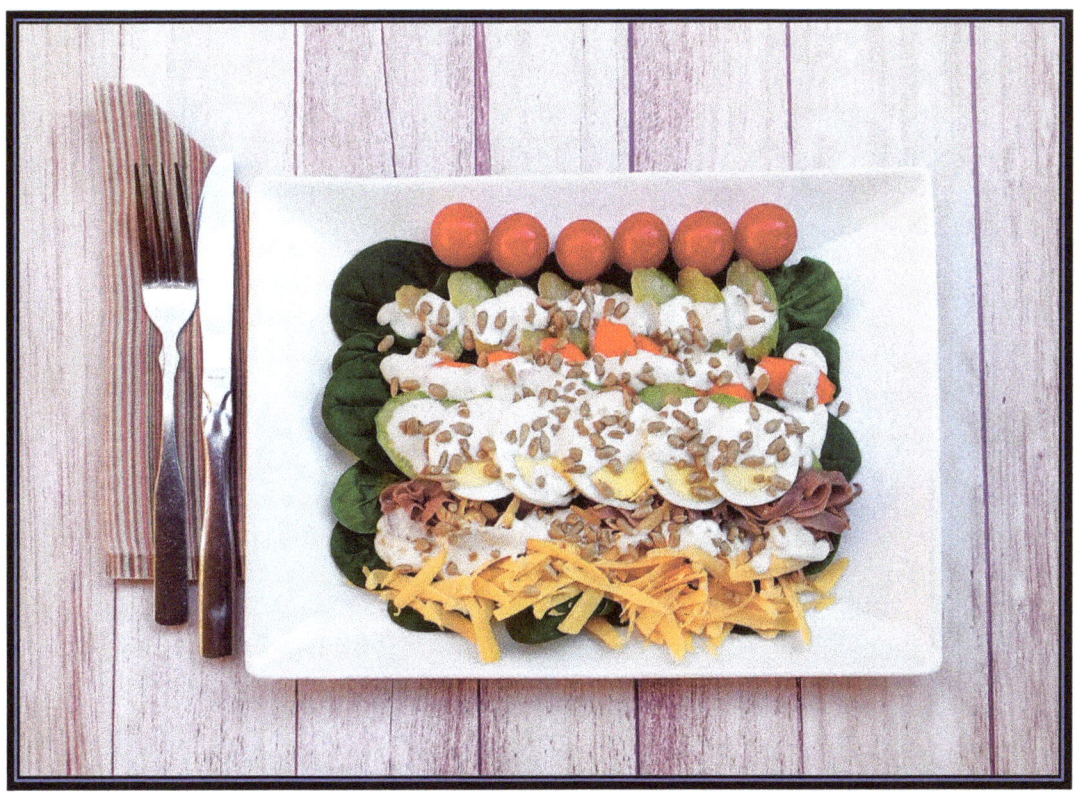

All Hail the Caesar Salad

START TO FINISH: ABOUT 22 MINUTES

Everyone assumes the Caesar salad originated in Italy, but it was actually invented in Mexico in 1924 by an Italian immigrant named Caesar Cardini, who owned a restaurant in Tijuana. Or the salad could be attributed to his brother, Alex. It might even be attributed to various employees of the restaurant. Food history anecdotes tend to resemble tall tales after a dish becomes famous. Anchovies or not? Worcestershire, instead? Leave the leaves whole or chop them or tear them? Lemon or lime? Hard to make? Hardly at all. I'm kind of disappointed this salad has nothing much to do with Julius, however.

A good-sized head of Romaine lettuce (one that weighs about a pound)
2 ounces Parmesan or Romano cheese, shredded
2 cups seasoned croutons (purchased or homemade; you'll need 3 ounces)

Hail Caesar Dressing

¾ cup olive oil
2 tablespoons lemon juice (or lime)
1 anchovy fillet (or ½ teaspoon anchovy paste OR 1 teaspoon
    Worcestershire sauce; if you like a stronger flavor,
    increase the fillets to 2 or even 3)
2 large garlic cloves
1 tablespoon Dijon mustard
1 large egg yolk
1 ounce Parmesan or Romano cheese, finely shredded
½ teaspoon salt
½ teaspoon black pepper

GARNISH: additional black pepper, freshly ground

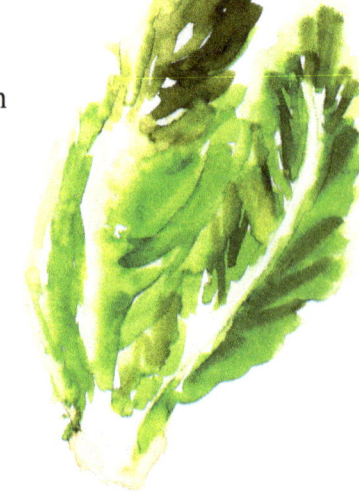

DECIDE how you would like to present your lettuce. You may cut off the stem, wash the leaves, and shake them off to dry. Place on a towel to dry further. Toss them with the dressing in a very large bowl. Place all on a large platter. Sprinkle the shredded Parmesan over all, followed by the croutons. Then you would pick each leaf up with your fingers.

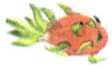

PREFERRED METHOD: Conversely, you (and your fellow diners!) might prefer to use a tidier technique. Cut off the lettuce's stem, wash, shake off, then either tear or chop the leaves into smaller chunks, or about 1" strips. Place on a towel. Set another towel on top and roll it all up to let the lettuce dry. Place in a very large bowl. Combine the cheese and croutons with the lettuce and toss.

COMBINE all the dressing ingredients in a small processor and blend well. Season. Pour the desired quantity over the salad and toss well. Garnish, as desired. Serve immediately, though if the salad stands for a short while, it will still be okay; the croutons will absorb some of the dressing and lose a bit of their crispiness. Not recommended for leftovers. Makes 4–6 servings. The dressing makes a little over 1 cup.

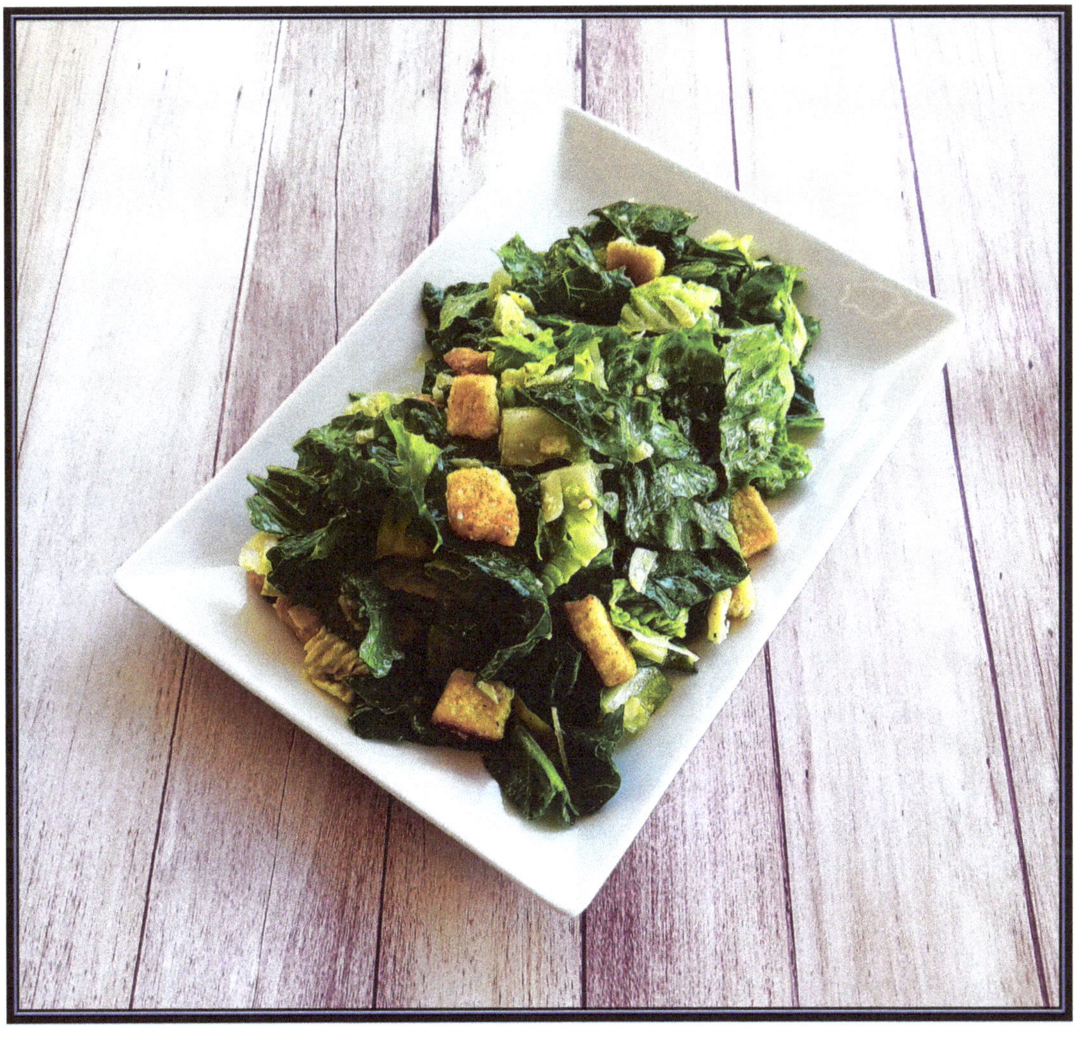

Chapter Four: Cold Salads 67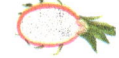

Naked Ambrosia

IN ADVANCE: TOASTING NUTS, COOLING, AND CHOPPING
IN ADVANCE: TOASTING COCONUT AND COOLING
PREP: 15 MINUTES
OPTIONAL CHILLING TIME: 1 HOUR OR SO

Leave it to American cuisine to reduce the concept of ambrosia (which literally means *food of the gods*) to a sickeningly sweet "salad" which is generally filled with canned fruit, mayonnaise, and the dreaded addition of marshmallows (I dread them, at least). Then you take it to every potluck you are ever invited to. I suppose marshmallows are like clouds and fit for the gods? I don't think so. Here is a naked version, which is a nice closing to this cold salad chapter. Cinnamon is the safest flavor to use, but if you really want to punch up the flavor, try cardamom.

1 ounce pecan halves, lightly toasted, cooled, and chopped finely in advance
1 ounce sweetened coconut flakes, lightly toasted and cooled in advance
A large apple, any variety
A large navel orange
A large banana
2 small mangos
1 tablespoon lemon juice
1 tablespoon sugar
1 teaspoon ground cinnamon

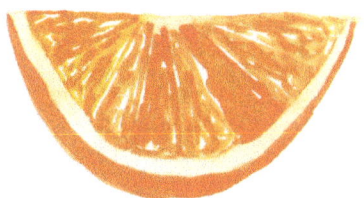

CORE the apple, cut it into ¾" chunks, and place in a large bowl. Peel the orange, section it, cut it into ¾" chunks, and add to the bowl. Peel the banana, cut it into ½" slices, and add to the bowl. Peel and cut the mangos into ¾" chunks; add them to the bowl.

MIX the lemon juice into the fruit. Combine the sugar and cinnamon in a tiny bowl. Sprinkle over all and mix in. Add the prepared nuts and coconut and mix well. Place in a 6-cup container; cover and refrigerate an hour or so, or you can serve immediately. Cover and refrigerate the leftovers, but not for too long. Your bananas will turn rather brown on the second day. Makes 5–6 cups.

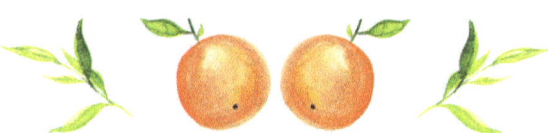

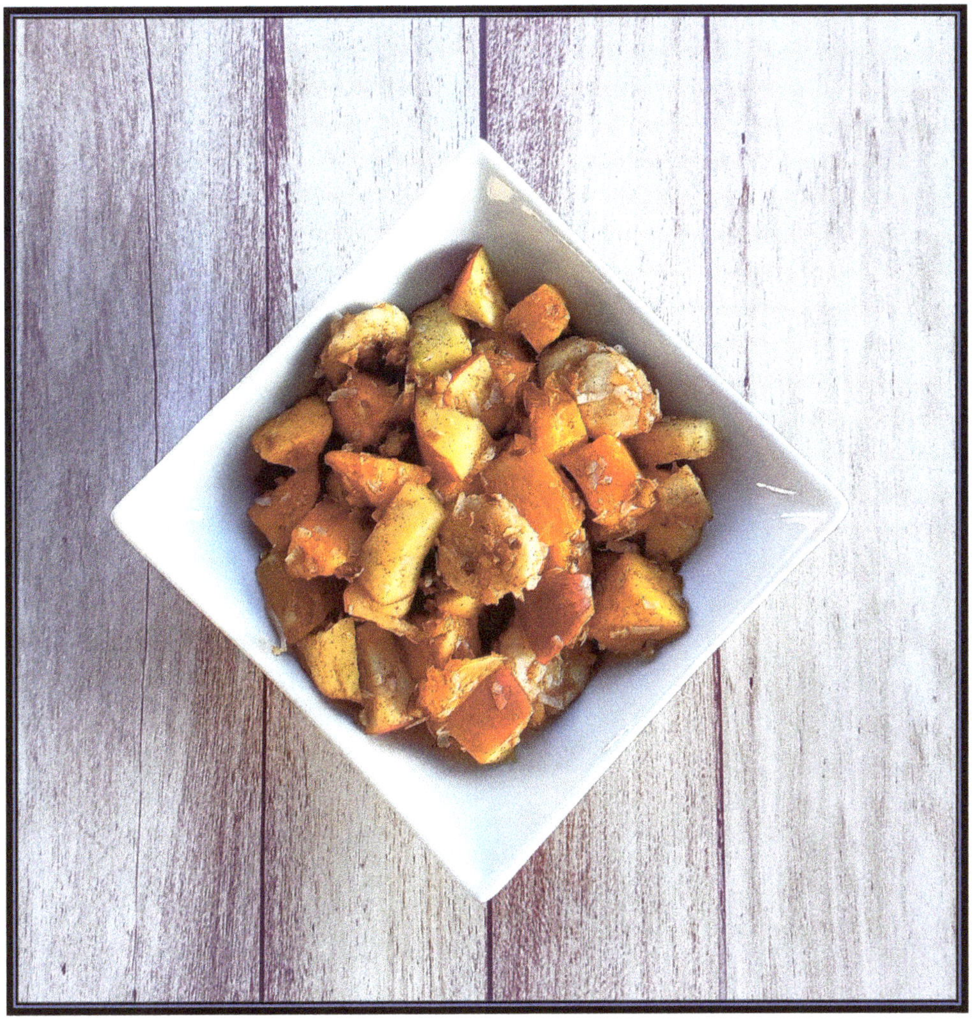

Chapter Five

Valentine's Day

Steaks with Benefits

Valentine's Day Taters

Cupid Cocktail

XOXO

The Evening-After Salad

Valentine's Day

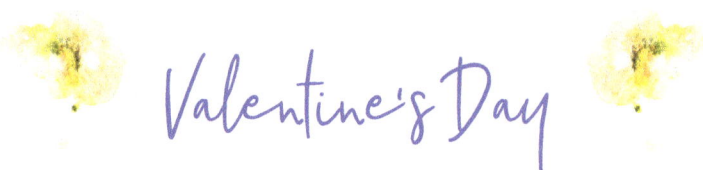

HERE'S A DECADENT Valentine's Day dinner to make at home. Bob and I hate crowds, so we usually celebrate this day at home. We'll often plan a Valentine's meal out a few days before or even after. I like to purchase a giant beefsteak tomato to slice and serve along with the steak and potatoes. If you imbibe, you can whip up the cocktail while the steaks rest. Set aside around a half a pound of the steak for The Evening-After Salad.

Or serve this anytime as a classy dinner. We had this for a Father's Day celebration in 2011. I used the steak recipe as is, doubled the potato recipe, cooked four ears of fresh corn (cut in half), and had two giant tomatoes on the side. Six people demolished all of this, with some strawberry shortcake for dessert.

Bob might put A.1. sauce on the steak. Part of being a "valentine" is learning to be okay with culinary idiosyncrasies, right?

Steaks with Benefits

ACTIVE PREP: ABOUT 28–34 MINUTES

This is so named because you will end up with enough to make The Evening-After Salad (page 79). Unless, of course, you eat massive amounts of steak. Which you shouldn't because you should save room for the potato recipe below. And the dessert...

2¼ pounds beef tenderloin steaks, 1½" to 2" thick (filet mignon)
Coarse kosher salt
Freshly ground black pepper
1 tablespoon salted butter
1 tablespoon olive oil
2 tablespoons cream sherry (or low-sodium beef broth)
1 tablespoon soy sauce
1 tablespoon balsamic vinegar
1 tablespoon water

GARNISH:

Place a thin slice of salted butter on top of each cooked steak.

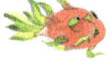

LET the steaks stand at room temperature for 30–60 minutes or so. Generously sprinkle the top sides of all the steaks with salt and pepper. Melt the butter and oil in a 3-quart deep skillet over rather high heat. Place the seasoned sides of the steaks down in the pan. Generously season the top sides of the steaks with more salt and pepper. Fry 5 minutes. With tongs, turn the steaks over and fry 5 minutes. Shake the pan gently a few times.

MEANWHILE, combine the cream sherry, soy sauce, vinegar, and water in a 1-cup glass measuring cup. Pour over the steaks. Cover and cook on medium heat 3 minutes. With tongs, turn over all the steaks and cook over moderately high heat, uncovered, another 1–3 minutes, depending on how well you like your steaks to be cooked (you might remove smaller steaks a bit earlier).

REMOVE the steaks to a plate and cover them with the pan lid. Let them rest 5–8 minutes. They should be *around* medium. Discard pan juices. Set aside a steak that appears to be around 6–8 ounces or so if you plan to make the salad for another meal. Place a thin slice of salted butter on top of each steak to serve. Cover and refrigerate the leftovers. Makes 2 servings, with extra to spare.

Valentine's Day Taters

IN ADVANCE: POTATO PREP, ABOUT 1 HOUR
PREP: ABOUT 25 MINUTES
BAKE: 15 MINUTES
STAND: 8–10 MINUTES
OVEN: 425°

Deluxe potatoes in a bowl to share with that certain special someone. If you anticipate being stressed about the day, you may prepare these the night before you need them. Refrigerate them overnight and let them stand at room temperature 30 minutes before baking.

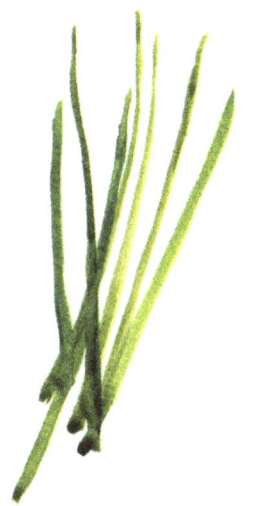

Chapter Five: Valentine's Day

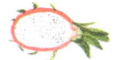

1 pound small red potatoes (do **NOT** exceed 1 pound!)
4 strips premium precooked bacon
3 tablespoons salted butter, divided
3 ounces garlic/herb cheese, softened (such as Alouette or Boursin)
3 tablespoons 1% milk
2 tablespoons sour cream (light is okay)
2 tablespoons heavy cream
½ teaspoon salt
½ teaspoon black pepper
¼ cup scallions (or fresh chives), finely chopped
1 teaspoon seasoned breadcrumbs

WASH the potatoes; poke each with a fork once. Microwave on HIGH until they are done (sharp-knife tender). This will take anywhere from 6–12 minutes depending on the relative sizes of the potatoes. Let them stand until they cool off for a while. Fry the bacon over rather high heat in a medium skillet until crispy but not burned. Set aside on a paper towel.

PREHEAT the oven to 425°. Coat 2 (1-cup) ramekins with cooking spray or grease lightly and place them on a medium baking sheet; set aside. In a medium glass bowl, microwave 2 tablespoons butter on HIGH briefly, just until melted, 30 seconds or so. Add the cheese, milk, sour cream, cream, salt, and pepper and mix thoroughly. Add the scallions and mix. With your hands, break the potatoes (with the peel) into rather small chunks and add to the bowl. Crumble the bacon and add this to the bowl. Mix well. Season, if desired.

DIVIDE evenly into the prepared ramekins. Sprinkle each with ½ teaspoon of the breadcrumbs. Cut the remaining 1 tablespoon of butter in half and place one portion on top of each. Bake 15 minutes. Let stand 8–10 minutes before serving. Cover and refrigerate the leftovers. Makes 2 servings.

Halfling alert:

If you are trying to satisfy the various hobbity-types of people you might have in your life, you'll want to double this recipe; then, you can easily serve 4–6. Double all the ingredients and place them in a 1½-quart casserole dish (coated with cooking spray or greased lightly) and bake for 25 minutes.

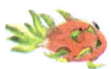

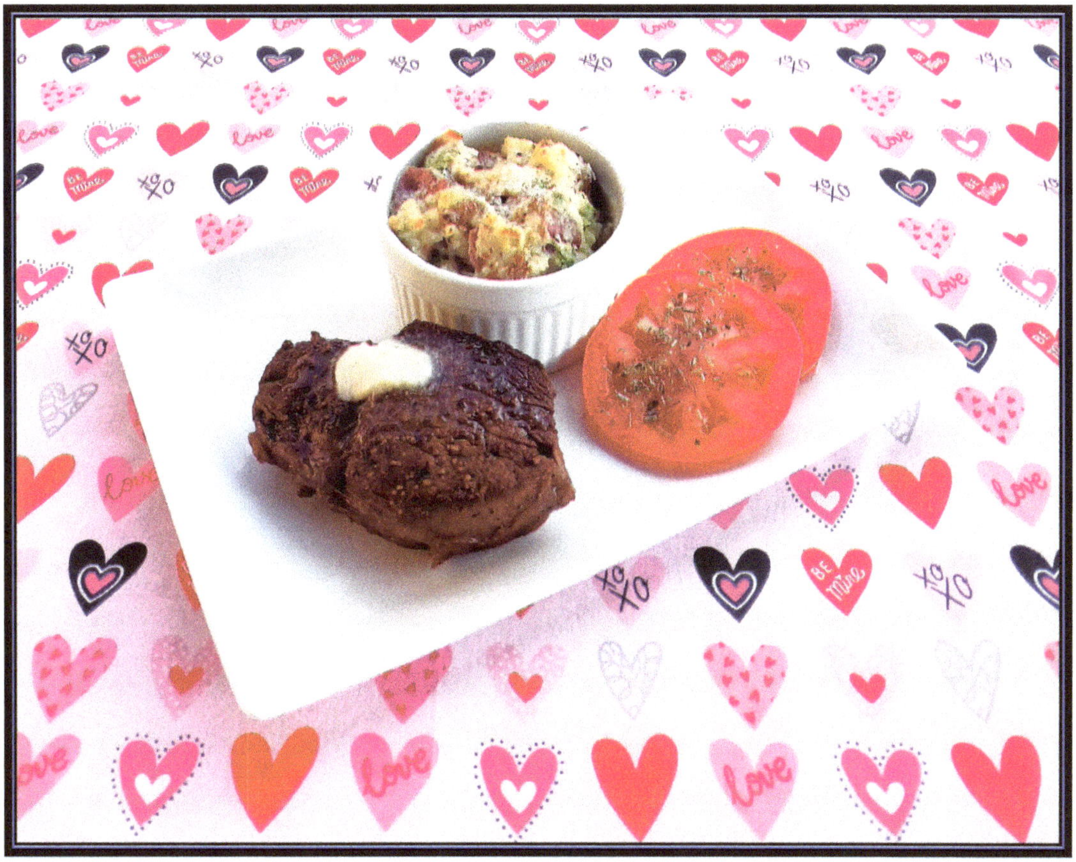

Top:
Valentine's Day Taters, page 73

Left:
Steaks with Benefits, page 72

Chapter Five: Valentine's Day   75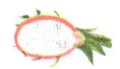

Cupid Cocktail

START TO FINISH: 5 MINUTES

This might knock off your socks... and bra... and panties... or whatever fun stuff you might be wearing. You can easily mix this up while the steaks and potatoes are cooking, or you might want to time it differently. Flavored vodkas (vanilla or whipped cream are best) can substitute for the rum; other bitters will be fine, depending on their flavor.

2 ounces coconut rum
2 ounces clear crème de cacao
2 ounces Chambord
1 tablespoon grenadine syrup
1 tablespoon half-and-half
8 drops (Angostura) bitters
A few ice cubes

GARNISH:

> Skewer a few perfect blueberries and/or raspberries on a pretty cocktail pick.

COMBINE all the ingredients in a cocktail shaker. Shake for 20–30 seconds. Strain into 2 coupe or martini glasses. Garnish, if desired. Makes 2 servings.

> **YOU COULD ALSO MAKE THIS A SUBSTANTIAL DESSERT INSTEAD.**
>
> Omit the ice cubes. Place all the ingredients in a blender. In heaping spoonfuls, add a full pint of vanilla ice cream that has been softened a bit. Blend well. Pour into two 12–14-ounce glasses. Serve immediately, or you can freeze the shakes about an hour or so in advance.

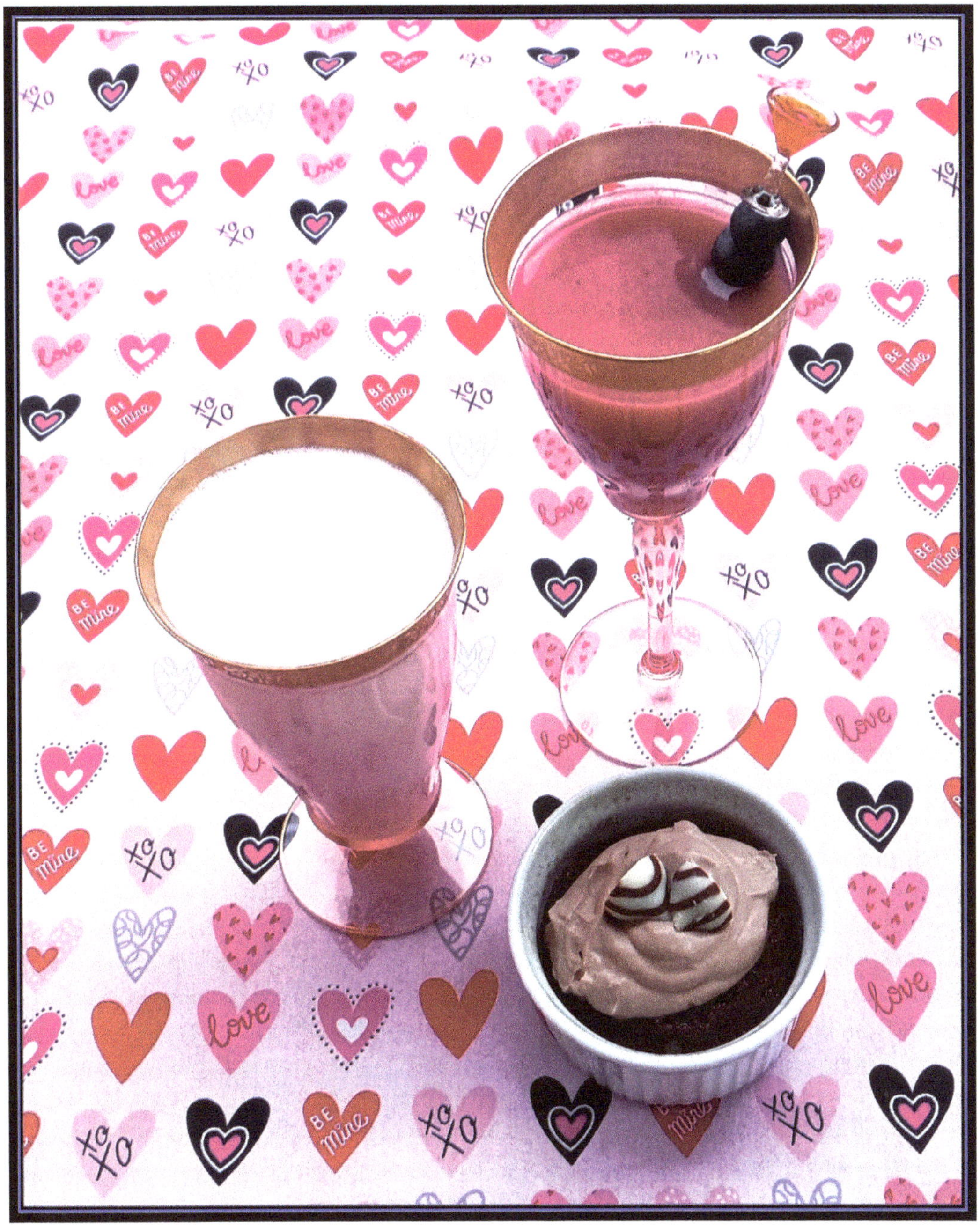

Clockwise, from top right:
Cupid Cocktail, page 76
XOXO, page 78
Cupid Cocktail (ice cream version), page 76

Chapter Five: Valentine's Day 77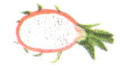

XOXO

ACTIVE PREP: ABOUT 18 MINUTES
CHILL: OVERNIGHT
BAKE: 12 MINUTES
STAND: 1 HOUR
OVEN: 450°

Fortunately, this almost flourless, lava-like dessert is started **the night before serving**, so you can save some time. It's just enough for two, so it is perfect for a Valentine's Day meal.

¼ cup half-and-half
1 ounce bittersweet chocolate chips
1 ounce white chocolate chips
1 tablespoon plus 2 teaspoons sugar
¼ teaspoon salt
2 tablespoons all-purpose flour
2 tablespoons clear crème de cacao
¼ cup liquid egg substitute
14 Hugs and/or Kisses candies, unwrapped (any variety)
¼ cup heavy cream
1 teaspoon cocoa powder

GARNISH:

Place an additional Hug or Kiss on top of the cream.

THE NIGHT BEFORE SERVING: Place the half-and-half, all the chocolate chips, 1 tablespoon sugar, and salt in a medium glass bowl. Microwave on HIGH in 20-second intervals until melted, about a minute total. Whisk well. Add the flour, crème de cocoa, and egg substitute and whisk well. Spray 2 (¾-cup) ramekins and place them on a small baking sheet. Pour the chocolate evenly into each. Cover both with a small sheet of foil. Refrigerate overnight.

SEVENTY-FIVE MINUTES BEFORE SERVING: Remove the baking sheet from the refrigerator and let it stand for a total of 30 minutes. After standing 15 minutes, preheat the oven to 450°. Remove the foil, then place 7 candies in each, with the points facing up. Bake 12 minutes. Let stand on the sheet 30 minutes.

MEANWHILE, place the cream, 2 teaspoons sugar, and cocoa powder in a 1-cup glass measuring cup. Whisk well by hand until rather firm. Refrigerate until needed.

TO SERVE: Divide the cream evenly on top of each and garnish, if you like. Makes 2 servings.

The Evening-After Salad

START TO FINISH: ABOUT 35 MINUTES

This vibrant salad is rather low fat and full of vegetables to counteract your previous Valentine's Day debauchery. This can stretch to serve three or even four if you add some crusty bread. Any other cooked, leftover protein works nicely here, as well. For a vegetarian option, you could certainly omit the meat and substitute cheese, beans, tofu, lentils, etc. Serve it all on a platter for more of a buffet presentation.

EVENING-AFTER DRESSING

2 tablespoons vegetable oil
2 tablespoons red wine vinegar
3 fairly large cloves fresh garlic
1 tablespoon lime juice
1 tablespoon orange juice
2 teaspoons sugar
½ teaspoon salt
½ teaspoon black pepper
½ teaspoon dried oregano
¼ teaspoon ground cumin
¼ teaspoon cayenne pepper

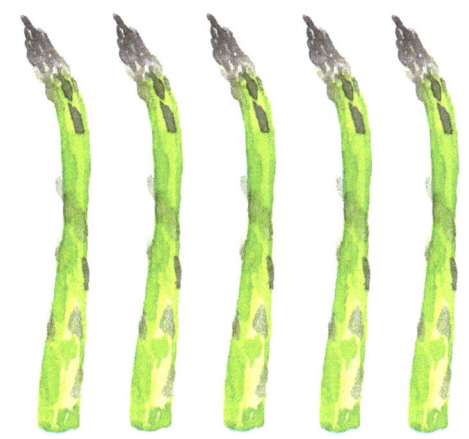

SALAD (PROPER)

1 ounce pine nuts
8 ounces pencil-thin fresh asparagus
3 cups water
8 ounces cooked and chilled leftover beef tenderloin
    (see Steaks with Benefits, page 72)
3 ounces greenery (any type of lettuce; spinach and/or arugula
    would also be fine)
8 grape tomatoes, cut in half
½ cup carrot, peeled and shredded
4 average radishes, thinly sliced

FOR the dressing, combine all the ingredients in a small food processor or blender and mix until smooth. Pour into a 1-cup glass measuring cup or a small bowl, to facilitate mixing with the salad. Season and set aside.

    PLACE nuts in a 9" by 5" metal loaf pan. Cook over moderate heat for about 1–2 minutes, shaking the pan frequently, just until they become lightly toasted. Pour into a small bowl and set aside; you will use the pan again in the next step.

    LINE up asparagus evenly by their tops on a cutting board. Cut the stems off at the bottom so the stalks end up about 7–8" long. Place in the 9" by 5" pan. Add the water. Bring to a boil, then cook on a gentle boil 5 minutes until they are crisp-tender. Drain and rinse in cold water. Set aside to drain.

    MEANWHILE, thinly slice the steak and spread it out on a dinner plate. Microwave on HIGH 30 seconds; set aside. Tear or chop your chosen greenery into bite-sized pieces (if necessary; some greens are already bite-sized) and place in a large bowl. Toss with 2 tablespoons of the prepared dressing. Arrange on 2 dinner plates. In the same bowl, toss an additional 1 tablespoon dressing with the asparagus. Arrange nicely on the plates. In the bowl, toss another 1 tablespoon dressing with the steak and arrange. Combine the tomatoes, carrot, and radishes with the remaining dressing in the same bowl and arrange on top of all. Sprinkle both with the pine nuts. Serve immediately. Makes 2 servings. Not recommended as leftovers.

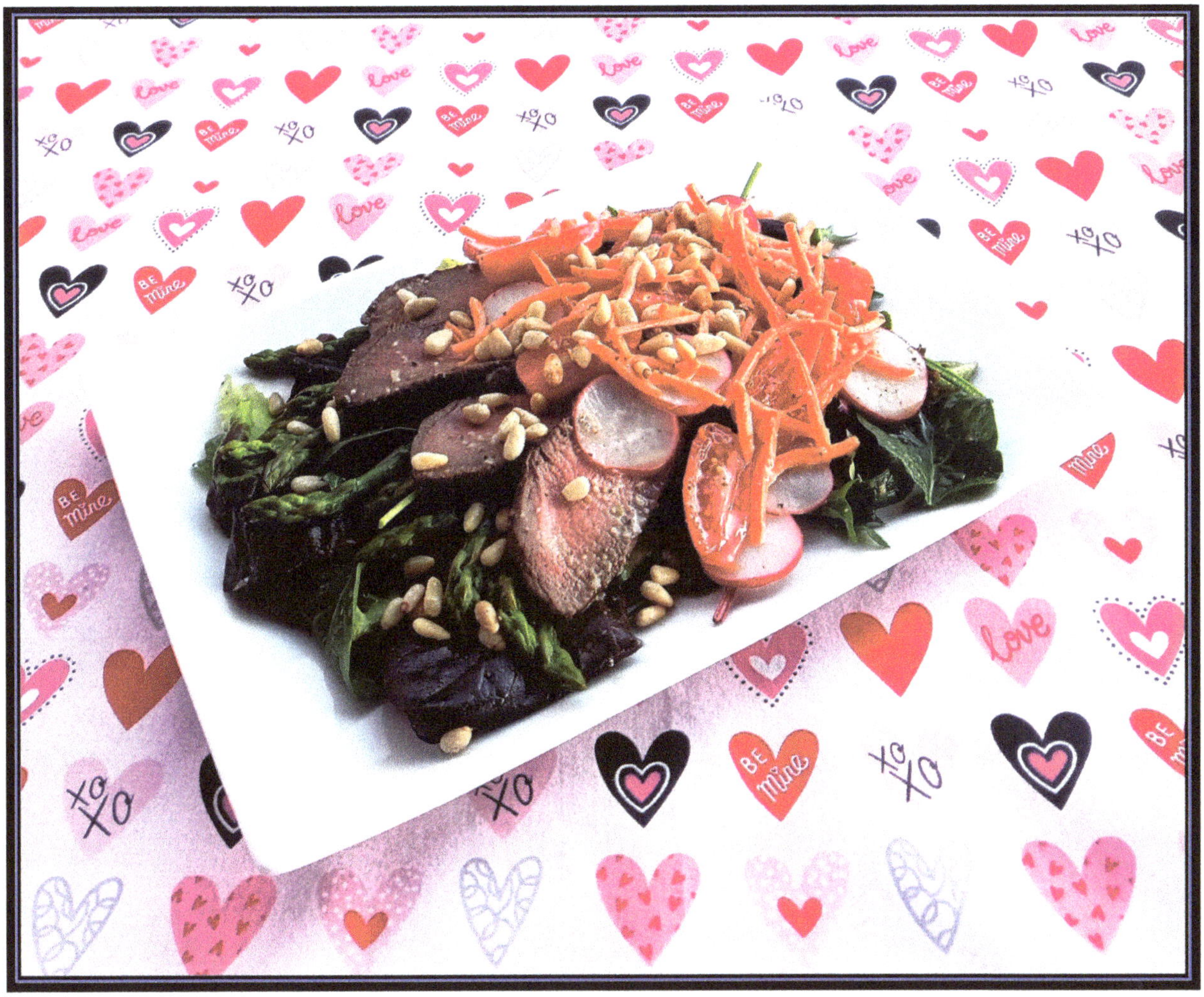

CHAPTER SIX

HOT SIDES

Mellow Mexican Rice

Tequila Peppers

Sandia Spoon Bread

Roasted Tiny Trees

Halfling Alert Taters

Lobo Beets & Greens

Búho Beans

Very Versatile Vegetables

Hot Sides

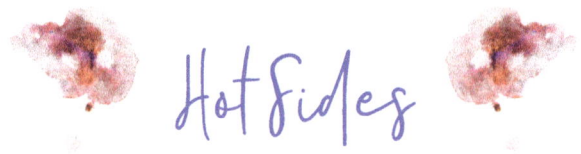

HERE IS ANOTHER assortment of sides to mix with many items within the cookbook.

Mellow Mexican Rice

START TO FINISH: ABOUT 48 MINUTES

We used to have a restaurant in town that served this type of rice as a side dish. They are no longer in business, so I invented my own. It is meant to be plain and savory, definitely not a Spanish-type rice recipe.

14.5-ounce can low-sodium chicken broth
¼ cup water
2 tablespoons tomato paste
2 tablespoons salted butter
1 teaspoon garlic powder
½ teaspoon salt
1 cup long-grain rice

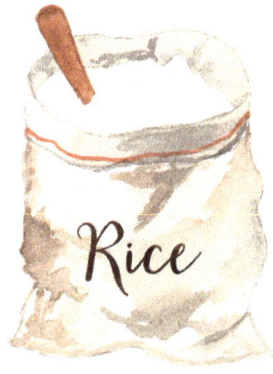

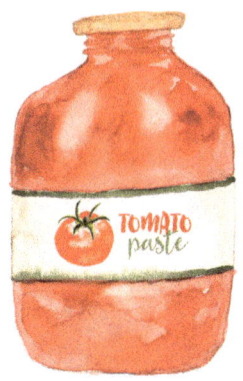

PLACE the broth, water, tomato paste, butter, garlic powder, and salt in a 2-quart saucepan. Bring to a boil; whisk well to combine. Add the rice and stir once. Turn the heat to the lowest setting. Cover and cook, undisturbed, 18 minutes. Turn off the heat and let stand, covered, 15–20 minutes. Season as desired. Stir well and serve. Cover and refrigerate the leftovers. Makes 4–6 servings.

Tequila Peppers

START TO FINISH: ABOUT 18 MINUTES

This is a colorful dish suitable to accompany many entrees. Feel free to substitute a flavored broth for the tequila, such as chicken or vegetable.

2 tablespoons tequila (any variety)
2 tablespoons heavy cream
1 tablespoon orange juice
½ tablespoon sugar
½ teaspoon salt
½ teaspoon chili powder
3 large bell peppers (preferably three different colors)
1 tablespoon vegetable oil

COMBINE the tequila, cream, orange juice, sugar, salt, and chili powder in a 1-cup glass measuring cup. Whisk well and set aside.

CUT the bell peppers in half vertically and remove the cores and seeds. Cut into ½″ slivers. Heat the oil in a large skillet over rather high heat. Add the peppers and sauté 3 minutes. Add the tequila mixture and boil 3 minutes, stirring frequently, until the vegetables are glazed. Season as needed. Cover and refrigerate the leftovers. Makes 3–4 servings.

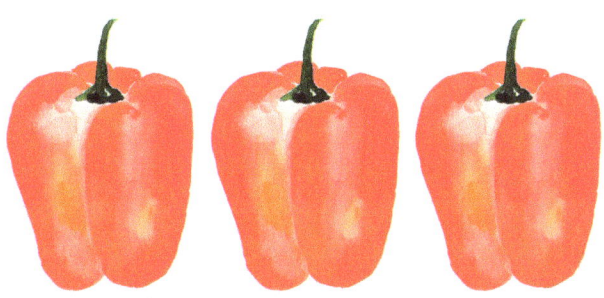

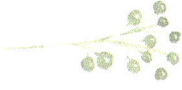

Chapter Six: Hot Sides   85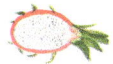

Sandia Spoon Bread

ACTIVE PREP: 15 MINUTES
BAKE: 1 HOUR
STAND: ABOUT 25 MINUTES
OVEN: 350°

One of our favorite Mexican restaurants often served a small scoop of corny goodness alongside some of their dishes. I always liked it quite a bit, but Bob didn't. But then I took it upon myself to come up with my own version, and he ended up liking that. The restaurant version was rather firm and much sweeter than mine, so maybe that was the problem for him. This dish ends up being slightly mushy in a deliciously pleasing way.

1 cup sour cream (or crème fraiche; light sour cream is okay)
2 large eggs
¼ cup salted butter
2 tablespoons sugar
½ teaspoon salt
4 ounces green chile, roasted and chopped, with juice
15.25-ounce can corn, drained
14.75-ounce can creamed corn
8.5-ounce box Jiffy corn muffin mix

NINETY MINUTES BEFORE SERVING: Remove the sour cream and eggs from the refrigerator and let stand. Place the butter in a large glass bowl and microwave on HIGH in 20-second intervals, just until melted. Let stand 15 minutes.

 MEANWHILE, preheat the oven to 350°. Coat an 8" square baking dish with cooking spray or grease lightly. Whisk the sugar, salt, and green chile into the butter. Whisk in the sour cream and eggs. Whisk in the remaining ingredients well. Pour into the prepared dish. Bake 1 hour. Let stand about 10 minutes before serving. Cover and refrigerate the leftovers. Makes 9 servings.

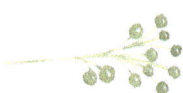

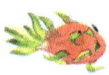

Roasted Tiny Trees

PREP: ABOUT 10 MINUTES
ROAST: 20 MINUTES
OVEN: 400°

Even I feel better about eating broccoli florets if I refer to them as tiny trees.

12 ounces fresh broccoli florets
2 tablespoons olive oil
1 tablespoon salted butter
1¼ teaspoons Savory Seasoning
    (page xi)
¼ cup pine nuts

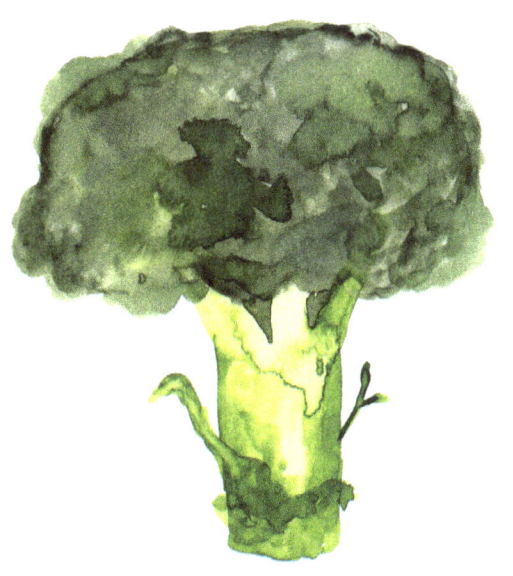

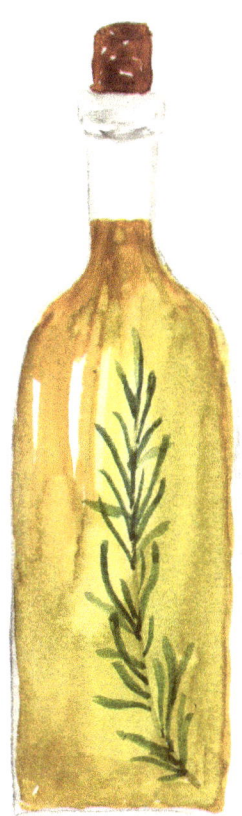

PREHEAT the oven to 400°. Coat an 11″ by 7″ baking dish with cooking spray or grease lightly. Cut any large florets into more manageable bites, around 1½″ pieces. Place in the prepared dish and set aside.

PLACE the oil and butter in a 1-cup glass measuring cup and microwave on HIGH in 10-second intervals, just until melted. Drizzle all over the broccoli. Sprinkle the seasoning over all evenly. Roast 10 minutes. Add the nuts and mix in. Roast another 10 minutes. Season. Stir and serve. Cover and refrigerate the leftovers. Makes 3–4 servings.

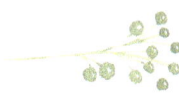

Chapter Six: Hot Sides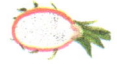

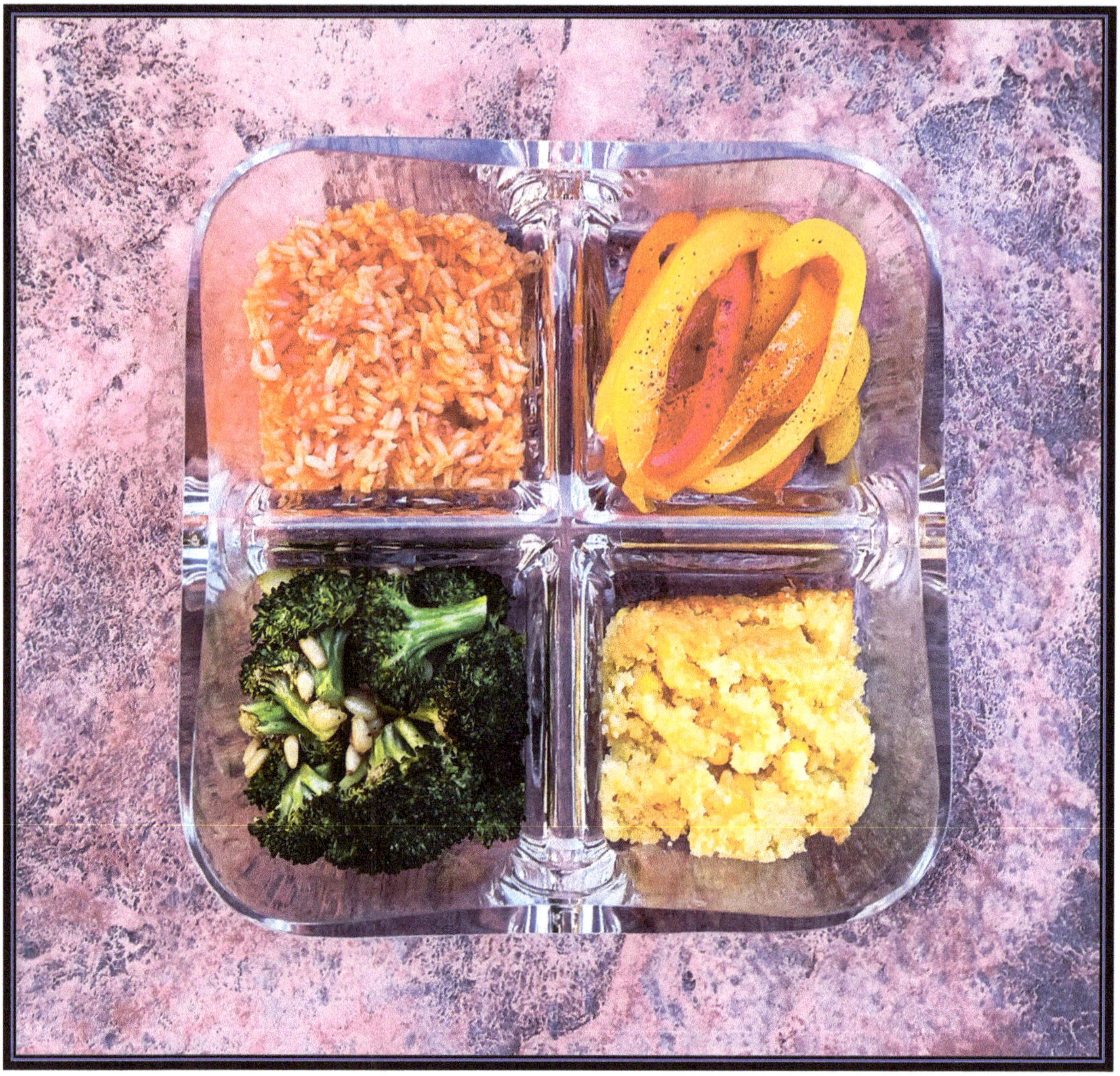

CLOCKWISE, FROM TOP LEFT:
Mellow Mexican Rice, page 84
Tequila Peppers, page 85
Sandia Spoon Bread, page 86
Roasted Tiny Trees, page 87

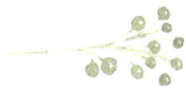

 88   Celebrating Comfy, Cozy Foods from North America: CH&M, Volume 3

Halfling Alert Taters

PREP: ABOUT 13 MINUTES
ROAST: 45 MINUTES
OVEN: 450°

Named so because a typical hobbit/halfling would probably eat these on a weekly basis. You can also use small red or fingerlings; neither need to be peeled, and you will need to cut them into ¾"–1" chunks. This recipe is also appropriate for those tiny marble-sized taters, if you can find them—no preparation for them besides washing!

1 tablespoon salted butter
1 tablespoon olive oil
½ teaspoon Savory Seasoning (page xi)
½ teaspoon crushed rosemary (2–3 tablespoons fresh, minced)
½ teaspoon salt
1½ pounds baby Dutch yellow potatoes (don't peel)

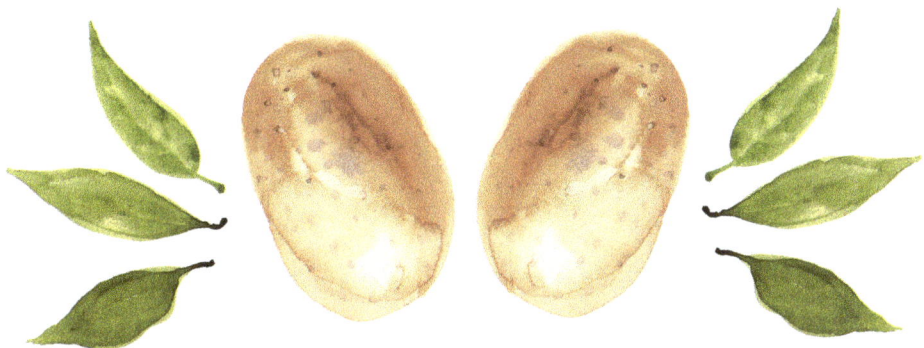

PREHEAT the oven to 450°. Coat a 9" square baking dish with cooking spray or grease lightly; set aside. Combine the butter, oil, and the 3 seasonings in a large glass bowl and microwave on HIGH about 30–40 seconds, until the butter has melted. Whisk to combine; set aside.

WASH the potatoes. Cut into about ¾"–1" chunks. Mix into the butter mixture, then pour into the prepared dish. Bake 45 minutes. Stir twice. They should be golden brown. Season, as desired. Cover and refrigerate the leftovers. Makes 3–4 servings, or enough for 1 hobbit.

Lobo Beets & Greens

ACTIVE PREP: ABOUT 40 MINUTES
ROAST: ABOUT 1 HOUR
STAND: ABOUT 1 HOUR
OVEN: 400°

Perhaps you have heard of Harvard Beets? Here's a Southwestern version. The University of New Mexico's (my alma mater) mascot is a wolf, or *lobo*. At sporting events (I never attended), the mascots are known as Lobo Louie and Lobo Lucy. In the '80s, apparently, the student body developed this chant: "Everyone's a Lobo: Woof! Woof! Woof!" A particular hand gesture supposedly accompanies this chant; nothing offensive, you somehow make your hand look like a wolf head. Yes, that's a rather silly ritual, isn't it? Whenever I hear that someone is going to attend UNM, however, I reflexively recite the chant in my head. Sometimes I even say it out loud…

Roast your beets earlier in the day and complete the final cooking preparations about 15 minutes before you want to serve them. You can simplify this recipe, if you like. You may use a 15-ounce can of sliced or diced beets, drained. If you do this, you may substitute 5–6 ounces of baby spinach and/or kale for the greens. But roasting beets isn't difficult, and greens are underrated. Give the original recipe a try!

1–1½ pounds fresh beets, with greens
1½ tablespoons olive oil, divided
3 tablespoons salted butter, divided
1 cup shallots, cut into ¼" slivers
1 tablespoon lime juice
1 tablespoon orange juice
1 tablespoon sugar, divided
½ teaspoon plus ⅛ teaspoon salt
½ teaspoon plus ⅛ teaspoon black pepper
½ teaspoon ground cumin
½ teaspoon chili powder
1 teaspoon minced garlic
¼ teaspoon crushed red pepper flakes
2 tablespoons water
1 tablespoon cider vinegar

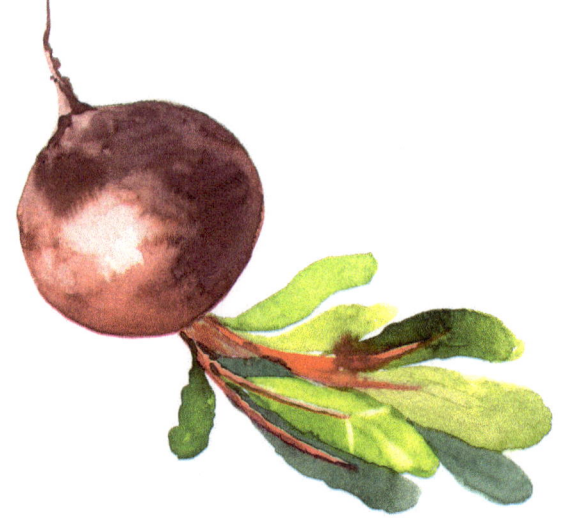

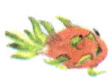

AT LEAST THREE HOURS BEFORE NEEDED: Preheat the oven to 400°. Cut the stems and roots of the beets down to 1". Place the greens back in your plastic grocery bag or in a covered container and store them in the refrigerator for later use. Wash the beets well and place them on a sheet of heavy-duty foil. Drizzle with 1 tablespoon oil. Enclose loosely, then bake 60 minutes, until they are sharp-knife tender. The total time will depend on the relative size of the beets; you might need some extra time for larger ones. Let them stand in the foil for an hour or so. Cut off the stems and roots and peel them. Cut into ¼" strips and set aside.

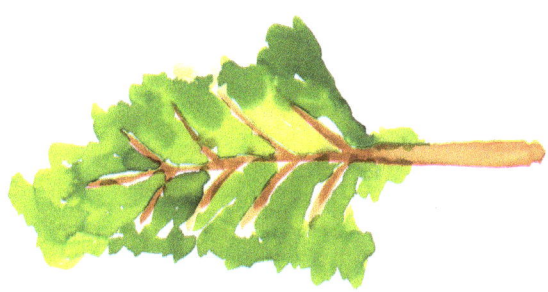

BREAK off the stems from the greens right below the leaves. Wash well and shake off the water. Cut into 1" slices and set aside.

MELT 2 tablespoons butter in a medium skillet over rather high heat. Add the shallots and sauté 2 minutes. Add the beets and sauté another minute. Add the 2 juices, 2 teaspoons sugar, ½ teaspoon salt, ½ teaspoon pepper, cumin, and chili powder. Sauté until the beets are glazed nicely. Season, if necessary. Cover and refrigerate the leftovers. Makes 3–4 servings.

TO PREPARE THE GREENS: Melt the remaining butter and oil over very high heat in a large skillet. Add the garlic and crushed red pepper. Add the water, the remaining sugar, and the greens. Cover and cook over very high heat for 2 minutes. Stir once, halfway through cooking. Add the vinegar and the remaining salt and pepper and boil, uncovered, 1–2 minutes, stirring almost constantly until the greens are almost dry (don't burn them). Season, as desired. Serve with the beets. Cover and refrigerate the leftovers. Makes about 1½ cups.

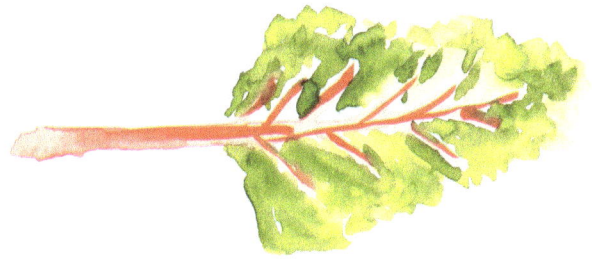

Búho Beans

ACTIVE PREP: 10 MINUTES
COOK: UP TO 3 HOURS
STAND: OVERNIGHT, 10–11 HOURS

We've got this popular restaurant in Albuquerque called the Owl Café. When you sit at your table, the wait staff will immediately present you with a small bowl of pinto beans topped with green chile, with a couple of saltine cracker packets on the side. It's kind of the perfect starter to a meal at this diner, especially since (you might recall from the chile section) pinto beans and green chile are the official state vegetables of New Mexico (a culinary designation established in 1965).

On a relatively recent visit, we were seated next to a table with a few people who were obviously tourists to the state. I overheard one of them say, when presented with the little bowl of beans and chile, that she had no idea what it was. I could understand not knowing about the chile, but the beans? It seems to me that beans must be sort of a ubiquitous North American food, but maybe that is a weird assumption to make. Regardless, I hope she liked them!

By the way, the word *búho* is Spanish for "owl." At least, it can be used for the word "owl" in general; many other words are used for more specific kinds of owls and owlets.

Pinto beans are a deceptively simple food to prepare and everyone has little secrets and details involved in their cooking. I have one daughter who adds a couple tablespoons of butter to her final product. My other daughter starts her dish with a sauté of something like chopped bacon, onion, and garlic; then she adds her beans (which were previously cooked for a brief time and left to stand), water, and seasonings for the secondary cooking. She then takes out a couple cups of beans, purees them, then adds them back to the pot for a creamier product. My own recipe here reflects the absolutely unadorned version offered at the Owl Café.

Start this recipe the night before you need them. If done sooner than expected, they can sit on the stove and be reheated later. Altitude, bean freshness, hard water, and your overall cooking temperature will affect this recipe. Add extra water if the beans have absorbed too much liquid. Also, keep in mind that homemade beans can be somewhat firmer than the ones you will find in cans (which have been sitting in a starchy liquid for who knows how long), even when they are quite tender. They may also split their skins, which is nothing to worry about.

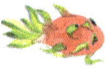

Early in the pandemic, when there were various food and supply shortages, I bought a 20-pound bag of pinto beans. I really thought I would cook more beans than I actually did. Lessons learned from this experience: Old beans take a much LONGER time to cook and buying in bulk is not necessarily a good idea. When you want to make pinto beans, be sure to buy fresh ones!

If you want to make refried beans (*refritos*), puree your pintos or mash them with a potato masher. Heat a couple tablespoons of oil or lard (a more traditional fat) in a large skillet and fry your beans over a rather high heat, stirring frequently. You just want to brown the edges a bit.

1 pound pinto beans
3½ quarts water, divided
1 teaspoon salt
1 teaspoon black pepper
1 teaspoon ground cumin
1 teaspoon onion salt
1 teaspoon garlic salt

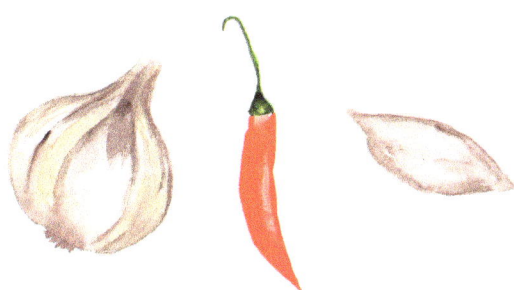

MANDATORY GARNISH: at least 1 cup of roasted and chopped green chile, with juice

OPTIONAL GARNISH:

Whole cloves of roasted garlic have occasionally been seen at this restaurant (see pages xvii and xviii for roasting garlic).

ALSO OPTIONAL GARNISH, IF YOU LIKE THEM: saltine crackers

THE NIGHT BEFORE SERVING: Combine the beans and 2 quarts water in a 4-quart saucepan. Cover and let stand overnight, about 10–11 hours. In the morning, drain them, and rinse and sort. Rinse out the pot and put the beans back in. Cover and let stand until you are ready to cook them.

THREE HOURS BEFORE SERVING: Add the remaining 6 cups water to the beans. Bring to a boil. Then cook on the lowest heat, covered, for 2 hours. Stir a couple of times. Add the 5 seasonings and raise the heat to get another boil going. Lower heat and cook, uncovered, on a gentle boil another 30–60 minutes until the beans are tender. Stir a few times. You want tender beans that are rather moist, with some liquid. Season, as desired. Cover and let stand or serve when ready.

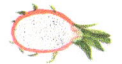

TO SERVE: Place a portion of beans in a bowl. Top with green chile. If you like garlic, throw a couple or a few cloves on top. You may serve with saltine crackers on the side (tortillas or cornbread also make nice accompaniments). Cover and refrigerate the leftovers; you can also freeze the beans. Beans will absorb their cooking liquid and will probably need a bit of water added to them when you reheat. Makes about 6 cups.

> **ALTERNATIVE TREATMENT:**
>
> Perhaps you would like to cook your beans in a slow cooker or a Crock-Pot kind of thing. You'll need something with at least a 5-quart capacity. Soak the beans with 2 quarts of water overnight in the pot, covered. Earlier in the day (say, early- to mid-morning), drain, rinse, and sort the beans. Rinse out your slow cooker a bit. Add the beans back. Add 5 cups of water and all the seasonings. Cover and cook on HIGH for 4 hours; then cook on LOW for about 2–3 hours, until the beans are tender. Stir a few times. Garnish and store the same as the original recipe.

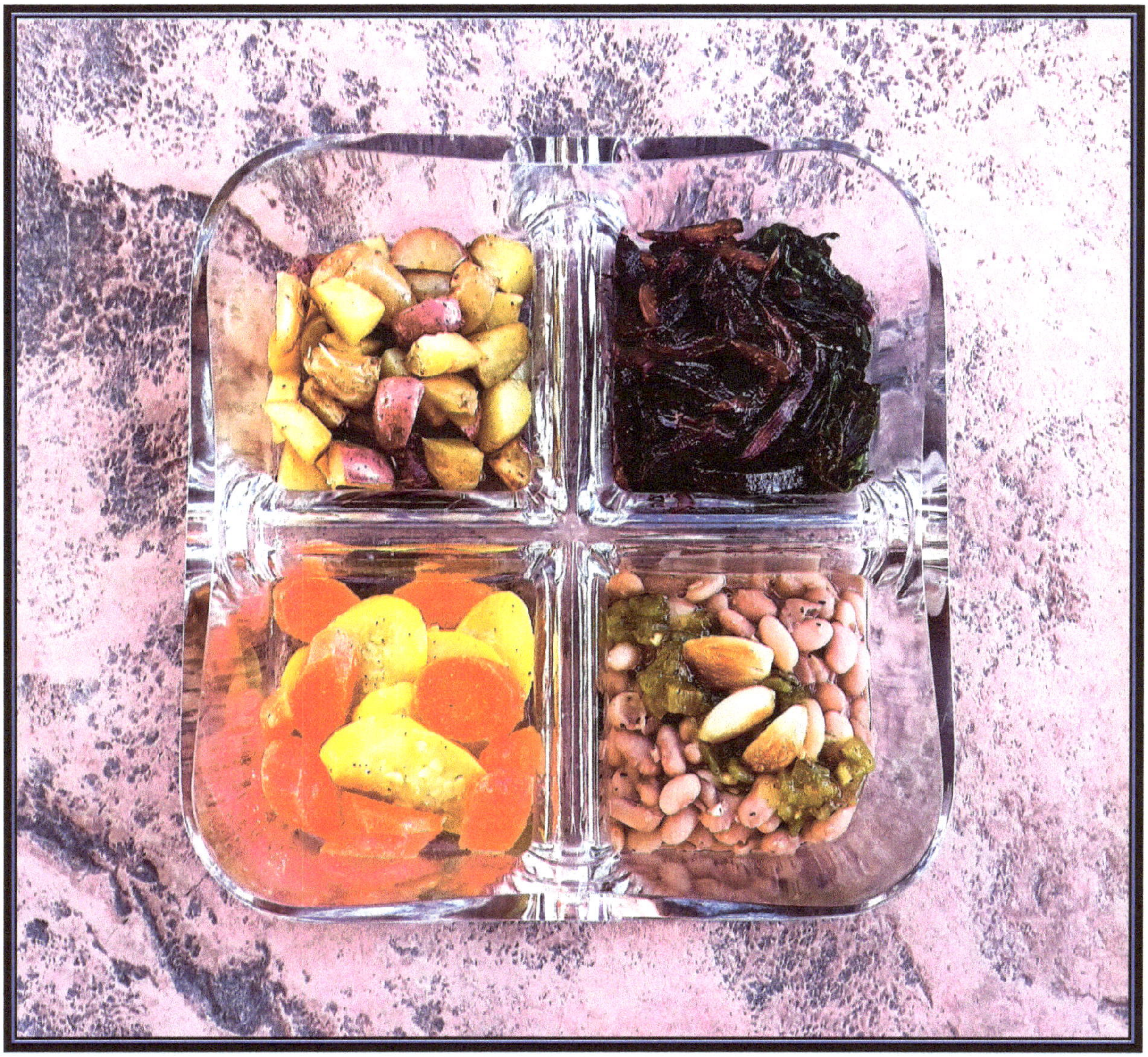

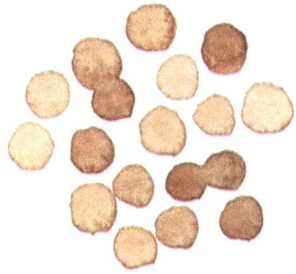

Clockwise, from top left:
Halfling Alert Taters, page 89
Lobo Beets & Greens, page 90
Búho Beans, page 92
Very Versatile Vegetables, page 96

Chapter Six: Hot Sides   95

Very Versatile Vegetables

START TO FINISH: ABOUT 15–25 MINUTES

I'm closing this chapter with an easy recipe that can utilize pretty much any kind of vegetable that lends itself to being boiled, either fresh or frozen. My favorite frozen option here is a mix of broccoli, cauliflower, and carrot (otherwise known as the Normandy mix from Costco). You want to use firm vegetables here, not fruity ones such as tomatoes or cucumbers. Probably not onions, mushrooms, or leafy items either. I mean carrot, squash, green beans, broccoli, cauliflower, peas, lima beans, etc. So, you can see you have options here. I usually cook half the recipe and it's just enough for two or three people, usually without leftovers (it depends on the vegetables you have chosen). Just use a quarter-cup of butter and skip the oil, if you want your veggies to bathe in buttery goodness. You can also steam your vegetables, instead of boiling them.

1½ pounds of fresh or frozen vegetables
    (you can use one type or a combination)
4 cups water
2 tablespoons olive oil
2 tablespoons salted butter
1½ teaspoons Savory Seasoning or Just the Basics
    (page xi and xiv, or use 2 teaspoons of any other savory
    seasoning mix listed in the **FEW ESSENTIALS** section)

PEEL and stem your fresh vegetables, if using. Cut into thin slices or chunks, whatever you prefer, depending on the vegetable. Combine the vegetables and water in a 4-quart saucepan and bring to a boil. Cook as long as directed (if using frozen) or until tender, over medium heat (so you might end up cooking anywhere from 5–15 minutes after the initial boil). If you are combining vegetables, you might need to cook one firmer type (say, sliced carrot) a bit longer than a softer type (such as zucchini), so you can add the softer vegetable after the first one has cooked a few minutes. Drain. Place the oil, butter, and seasoning in the pot and melt over rather high heat. Add the vegetables and stir to coat. Season, as desired. Cover and refrigerate the leftovers. Makes 4–6 servings.

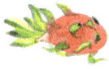

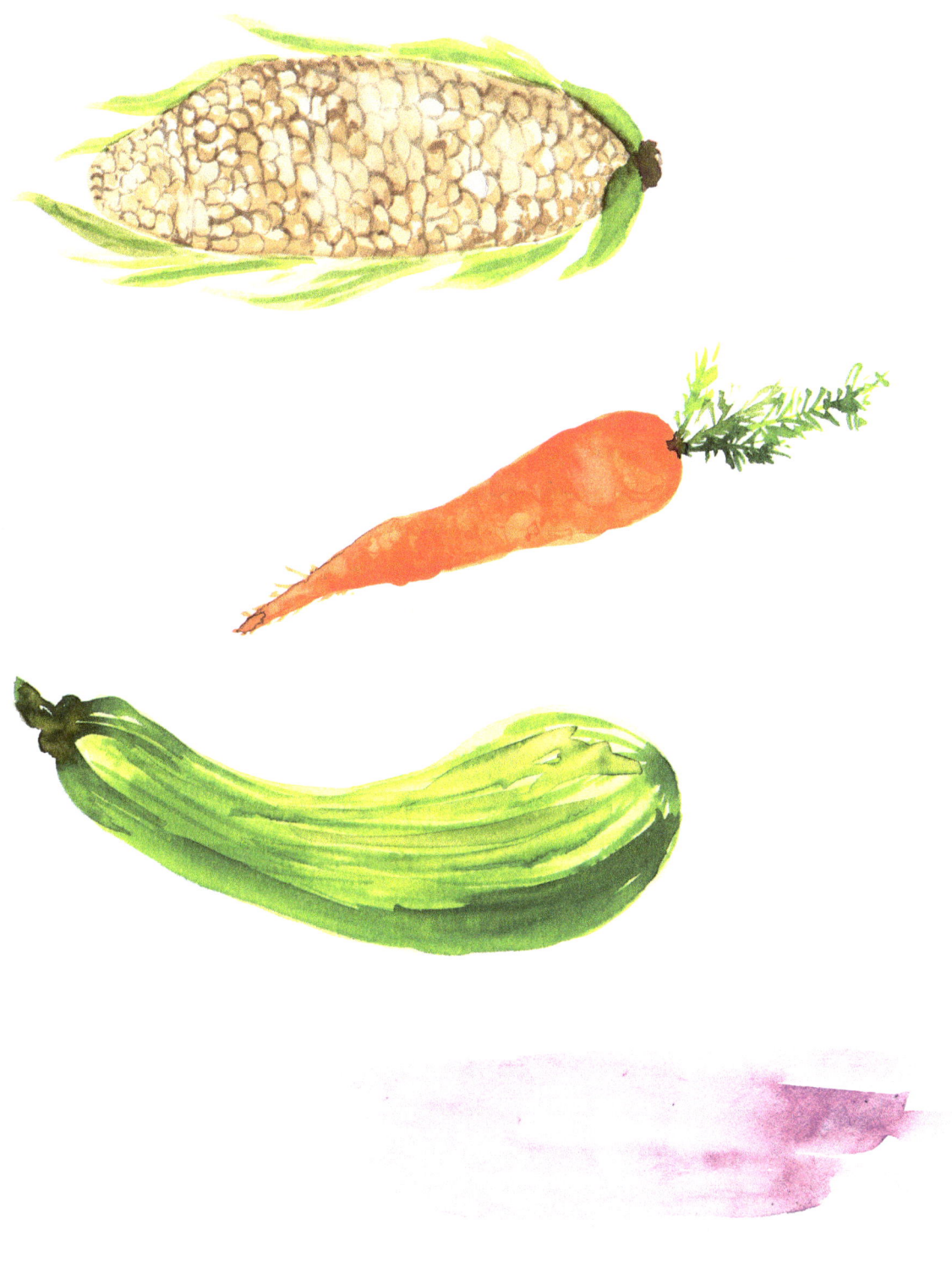

Chapter Seven

Cinco de Mayo

Zaragoza's Lasagna

Agave Shrimp

Calabacitas

Puebla Coleslaw

Biscochitos

Cinco de Mayo

MANY AMERICANS MISTAKENLY believe that Cinco de Mayo is the Mexican Independence Day (which is celebrated on September 16). Cinco de Mayo, or the Fifth of May, actually commemorates the Mexican army's victory over the French forces at the Battle of Puebla in 1862. This happened after a civil war (the War of the Reform) in Mexico, with conservatives and liberals fighting for control of the country. Wars cost money, of course, and Mexico had quite a few debts to pay. The French figured it was a good time to invade. The short Battle of Puebla held the French off temporarily, but afterward, Mexico was under French control for a while. Cinco de Mayo is a good example of underdogs achieving victory against imperialist oppressors. And everybody loves an underdog story, right?

While it is moderately celebrated in Mexico, its popularity as a holiday where one can over-indulge in margaritas and enchiladas has definitely grown in scope in the United States, in the same way St. Patrick's Day has expanded its reach to include anyone looking for a secular good time in the month of March.

I've obviously taken some license with my menu here, combining New Mexican and Italian influences, but your guests probably won't mind (you might recall I am not writing a cookbook based on historical dishes, just sharing delicious foods that happen to go together well, in a regional kind of way). You can always swap out various other recipes from other chapters if you like. Guacamole (page 5) and salsa are always welcome on the table, or make my Truth or Consequences Stuffed Peppers (page 165) instead of the lasagna.

Zaragoza's lasagna

PREP: ABOUT 48 MINUTES
BAKE: 1 HOUR AND 25 MINUTES
STAND: 10 MINUTES
OVEN: 400°

The Battle of Puebla was led by General Ignacio Zaragoza, who happened to have been a native Texan. He was a man of military and political promise with a bright future. Tragically, he contracted typhoid fever soon after May 5 and died at the age of 33 on September 8.

2 (10-ounce) cans diced tomatoes with green chiles (such as Ro*Tel)
1 pound chorizo, skins removed (or any Italian sausage, mild or spicy)
1 cup onion, coarsely chopped
1 tablespoon minced garlic
15-ounce can tomato sauce
16-ounce jar red chile sauce (or 2 cups of Red Chile Sauce, page xxviii)
1½ cups mild olives, pitted, drained, and sliced (green or black)
15.5-ounce can pinto beans, drained and rinsed
10 ounces queso panela (or fresco)
5 ounces sharp cheddar cheese, finely shredded
3 large eggs
½ cup table cream (or heavy cream)
1½ cups sour cream (light is okay)
½ teaspoon salt
½ teaspoon black pepper
12 no-cook lasagna noodles
   (I use ones with curly edges)

GARNISH:

See the **NICE NEW MEXICAN & MEXICAN GARNISHES** list on page ii and choose a few of your favorites.

PLACE the diced tomatoes in a strainer to drain well. Press on them to squeeze out most of the liquid. Coat a 5-quart deep skillet with cooking spray. Sauté the chorizo, onion, and garlic over very high heat until the pink is gone, breaking up the meat. Drain only if it's exceptionally greasy (it probably won't be). Mix in the drained tomatoes. Add the tomato sauce and red chile sauce and combine well. Let stand.

PLACE the prepared olives and pinto beans in a medium bowl and combine well. Set aside. Crumble the queso panela and place in a medium bowl. Add the cheddar, mix well, and set aside. Place the eggs, cream, sour cream, salt, and pepper in a large bowl. Combine well with a whisk. Set aside.

PREHEAT the oven to 400°. Coat a 13" by 9" baking dish with cooking spray or grease lightly and set the pan on a large baking sheet. Spread 1½ cups of the prepared meat sauce in the pan. Place 4 lasagna noodles in the dish—lay 3 the long way, then the final one crosswise. You will break off part of this final noodle, and break this portion into small pieces to fit in the empty spots. Don't overlap the noodles; they need room to expand while cooking. Now layer:

Chapter Seven: Cinco de Mayo

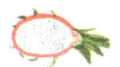

One-third of the sour cream mixture (spread to cover fairly well)
Half of the olive mixture (sprinkle over evenly)
1 cup sauce (spread to cover fairly well)
One-third of the cheese mixture (sprinkle over all evenly)
4 more noodles, placed as instructed above
    (press down gently on all)
One-third sour cream
Remaining olives
1 cup sauce
One-third cheese
Remaining noodles (press down gently on all)
Any remaining sour cream
Any remaining sauce
Any remaining cheese

BE sure the final layer of sour cream/sauce covers to the edge of the pasta. Cover loosely with light foil—crimp at the edges, but leave a little loose at the top. Bake 70 minutes. Remove the foil and bake 15 more minutes. Remove from the oven and let it stand 10 minutes before cutting. Garnish, if you like. Cover and refrigerate the leftovers; they freeze well. Makes 8–12 servings, more or less.

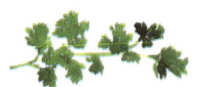

Agave Shrimp

PREP: ABOUT 25–30 MINUTES
CHILL: 2–3 HOURS

This is a lighter take on a typical shrimp salad.

4 quarts water
¼ cup Old Bay Seasoning
6 teaspoons hot sauce, divided
2 pounds medium or large raw shrimp (if frozen, thaw as directed; tails OFF)
¼ cup vegetable oil
¼ cup tomato paste
¼ cup lime juice

¼ cup light agave syrup
2 teaspoons celery salt
2 teaspoons garlic salt
1 cup scallions, thinly sliced

Garnish: chopped fresh cilantro

Place the water, Old Bay, and 4 teaspoons hot sauce in an 8-quart saucepan. Bring to a boil. Add the shrimp and cook just until the shrimp turn pink, which could take anywhere from 1–3 minutes, depending on the size of your shrimp. Stir a couple of times. Drain and set aside; reuse the pot.

Place the oil, tomato paste, lime juice, agave, the 2 salts, and the remaining hot sauce in the saucepan. Whisk well. Mix in the scallions, then the shrimp. Place in a 6-cup container, cover, and refrigerate 2–3 hours before serving. Mix a couple of times. Garnish before serving, if desired. Cover and refrigerate the leftovers. Makes 4–6 servings.

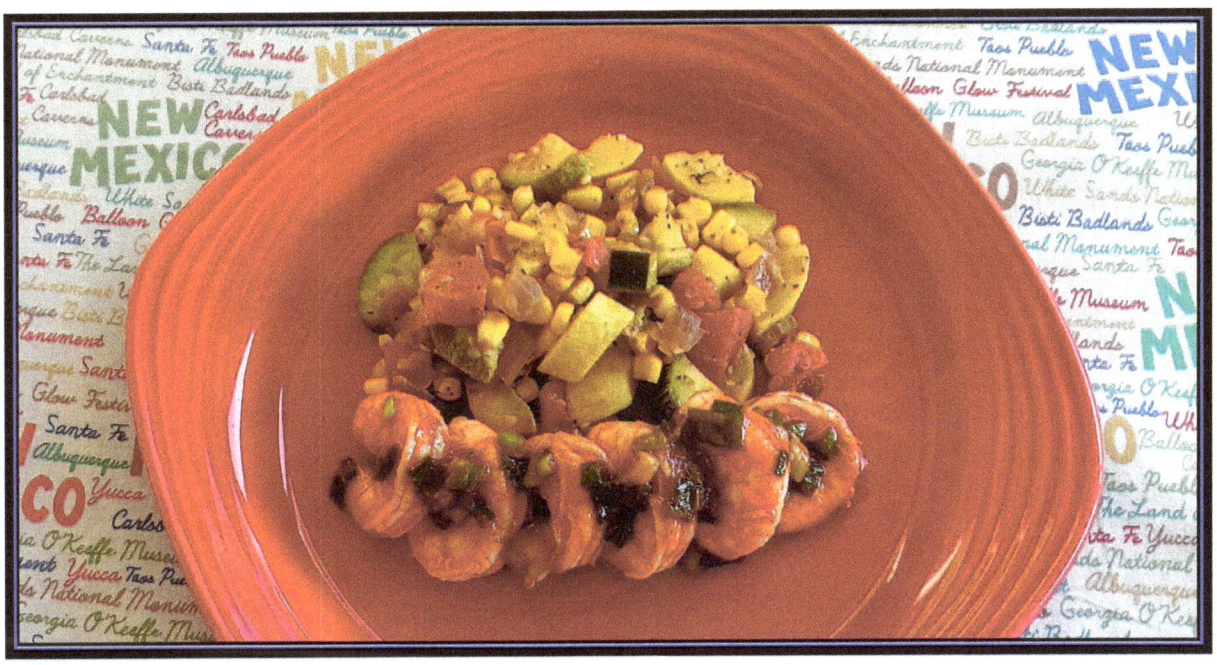

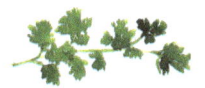

Top:
Calabacitas, page 104

Bottom:
Agave Shrimp, page 102

Chapter Seven: Cinco de Mayo

Calabacitas

START TO FINISH: ABOUT 42 MINUTES

Calabaza is the Spanish word for winter squash. *Calabacitas* means "little squash." Any kind of summer squash can qualify as a little squash, though around my neighborhood grocery stores, we do have a variety of squash actually called *calabacitas* that has a pale green skin, with some subtle stripes. It has a mild flavor, as opposed to zucchini (otherwise known as courgette), which can occasionally be on the bitter side. I like to use a combination of three squashes to make this hearty side dish. If you have trouble locating a particular variety of summer squash, feel free to use just zucchini or yellow squash, or a combination of the two.

This dish is a lovely and low-carb alternative to rice and beans. You may also use it as a filling for burritos or enchiladas, or just serve it in a bowl as a stew.

12 ounces calabacitas
12 ounces yellow squash
12 ounces zucchini, partially peeled
1 tablespoon salted butter
1 tablespoon olive oil
2 tablespoons minced garlic
1 cup red onion, coarsely chopped
14-ounce can stewed tomatoes
2 cups fresh or frozen corn
4 ounces roasted and chopped green chile, with juice
1 teaspoon salt
1 teaspoon black pepper
1 teaspoon dried oregano (2–3 tablespoons fresh, minced)

GARNISH:

A sprinkling of cheese is nice, such as shredded cheddar, or crumbled Mexican cheeses, such as panela, fresco, or cotija.

CUT the stem ends off all the squash. Cut in quarters lengthwise, then cut into ½" chunks; set aside. Melt the butter and oil over rather high heat in a 5-quart deep skillet. Add the garlic and onion and sauté 3 minutes. Add all the squash to the pan and sauté another 5 minutes.

MEANWHILE, drain the tomatoes, then cut into ½" bits. Add to the pan. Add the remaining ingredients and bring to a boil. Cook on medium heat, covered, 15 minutes. Stir a couple of times. Then cook over rather high heat, uncovered, another 3–4 minutes. Stir often until it is a bit drier and the vegetables are tender. Season, if desired. Garnish if you like. Cover and refrigerate the leftovers; they freeze well. Makes 6–8 servings.

Puebla Coleslaw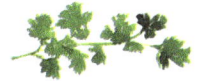

START TO FINISH: 17 MINUTES

The Battle of Puebla took place on Cinco de Mayo, so I figured I would commemorate the town and the battle with this light, slightly spicy slaw.

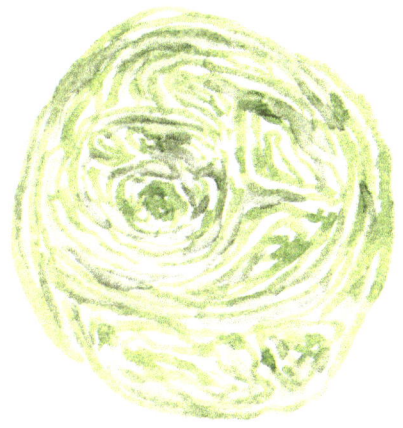

2 tablespoons sugar
3 tablespoons vegetable oil
2 tablespoons mayonnaise (sour cream will also work, light or regular)
2 tablespoons red wine vinegar
1 tablespoon lime juice
½ teaspoon salt
¼ teaspoon cayenne pepper
4-5 cups cabbage, cored and coarsely chopped
⅓ cup red bell pepper, cored and coarsely chopped
⅓ cup red onion, coarsely chopped
⅓ cup frozen corn, thawed
1 large jalapeño, cut off stem, remove seeds with a spoon, and chop finely

IN a large bowl, combine the sugar, oil, mayonnaise, vinegar, lime juice, salt, and cayenne well with a whisk. Season, as desired. Add the remaining ingredients and mix well. Cover and refrigerate the leftovers. Makes 6–8 servings.

Chapter Seven: Cinco de Mayo

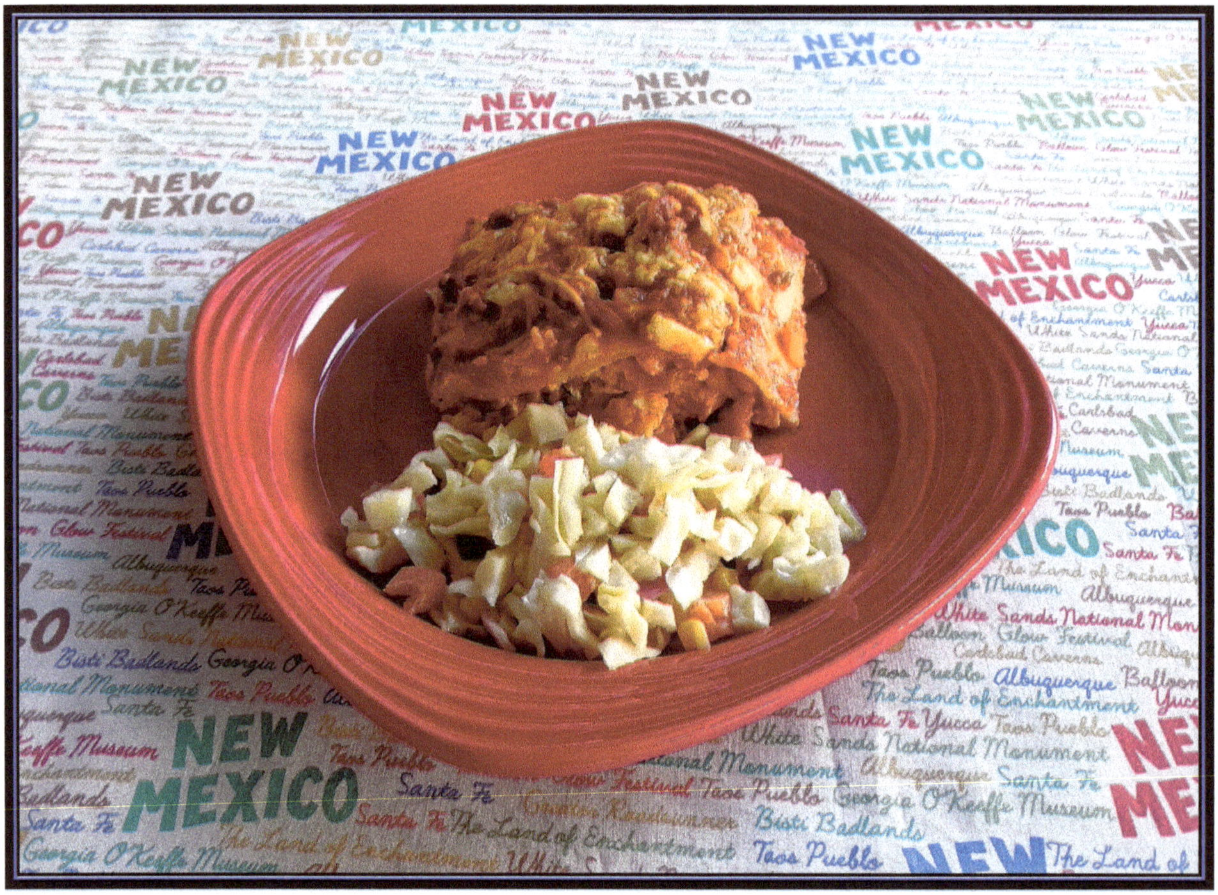

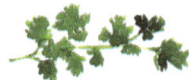

TOP:
Zaragoza's Lasagna, page 100

BOTTOM:
Puebla Coleslaw, page 105

Biscochitos

ACTIVE PREP: ABOUT 30 MINUTES
STAND: 30 MINUTES
CHILL: 2 HOURS
BAKE: 10 MINUTES PER BATCH
COOL: 20 MINUTES
OVEN: 375°

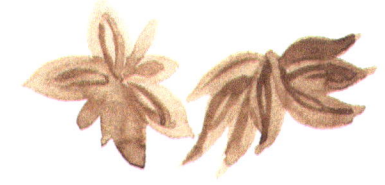

These cookies are New Mexican in origin (they are our official state cookie!) and traditionally served around Christmastime, but that shouldn't stop you from adding them to your springtime Cinco de Mayo celebration or any other time of year.

Lard is the traditional fat required for these sweets. You could probably substitute butter or vegetable shortening, but they really will not taste as good. You may also roll the dough out and cut various shapes, if you like. This will change your yield and your baking time, so you will need to experiment. I like my biscochitos to be a bit on the thicker side, so a roll and a cut works well.

¼ cup half-and-half
1 tablespoon anise seed
1 tablespoon vanilla extract
8 ounces lard, rather soft
1 cup sugar
1 large egg
3 cups all-purpose flour
2 teaspoons baking powder
½ teaspoon salt
⅓ cup cinnamon sugar
    (see page xvi for a recipe)

COMBINE the half-and-half, anise seed, and vanilla in a 1-cup glass measuring cup and let stand for 30 minutes or so.

COMBINE the lard and sugar in a very large bowl and cream together well; scrape sides down. Add the egg and the half-and-half mixture and combine well on medium speed for 2 minutes. Add the flour, baking powder, and salt and combine on lowest speed, then mix on medium speed for 2 minutes; scrape down sides halfway through to mix thoroughly. Place on a lightly floured surface. Divide the dough into 2 portions. Form each half into a 12″ long cylinder. Press on the ends gently to straighten them. Place on a large baking sheet and refrigerate around 2 hours.

PREHEAT the oven to 375°. Coat 2 large baking sheets with cooking spray or grease lightly; set aside. Place the dough portions on a cutting board. Place the cinnamon sugar in a shallow bowl. Cut one cylinder into 20 slices. Dip each side, top and bottom, in the cinnamon sugar. Place 10 on each prepared baking sheet. Bake 10 minutes. Let stand on pans 2 minutes, then carefully remove the cookies to racks to cool. Repeat with the remaining dough (any extra cinnamon sugar can be used in other recipes). Keep them covered at room temperature. Makes 40.

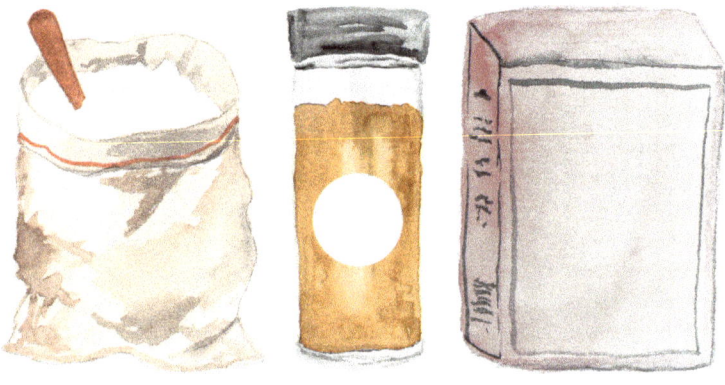

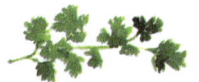

NEW MEXICO
The Land of Enchantment
White Sands National Monument
Albuquerque
Santa Fe
Taos Pueblo
Bisti Badlands
Georgia O'Keeffe Museum
Carlsbad Caverns
Balloon Glow Festival
Yucca

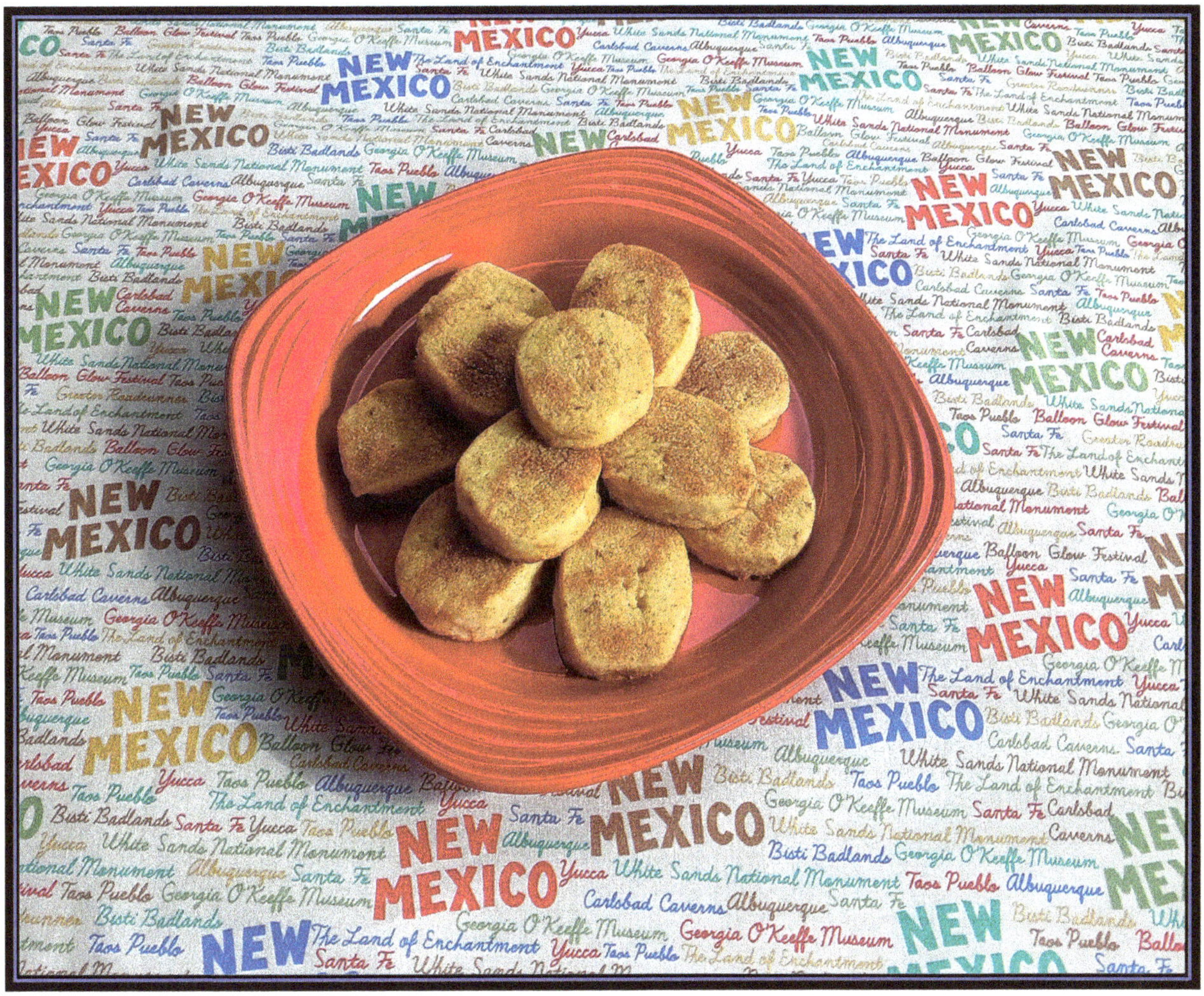

CHAPTER EIGHT

LUNCHY STUFF

Mustards & Mayos

C.H.E.T.

Hasperat

Giant Funky Ham Sandwich

Jakkubano

Roast Beef & Gorgonzola Sandwich

Tauntaun Wontons

Chile Joes

Mom's Bell Pepper

Burque Turkey

Burqueño Beef

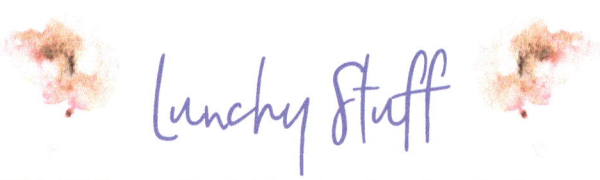

Lunchy Stuff

OUR LUNCHES ARE usually fairly simple, plus I often serve breakfast for lunch, such as a burrito or an English muffin egg sandwich (pancakes pop up occasionally). But I ended up with a few substantial sandwich items and some flavored mayonnaises and mustards. All of this evolved into a whole chapter.

What about those breakfast items mentioned above? I'm not going to supply exact recipes for those. Burrito—I use two strips of precooked and crumbled bacon, scramble an egg, mix some shredded cheese in it, then the bacon; pile this all on a medium-sized flour tortilla, pour a tablespoon of red chile sauce all over, fold like a burrito, and microwave for about 20 seconds. Done. Egg sandwich—I use a precooked sausage patty, scramble an egg, mix some shredded cheese in it, use a spatula to make it sort of a square size. While the egg is cooking, toast a sliced English muffin. Place the sausage on one half and place the egg on top. Then, place the other half of the muffin on top. I usually serve this with Sriracha sauce. Done. You have now saved yourself two trips to fast food places.

Sometimes I get a hankering for fancier mustards and mayonnaises, so let's start with those. These will work on sandwiches, or with those ubiquitous chicken nuggets, or as dips for various vegetables, whatever you like. You will also find additional mayo/mustard spreads scattered within the recipes below; all are easy to increase, if needed.

MUSTARDS & MAYOS

These items are great as dips or spreads for any sort of fried nugget you might like—chicken, fish, zucchini, French fries, etc. Some of the items could be thinned with a bit of milk to convert them into salad dressings. I have based many of the mayonnaise recipes on half a cup of mayonnaise as your starting ingredient, but they are easy to double or triple as needed. All are perfectly suited to be spread on many sorts of sandwiches. You could also try mixing these flavored mayonnaises into the salads in the C.H.E.T. section below for variety, or whatever cold salad you like.

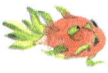

Smoky BBQ Sauce

START TO FINISH: 7 MINUTES

2 tablespoons 1% milk
¼ cup sour cream (light is okay)
¼ cup mayonnaise
¼ cup barbecue sauce (any variety is fine)
1 teaspoon chipotle powder
¼ teaspoon salt

WHISK all the ingredients well in a medium bowl. Cover and refrigerate the leftovers. Makes almost 1 cup.

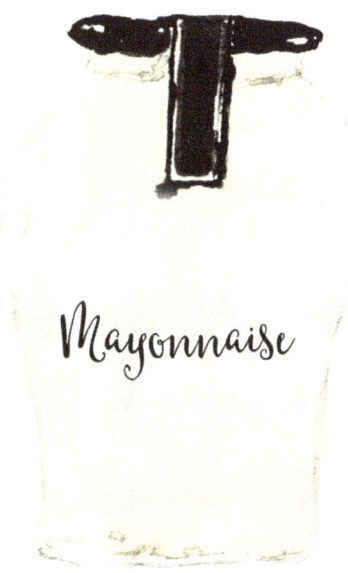

Honey Mustard Sauce

START TO FINISH: 7 MINUTES

⅓ cup sour cream (light is okay)
¼ cup Dijon mustard
3 tablespoons honey
1 teaspoon chili powder
¼ teaspoon salt

WHISK all the ingredients well in a medium bowl. Cover and refrigerate the leftovers. Makes about ¾ cup.

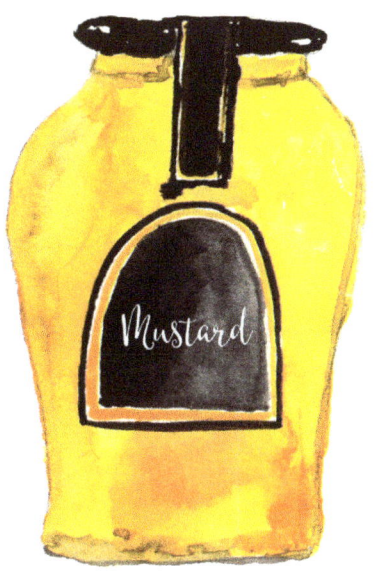

Chapter Eight: Lunchy Stuff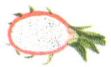

Horsey Mayo

START TO FINISH: 5 MINUTES

½ cup mayonnaise
¼ cup prepared horseradish
2 tablespoons Dijon mustard
½ teaspoon salt
½ teaspoon white pepper

WHISK all the ingredients well in a medium bowl. Cover and refrigerate the leftovers. Makes about ¾ cup.

Pesto Mayo

START TO FINISH: 5 MINUTES

½ cup mayonnaise
½ cup pesto sauce (any variety)
1 teaspoon garlic powder
1 teaspoon crushed red pepper flakes
½ teaspoon salt

WHISK all the ingredients well in a medium bowl. Cover and refrigerate the leftovers. Makes about 1 cup.

Sriracha Mayo

START TO FINISH: 5 MINUTES

½ cup mayonnaise
2 tablespoons Sriracha sauce
1 teaspoon garlic powder
1 teaspoon lime juice
½ teaspoon salt

WHISK all the ingredients well in a medium bowl. Cover and refrigerate the leftovers. Makes about ⅔ cup.

Tomato Mayo

START TO FINISH: 8 MINUTES

½ cup mayonnaise
½ teaspoon salt
½ teaspoon garlic powder
½ teaspoon crushed red pepper flakes
⅓ cup julienned sun-dried tomatoes packed in oil

Whisk the mayonnaise and the 3 seasonings well in a medium bowl. Remove the tomatoes from the oil and place on paper towels. Pat dry, then chop finely. Measure them now to make ⅓ cup. Add to the bowl and mix well. Cover and refrigerate the leftovers. Makes about ¾ cup.

Chipotle Mayo

START TO FINISH: 6 MINUTES

½ cup mayonnaise
¼ cup chipotle peppers in adobo sauce, minced
½ teaspoon salt
½ teaspoon garlic powder

Whisk all the ingredients well in a medium bowl. Cover and refrigerate the leftovers. Makes about ¾ cup.

C.H.E.T.

This stands for Chicken, Ham, Egg, and Tuna. These are incredibly easy salads, but I really like them because of their simplicity. For each recipe, you can substitute/exchange the seasonings from the **FEW ESSENTIALS** part of the cookbook. They are also designed to make about one and a half cups each. This might serve anywhere between two to four people, depending on various circumstances, such as how big you make a sandwich, or how many crackers you like to put your chicken salad on, etc. Yes, I'm obviously rather boring around lunchtime, but I kind of love having some predictable routines in my life.

Mix and match your dry seasonings, mustards, and mayonnaises in these salads for new flavor profiles. Don't have any celery hanging around? Sometimes I don't have any. Try chopping up some other rather firm vegetables, such as jicama, radishes, or bell peppers, any color. Cucumber? Maybe, but it might be a bit wet in your salad. Shredded carrot might be good. What about onion? You can use any color onion you like, or shallots, or scallions. Simplify even more by omitting the vegetables because sometimes you only really need the absolutely bare essentials on your cracker.

Chicken Salad

START TO FINISH: 10–12 MINUTES

6 ounces cooked chicken, finely chopped
¼ cup celery, finely chopped
¼ cup red onion, finely chopped
1½ teaspoons Mexican Mix (page xiv)
1 teaspoon stone ground mustard
⅓ cup mayonnaise

COMBINE the ingredients in a medium bowl. Season, if desired. Cover and refrigerate the leftovers. Makes about 1½ cups.

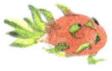

Ham Salad

START TO FINISH: 10–12 MINUTES

6 ounces ham, finely chopped
¼ cup celery, finely chopped
¼ cup white or yellow onion, finely chopped
2 tablespoons dill pickle relish
½ teaspoon black pepper
½ teaspoon salt
¼ teaspoon dried dill weed (1–2 tablespoons fresh dill, minced)
1 teaspoon spicy brown mustard
⅓ cup mayonnaise

IF the ham is rather wet, pat it dry with paper towels. Place in a medium bowl. Add the remaining ingredients and combine well. Season, if desired. Cover and refrigerate the leftovers. Makes about 1¾ cups.

Egg Salad

IN ADVANCE: HARD BOILING EGGS AND CHILLING (APPROXIMATELY 2 HOURS)
START TO FINISH: 10–12 MINUTES

3 large eggs, hard-boiled and chilled in advance
¼ cup celery, finely chopped
¼ cup red onion, finely chopped
¾ teaspoon Savory Seasoning (page xi)
1 teaspoon yellow mustard
⅓ cup mayonnaise

PEEL the eggs, rinse them off, then cut with an egg slicer. Turn them once and slice again. Place in a medium bowl. Add the remaining ingredients and combine well. Season, if desired. Cover and refrigerate the leftovers. Makes about 1½ cups.

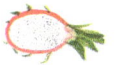

Tuna Salad

Start to finish: 10–12 minutes

7-ounce can of albacore tuna packed in water
¼ cup celery, finely chopped
¼ cup scallions, thinly sliced
2 tablespoons sweet pickle relish
1½ teaspoons Cajun Mix or New England Mix (both on page xv)
1 teaspoon Dijon mustard
⅓ cup mayonnaise

DRAIN the tuna well. Break it up and place it in a medium bowl. Add the remaining ingredients and combine well. Season, if desired. Cover and refrigerate the leftovers. Makes about 1¾ cups.

SANDWICHY SORT OF ITEMS

Once or twice a week, we usually have a cold cut, cheese, lettuce, and tomato kind of sandwich, but occasionally, I splurge and make something more substantial. A couple of the items in the following pages are appropriate for more crowded situations.

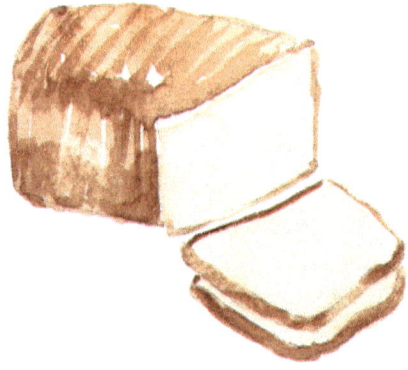

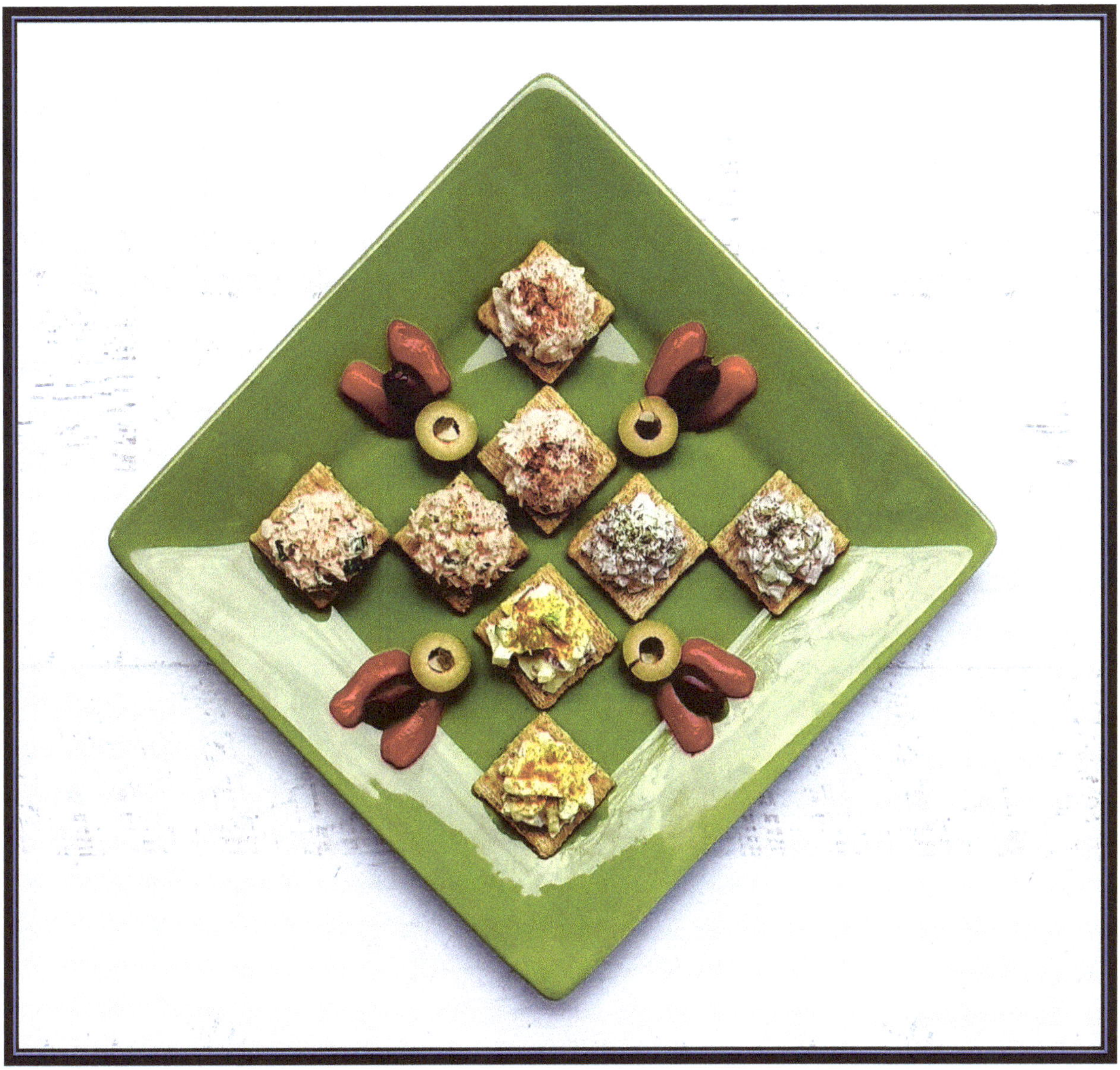

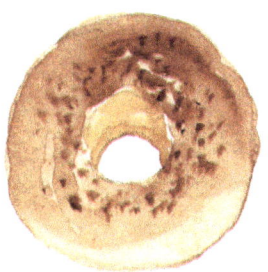

Clockwise, from top:
Chicken Salad, page 116
Ham Salad, page 117
Egg Salad, page 117
Tuna Salad, page 118

Chapter Eight: Lunchy Stuff   119

Hasperat

IN ADVANCE: MAKING PICKLES AND CHILLING OVERNIGHT
ACTIVE PREP: ABOUT 40 MINUTES

Besides hanging around Middle-earth, I often visit The Final Frontier. One of my favorite peripheral characters in *Star Trek: The Next Generation* is Ro Laren. Ro's loyalties may be torn between Starfleet and her fellow Bajorans' resistance to the dreaded Cardassians, but she is definitely NOT torn about her allegiance to the spicy sandwich, which is a specialty of her home planet, Bajor. Her father apparently made the "strongest" (meaning, spiciest) Hasperat she had ever tasted, and all others paled in comparison.

    This vegetarian sandwich is not for the faint of heart. It might even be more appropriate for Klingons, who like to live more dangerously with their food choices. If you are a bit faint, you can certainly reduce the spicy components of this recipe, or even leave them out altogether; it will still taste fine. Can you add some meat to this wrap? You can, but I would keep it to a bare minimum, say, a couple of tablespoons of some cooked chicken or bacon on each sandwich. This sandwich is also not conducive to being leftovers, because the tortilla ends up being sticky and chewy. I tried this once, and I wasn't pleased with the refrigerated leftovers. So, when I plan to serve this, I make all the pickles and the cream cheese mixture; then, I assemble two wraps right when I want to serve them. A couple of days later, I'll assemble two more wraps, using up the pickles and cheese.

    Start this recipe at least one night before serving so the pickles can soak in the spice.

½ cup water
½ cup cider vinegar
2 tablespoons sugar
1 tablespoon crushed red pepper flakes
1 tablespoon lemon juice
1 teaspoon salt
½ cup red bell pepper
½ cup green bell pepper
½ cup red onion
2 good-sized jalapeños

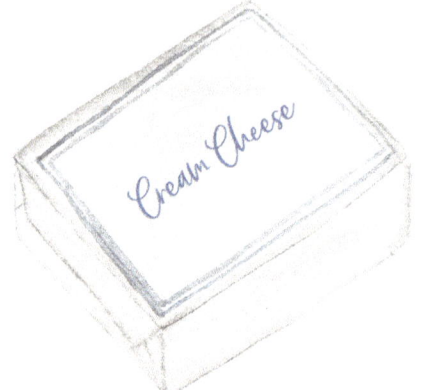

8 ounces light cream cheese (Neufchâtel)
2 tablespoons sour cream (light is okay)
3 tablespoons Sriracha sauce
4 large flour tortillas (11–12″ in diameter)
A total of 3 cups of assorted extra vegetables—choose 3 items from these
    suggested options and put about ¼ cup on each tortilla:

- shredded carrot and/or chopped or shredded cabbage
- chopped spinach, kale, or other greenery
    (cut larger leaves into smaller quantities)
- sliced avocado with a bit of salt sprinkled on it
- cucumber, peeled and sliced

START AT LEAST ONE NIGHT BEFORE SERVING (THE PICKLE CAN BE MADE A FEW DAYS IN ADVANCE): Combine the water, vinegar, sugar, crushed red pepper, lemon juice, and salt in a 1-quart saucepan. Bring to a boil, whisking to combine. Boil 1 minute; set aside. Remove any stems, seeds, and membranes from the following 4 vegetables. Finely chop them all and place them in a 4-cup container. Pour the prepared brine over, cover, and refrigerate at least overnight. Stir a few times.

TO ASSEMBLE: Drain the pickles well and set aside. Place the cream cheese in a medium glass bowl and microwave on HIGH in 20-second intervals until it is very soft, but not liquid, about 60 seconds total. Add the sour cream and Sriracha and combine well with a whisk; set aside. Prepare your extra vegetables as you like and set aside.

SPREAD ¼ of the cream cheese mixture on 1 tortilla, leaving about ½″ around the edges. Place ¼ of the pickles in the middle area. Place ¼ cup of each of your chosen 3 vegetables on top. Roll up like a burrito: Fold the right and left edges toward the center, then roll up the bottom until the filling has been enclosed. Place the seam side down and cut diagonally to serve. As stated above, your leftover wrap might not be completely satisfying, so wrap them as needed. Otherwise, you would want to cover and refrigerate any leftovers. Makes 4 servings, but you can also serve 6 or 8, depending on how you cut each wrap.

RO LAREN SAYS:

"I've spent the better part of my life fighting the Cardassians.
I never thought I'd be helping them out. Maybe some Hasperat will
give me the strength to deal with this situation… yes, that's much better.
Hmm… That is really spicy! YIKES! I love it!"

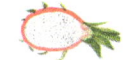

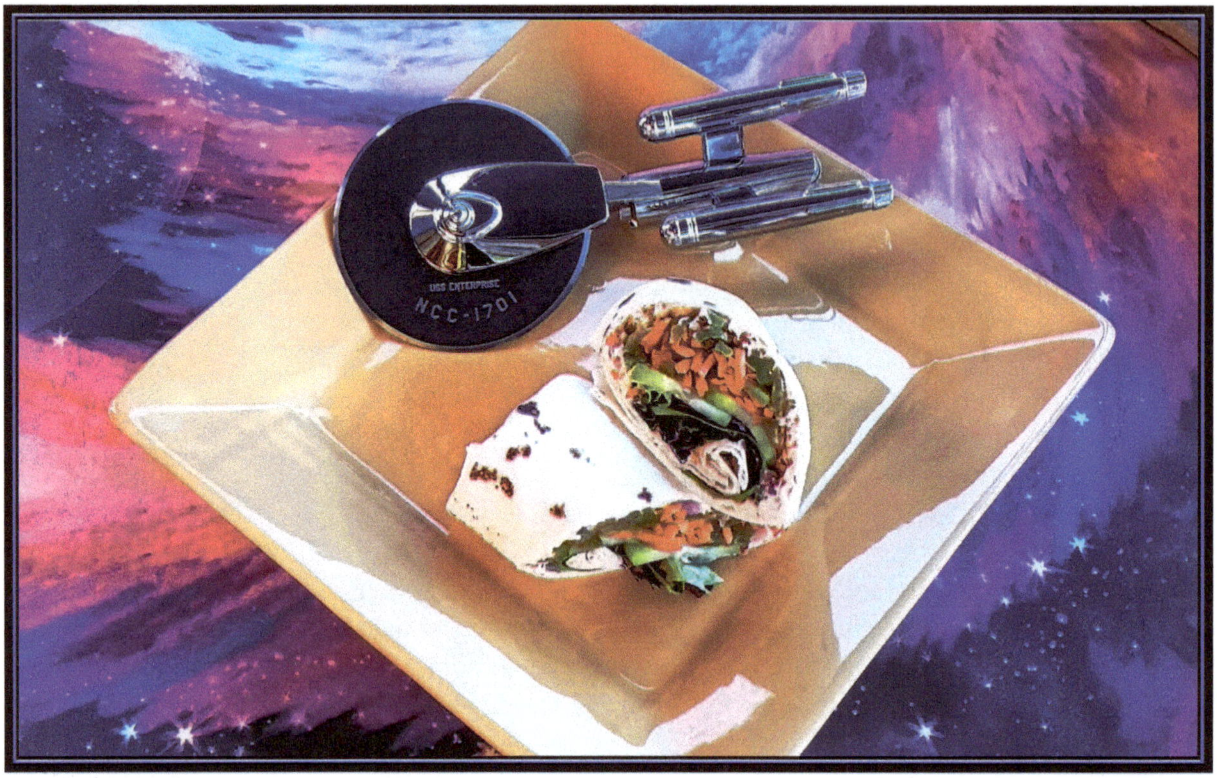

Giant Funky Ham Sandwich

START TO FINISH: ABOUT 25 MINUTES

Perfect to pair with some tomato soup! You can prepare this on a griddle, a skillet, or even on a panini press—just butter the top of the sandwich if you use this method, and press it for five minutes. You might only cook one at a time, depending on the size of your press.

5.2-ounce package Boursin cheese (any flavor, or ⅔ cup of your
    favorite soft, herby cheese)
1 ounce sun-dried tomatoes, minced (NOT oil-packed)
¼ teaspoon white pepper
4 slices of any good quality multi-grain sandwich bread
6 ounces smoked ham, sliced paper-thin
1 cup sliced sandwich pickles (any variety you like; dill, sweet, spicy/sweet)
Some soft salted butter or margarine

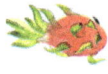

PLACE the cheese in a medium glass bowl and microwave on HIGH 30 seconds or so until it is soft enough to mix easily. Add the tomatoes and pepper and combine well. Spread this mixture equally on 2 slices of bread. Divide the ham evenly and fold the slices in half to place nicely on top of the cheese. Divide the pickles and place on top of the ham. Place the other slices of bread on top of the pickles. Spread butter on top.

HEAT a griddle or large skillet (or press) until moderately hot. Carefully place the buttered side down on the pan. Press down with a flat spatula. Spread more butter on the top. Cook until golden brown, about 3 minutes. Carefully flip over; press down. Cook this side until golden brown, another 3 minutes or so. Cut the sandwiches in half and serve. Wrap any leftovers in foil and refrigerate. Heat in the foil wrapping in a 350° oven for 8–10 minutes. Makes 2–4 servings.

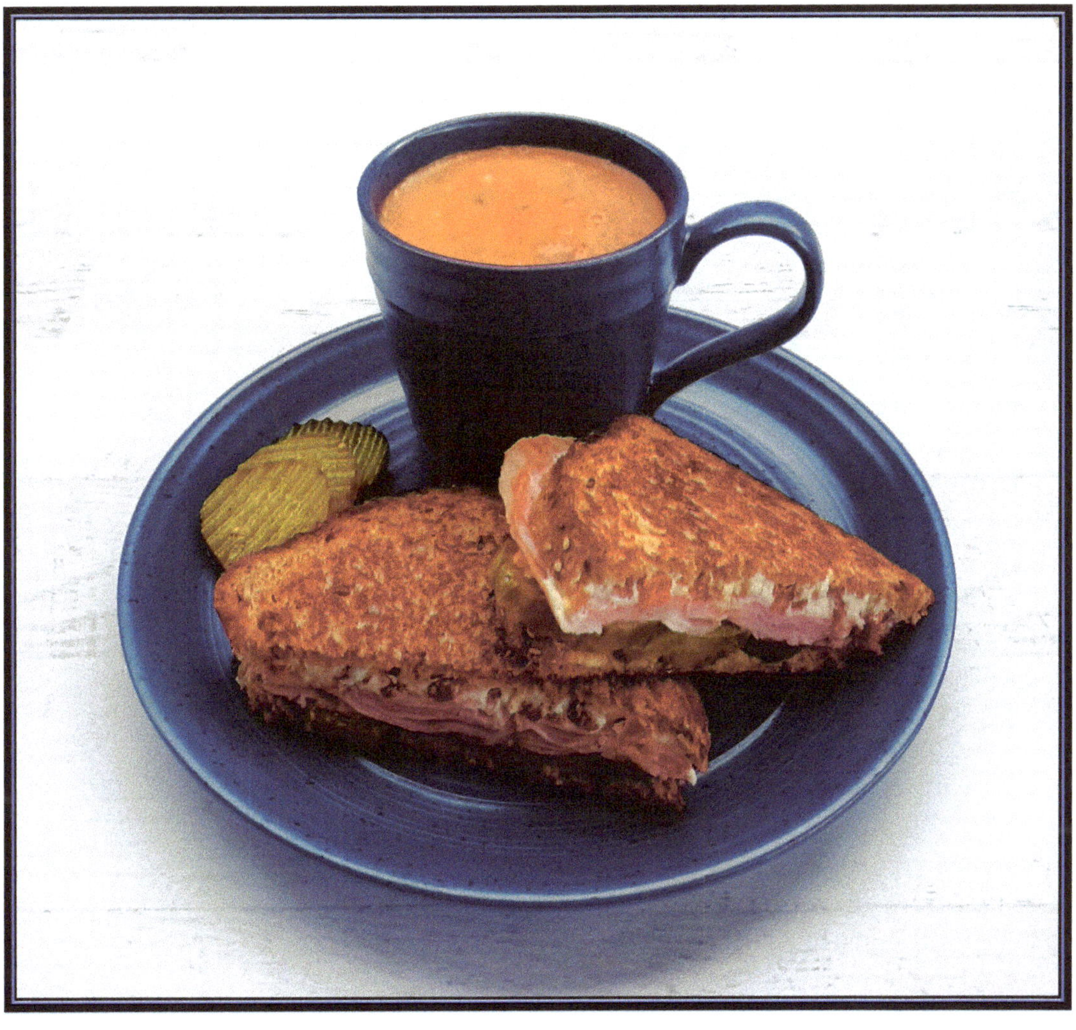

Chapter Eight: Lunchy Stuff   123

Jakkubano

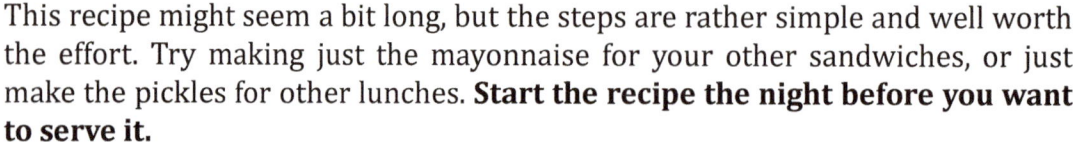

ACTIVE PREP: ABOUT 30 MINUTES
STAND: 1 HOUR
CHILL: OVERNIGHT
BAKE: ABOUT 20–30 MINUTES
COOK: 5–7 MINUTES
OVEN: 400°

This recipe might seem a bit long, but the steps are rather simple and well worth the effort. Try making just the mayonnaise for your other sandwiches, or just make the pickles for other lunches. **Start the recipe the night before you want to serve it.**

> In *The Force Awakens*, our plucky *Star Wars* heroine Rey was accustomed to slaving away in the sweltering Jakku sunshine, trying to earn enough credits to buy herself a "quarter-portion." This greenish, puffy bread product was not exactly an exciting food choice. If she ever had extra credits, however, she would treat herself to this wonderful sandwich. She could probably live off one of these for a few days.

1½ teaspoons chipotle powder, divided
1½ teaspoons garlic powder, divided
1 teaspoon onion powder
1 teaspoon salt, divided
½ teaspoon black pepper
8 ounces pork tenderloin
1 large seedless cucumber
½ cup water
½ cup white wine vinegar
1 tablespoon plus 1 teaspoon packed light brown sugar
½ teaspoon dried dill weed
½ teaspoon white pepper
½ cup mayonnaise
1 tablespoon yellow mustard

2 thin loaves of unsliced baguettes/bread, each about 11–13" long
(like Italian or sourdough; or you could use a really long loaf
of French bread, cut in half)
4 ounces honey ham, cut into paper-thin slices
4 ounces Gruyère cheese, cut into paper-thin slices
About 2 tablespoons olive oil

The night before serving: Combine 1 teaspoon chipotle powder, 1 teaspoon garlic powder, onion powder, ½ teaspoon salt, and ½ teaspoon pepper in a small bowl. Sprinkle all over the pork. Wrap tightly in plastic wrap; set on a dish and refrigerate overnight.

Also, on the night before serving: Cut off the ends of the cucumber and peel it. Cut into 3" long sections, then cut into julienned strips; set aside. Combine the water, vinegar, 1 tablespoon brown sugar, dill weed, white pepper, and ½ teaspoon salt in a 1½-quart saucepan. Boil 1 minute. Turn off the heat and add the prepared cucumbers. Cover and let stand 1 hour. Refrigerate overnight in the pot or another covered container.

And one more thing to prepare on the night before serving: Combine the mayonnaise, mustard, ½ teaspoon chipotle powder, ½ teaspoon garlic powder, and 1 teaspoon brown sugar in a small bowl. Whisk well; cover and refrigerate overnight.

The day of serving: Bake the bread as directed, if necessary, and set aside. Preheat the oven to 400°. Coat a small baking sheet well with cooking spray. Unwrap the pork and bake 20–25 minutes. Turn over halfway through cooking. The internal temperature should be about 160°. Let it rest on the pan while you assemble your other ingredients. Drain the cucumbers; set aside.

Heat a panini press. Split the loaves lengthwise carefully, leaving the bottom parts intact. Spread them open carefully. Spread the prepared mayonnaise all over the interiors of each loaf, top and bottom. Slice the pork very thinly. Lay it evenly on the bottom sides of each loaf. Lay the ham on top of the pork, evenly. Lay the cheese next. Lay some pickles on the cheese. Don't overstuff; just serve any extra pickles on the side. Press the top of the bread down. Brush tops lightly with some olive oil. Cut in half diagonally. Press 2 halves about 5–7 minutes, until golden brown. Serve with leftover pickles on the side. Cover and refrigerate any leftover pickles. Wrap the sandwich leftovers in aluminum foil and refrigerate. Reheat them in the foil wrap in a 350° oven for about 10 minutes. Makes 4 servings.

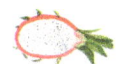

HAN SOLO SAYS: "Where'd you get this recipe?"

REY: "I stole it. From Unkar Plutt. He stole it from the Irving Boys, who stole it from Ducain."

HAN: "But he stole it from me! Well, you tell him that Han Solo just stole it back… for good."

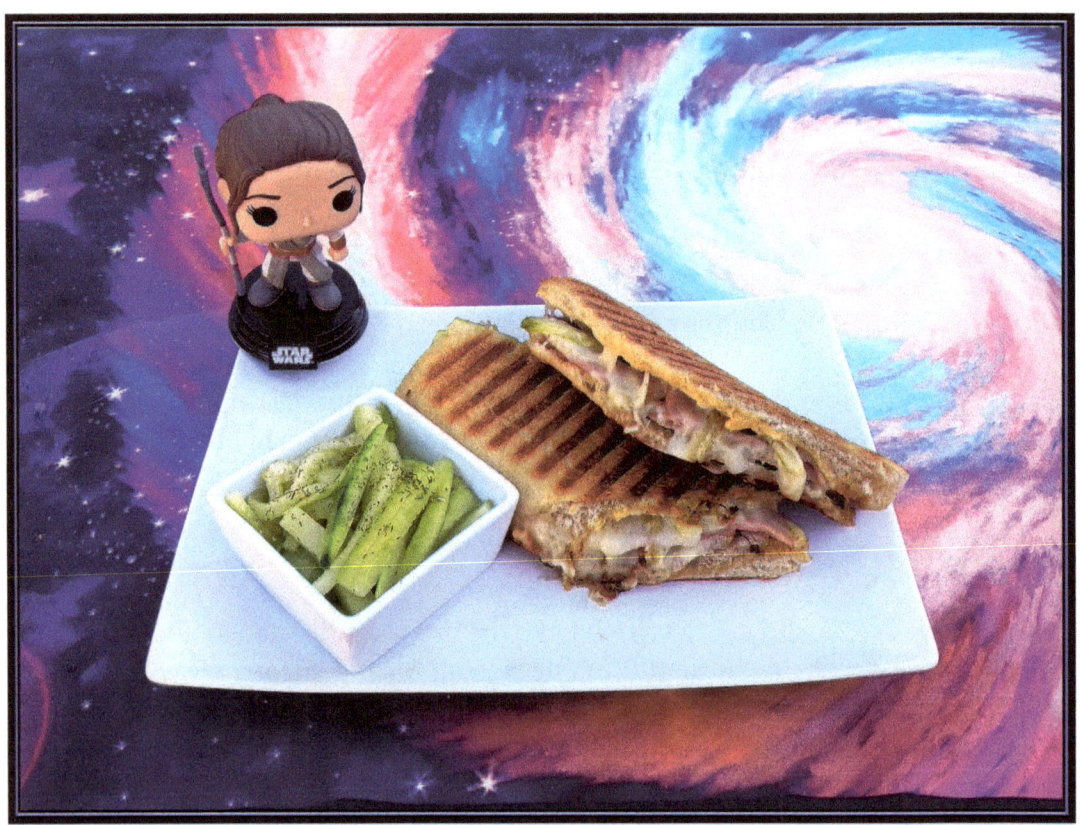

Roast Beef & Gorgonzola Sandwich

START TO FINISH: ABOUT 25 MINUTES

HALFLING ALERT! Well, I just think this hearty sandwich would really be appealing to your typical halfling, especially with a foamy pint for company.

2 ounces light cream cheese (Neufchâtel)
1 teaspoon prepared horseradish
½ teaspoon salt
½ teaspoon black pepper
2 ounces Gorgonzola cheese, crumbled
4 slices of good quality, highly flavored sandwich bread
    (such as pumpernickel, rye, or sourdough)
6 ounces roast beef, sliced paper-thin
A few thin slices of red onion
About 1 cup baby arugula, loosely packed
    (or baby spinach leaves, or a
    combination of both)
Some mayonnaise
Some soft salted butter or margarine

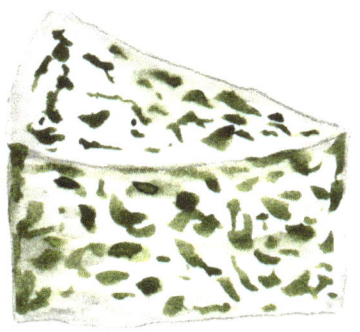

PLACE the cream cheese in a small glass bowl. Microwave on HIGH in 20-second intervals until very soft, about 40 seconds total. Mix in the horseradish, salt, and pepper well. Add the Gorgonzola and combine well; set aside.

PLACE 2 slices of bread on a cutting board. Divide the cream cheese mixture between both. Divide the roast beef evenly and fold the slices in half to place nicely on top of the cheese. Lay the red onion slices next. Divide the arugula between the 2 sandwiches. Spread mayonnaise lightly on the remaining bread slices and place this side down on the arugula. Press down on both sandwiches.

HEAT a griddle, large skillet, or panini press to moderately high. Spread some butter on top of each sandwich and place this side down on the heated pan. Press down on each, then spread more butter on top. Fry about 3 minutes, until golden brown. Carefully flip them over (you don't need to flip them if you use a press) and fry another 3 minutes or so. Cut in half to serve. Wrap the leftovers in foil and refrigerate. Heat in the foil wrapping in a 350° oven for 8–10 minutes. Makes 2–4 servings.

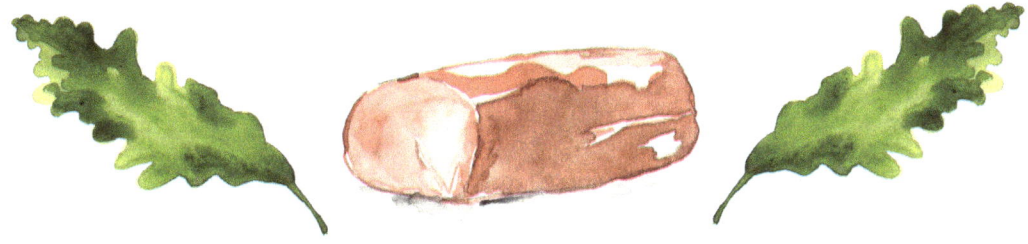

Chapter Eight: Lunchy Stuff   127

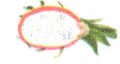

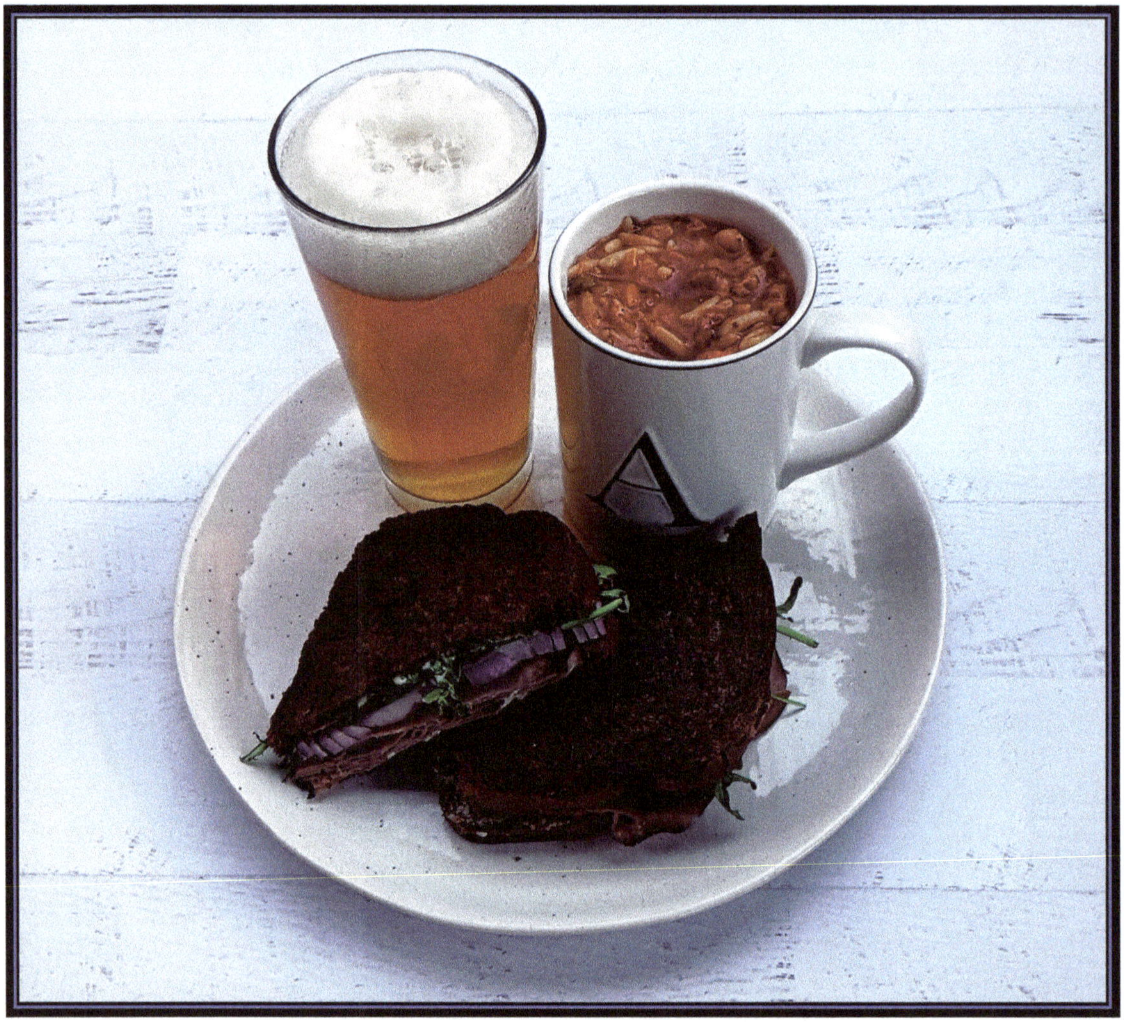

Tauntaun Wontons

Prep: about 35 minutes
Bake: 15 minutes
Stand: 5 minutes
Oven: 350°

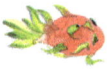 Celebrating Comfy, Cozy Foods from North America: CH&M, Volume 3

> This is the perfect food to serve at a pre-Battle of Hoth party (as seen in *The Empire Strikes Back*) if you ever feel the need to throw one of those types of shindigs. Spicy, crunchy, creamy, cheesy—all the qualities you want to eat before you head out to the frigid wasteland of the ice planet Hoth. Facing numerous AT-AT walkers will be a snap after you eat some of these! They are usually not made with actual tauntaun meat, you know, because the flesh of those beasties is a bit fragrant, to say the least.

1 pound hot Italian bulk sausage (or chorizo)
8 ounces light cream cheese (Neufchâtel)
2 large eggs, room temperature
¼ teaspoon salt
¼ teaspoon black pepper
½ cup prepared salsa (any variety)
1 cup scallions, thinly sliced
12-ounce package of wonton skins
4 ounces sharp cheddar cheese, finely shredded

Garnish:

> You can spoon items like sour cream or prepared guacamole on top of each, and crown each with a dab of Sriracha sauce, perhaps.

COAT a medium skillet with cooking spray. Break up and fry the sausage over rather high heat until the pink is gone. Drain and set aside. Place the cream cheese in a large glass bowl and microwave on HIGH in 20-second intervals until it is very soft, but not liquefied, about a minute total. Whisk the eggs, salt, and pepper into the cheese well. Mix the salsa and scallions into the cream cheese mixture well, then add the sausage; set aside.

PREHEAT the oven to 350°. Coat 48 miniature muffin cups with cooking spray. Carefully push a wonton skin into each cup. Try to keep them all opened up. Spray the wontons with additional cooking spray. Bake 5 minutes. Remove from the oven and open up any tips that have fallen over while they are hot. Divide the filling into each; start with approximately 1 tablespoon of cheese filling, then distribute the rest evenly. Sprinkle the cheddar cheese evenly over all of them, starting with a generous teaspoon on each, then distribute the rest of the cheese to any wontons that look a bit sparse. Bake 10 minutes. Let stand 5 minutes before serving. Garnish, if desired. Cover and refrigerate the leftovers; a reheat in a warm oven will help them stay crispy, rather than microwaving them. Makes 48.

FUN-LOVING STORMTROOPERS SAY:

"Hey girl—Hoth may have turned our deluded brains into mushy lasers, but face it. You just can't bear to let gorgeous guys like us out of your sight."

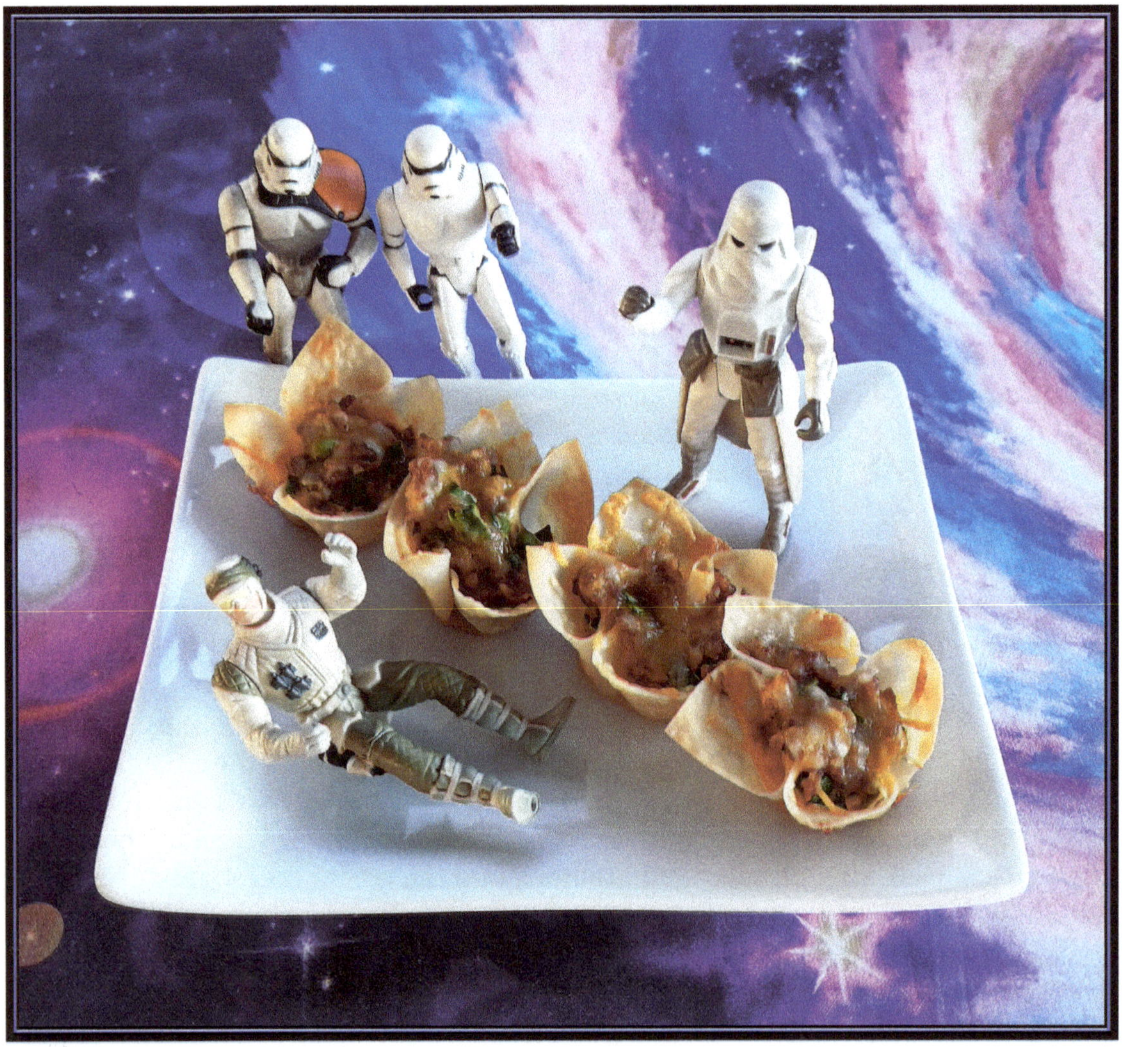

130   Celebrating Comfy, Cozy Foods from North America: CH&M, Volume 3

Chile Joes

START TO FINISH: ABOUT 35 MINUTES
BAKE: 7 MINUTES
OVEN: 350°

This is a great recipe for a moderate crowd, and it would also be a delicious addition to a Super Bowl party. If you use larger buns, you will probably serve eight people; then, you will only need eight slices of cheese.

1 pound ground beef sirloin
1 tablespoon minced garlic
1 cup onion, finely chopped
1 large green bell pepper, cored and finely chopped
4 ounces roasted and chopped green chile, with juice
¼ cup regular cream of wheat
1 teaspoon salt
1 teaspoon black pepper
1 teaspoon hot sauce
8-ounce can tomato sauce
⅔ cup water
12 regular-sized hamburger buns
12 rather thick slices of pepper jack cheese
    (use 24 slices if they are very thin)

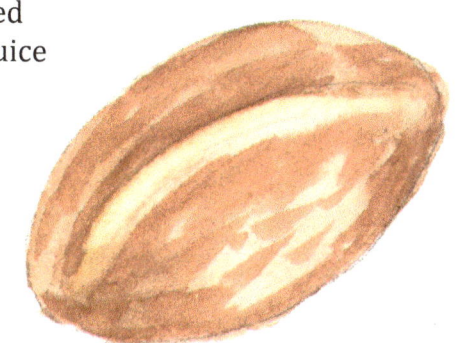

PREHEAT the oven to 350°. Coat a 3-quart deep skillet with cooking spray. Fry the beef, garlic, onion, and bell pepper over rather high heat until the pink is gone, breaking up the meat. Add the chile, cream of wheat, salt, pepper, hot sauce, tomato sauce, and water and combine well. Bring to a boil, then cook over the lowest heat, uncovered, about 15 minutes or so. Stir a few times until the mixture becomes thicker, but not too dry. Season, if desired.

MEANWHILE, open the buns and place them on 2 large baking sheets with the interior portions facing up. Lay a slice of cheese on each of the bun tops. Bake 7 minutes. To assemble, divide the meat into 12 portions and place on each bun bottom. Top with the cheese portion of the bun and serve. Wrap any assembled leftover sandwiches in foil and reheat in a 350° oven for 8–10 minutes. Makes 12.

A COUPLE OF EXTRA SUGGESTIONS…

We don't really need formal recipes for a couple of these items, and my mom's bell pepper dish doesn't require any sort of measuring, so I'll just suggest what to do for each item.

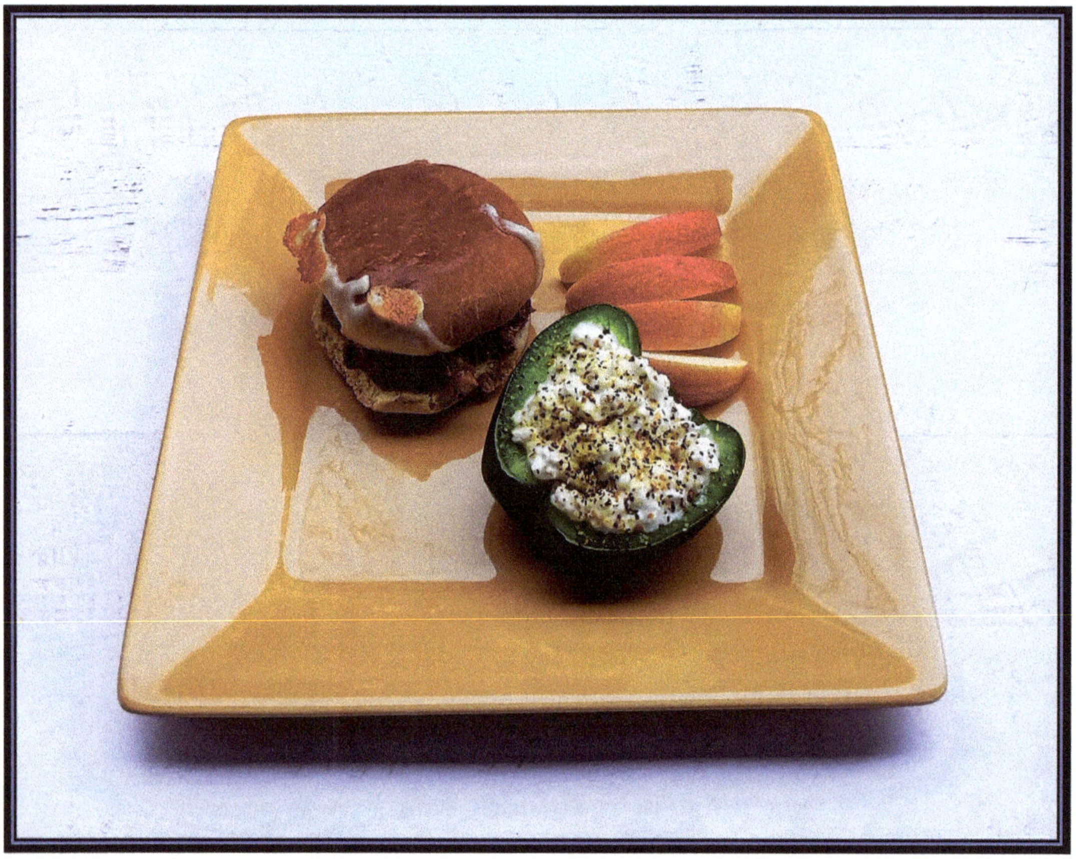

LEFT:
Chile Joes, page 131

RIGHT:
Mom's Bell Pepper, page 133

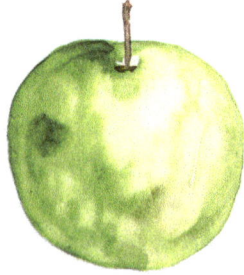

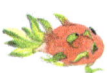

Mom's Bell Pepper

START TO FINISH: ABOUT 6 MINUTES

HERE'S a really quick lunch that is more satisfying than you might think. Take a rather symmetrical green bell pepper and cut it in half from stem to bottom. Remove all the seeds and membranes, and carefully cut the stem out with a small, sharp knife. Fill the cavity with small curd cottage cheese. Sprinkle a bunch of coarse lemon pepper all over the cottage cheese, pick it up, and enjoy. Talk about low-carb! Makes 2.

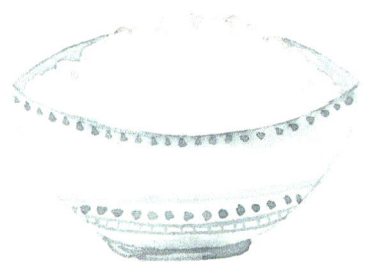

Burque Turkey

IN ADVANCE: TOASTING NUTS AND COOLING
PREP: ABOUT 15 MINUTES
PRESS: 6 MINUTES PER BATCH

Pretty much every Albuquerque restaurant offers a take on this kind of sandwich. You can use whatever high-quality bread or roll (or bagel, or naan, or croissant) you like, whatever flavor. Here's a chance to use any kind of flavored mayonnaise or soft cheese spread you like. The only mandatory ingredients are turkey and green chile. One of our favorite sandwich shops uses toasted and buttered sourdough. They build this sandwich with paper-thin slices of honey-roasted turkey, Havarti cheese, green chile, and tomatoes. Use a chipotle mayo (see page 115 for my recipe) as the spread. Any sandwich you build can be served cold, pressed, or griddled.

When my ex-son-in-law had a food truck, he would construct a Burque Turkey on sliced herbed focaccia bread and give it a press. However, any type of substantial sandwich bread will work with this creamy filling; you could even roll it up in flour tortillas and grill them on a skillet. Here is my version of his recipe:

Chapter Eight: Lunchy Stuff   133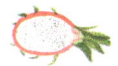

½ cup pine nuts, lightly toasted and cooled in advance
8 ounces light cream cheese (Neufchâtel)
½ cup red onion, finely chopped
8 ounces cooked turkey, diced
1 ounce sun-dried tomatoes, finely chopped (NOT oil-packed)
1 teaspoon salt
1 teaspoon black pepper
8 ounces roasted and chopped green chile, drained well
Focaccia bread (a 13″ by 9″ loaf will do the job)

HEAT a panini press. Place the cream cheese in a very large glass bowl and microwave on HIGH in 20-second intervals until soft enough to mix (around 60–90 seconds or so). Add the onion, turkey, tomatoes, salt, pepper, the toasted nuts, and chile and mix well. Season, if desired. Cut the bread into 6 or 8 portions, then slice each one in half carefully. Spoon a sixth (or eighth) of the cheese mixture on top of a slice of focaccia bread. Place the top of the bread on top and place in the heated press (you can probably fit 2 at a time in a typical press). Press for 5–6 minutes, until the bread is golden brown. Cut each in half to serve, if you want. Repeat with remaining bread and filling. Cover and refrigerate any leftover filling. Makes enough filling for 6–8 good-sized sandwiches.

Burqueño Beef

START TO FINISH: VARIABLE, BETWEEN 10–20 MINUTES

WITH this variation, you would use paper-thin roast beef slices, green chile, cheeses such as pepper jack or cheddar, maybe some tomatoes and onions if you like, and spicy or horseradish mayonnaise (see page 114 for my recipe). The bread is up to you—sourdough, rye, marble rye, multi-grain, bagel, etc. As mentioned above, this type of sandwich can be served hot or cold—press, griddle, or serve it on toasted or cold bread, any variety.

"TOO FEW PEOPLE UNDERSTAND A REALLY GOOD SANDWICH."
~ JAMES BEARD ~

YOU UNDERSTAND THEM BETTER NOW.

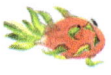

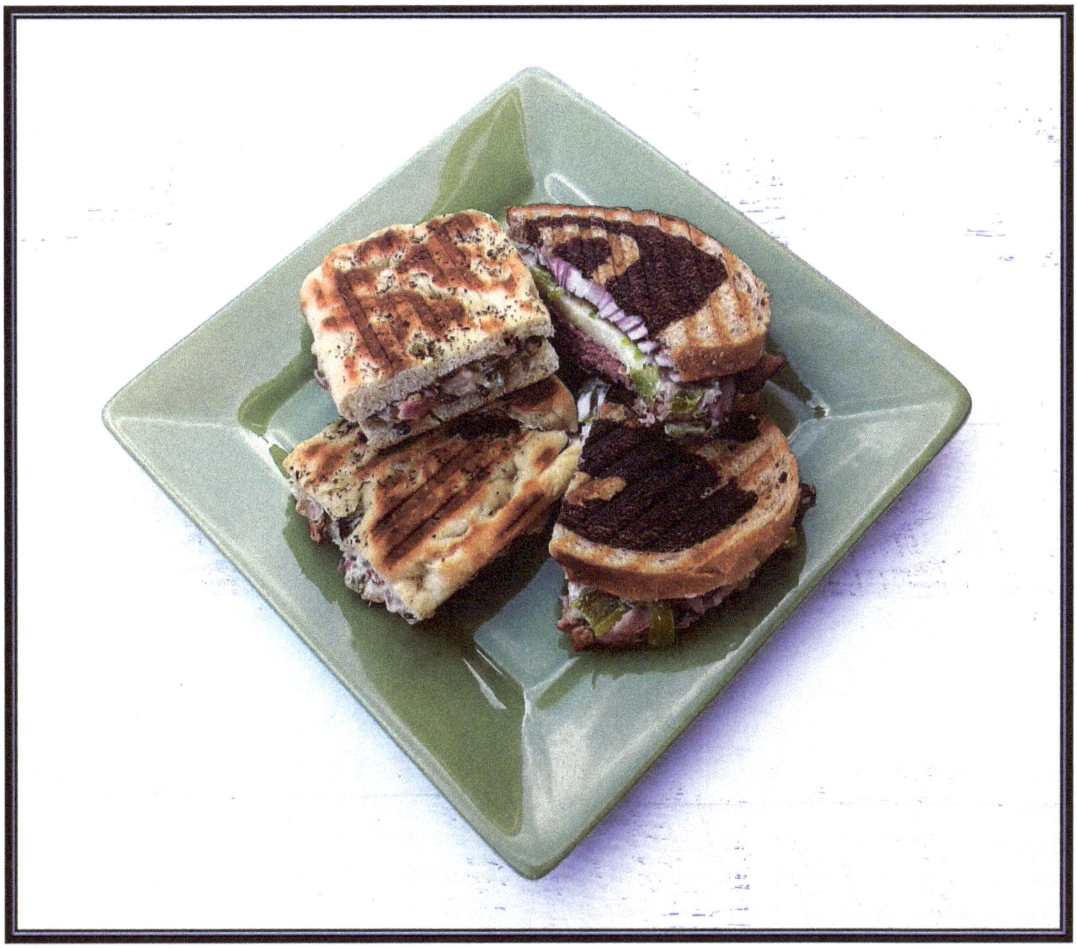

LEFT:
Burque Turkey, page 133

RIGHT:
Burqueño Beef, page 134

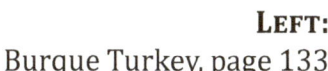

Chapter Nine

The Fourth of July

The Mile High Boil

Boil Bonus Soup

Cranberry Spinach Salad

Uncle Donny's Tropical Apple Cider Punch

Snickers Salad

The Fourth of July

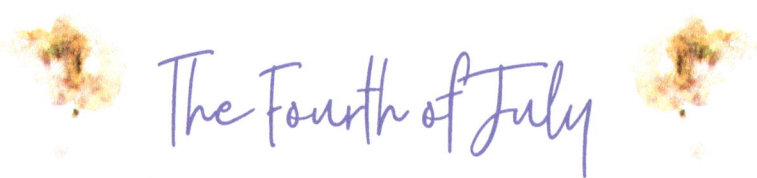

THIS USED TO be a more popular holiday around our household when my kids were small, and we would actually have a party occasionally. Or maybe it was just once. And I'm pretty sure it was a potluck. After we got a dog, however, we decided to stop setting off our own meager fountain-type fireworks because our lovely Lady (not a Cocker, but a lively Jack Russell terrier mix we rescued in 2004) was certainly traumatized by our neighbors' more explosive and illegal ones.

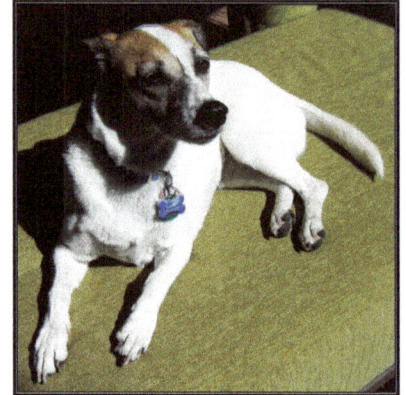

We started doing a boil for the holiday. This became an excuse to wrap newspapers all over the dining room table so you could toss your scraps on it, then wrap it all up for future garbage collection. My brother-in-law and my uncle (both elderly lifelong bachelors) were rather amused and bemused by this custom, respectively, though ultimately, they did enjoy the food.

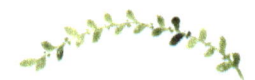

The Mile High Boil

PREP: 50–60 MINUTES

I have found that the seafood boil restaurants around Albuquerque (which sits at a mile high altitude) usually serve all the meat and vegetables in a plastic bag or a bowl, automatically coated with a bunch of messy (though delicious) sauce. I'm not sure if that is a traditional way of serving a low country boil or not. Inevitably, the restaurants don't really supply you with enough napkins, either. So, I like to serve the sauces on the side, then you can control how messy you want to be. I have occasionally found red, white, and blue fingerling potatoes for this recipe! How patriotic.

This will generally serve four, maybe six, depending on individual appetites. Be sure to double the recipe and use a 16-quart stockpot if you would like to have plenty of food, as well as leftovers for another meal or for the following soup recipe. Newspaper or butcher paper can be spread all over your table, if you want to toss

your tails and cobs off your plate. Be sure to make all the sauces to accompany your boil; they can be made in advance, or just make them while all your foods are cooking. If you do make them in advance, bring them to a spreadable room temperature for 30–60 minutes before serving, especially the Potato Sauce. All the sauces keep well for a while and can be used in other dishes.

12 cups water
¼ cup Old Bay Seasoning
1 tablespoon sea salt
1 tablespoon hot sauce
2 pounds fingerling potatoes or other small creamer types (don't peel)
4 ears of corn; shucked and cut in half (frozen is okay)
1 pound smoked sausage, cut into 1" chunks (any variety)
1 pound large raw shrimp, 20–25 per pound (thaw as directed,
    if using frozen; tails on or off)

GARNISH:

You can't go wrong with an extra sprinkling of Old Bay and extra hot sauce.

INDIVIDUAL SAUCE RECIPES ARE BELOW, WITH INDIVIDUAL PREP TIMES.

YOUR boil will cook uncovered on a VERY high heat and you will want to stir it occasionally, as you add ingredients.

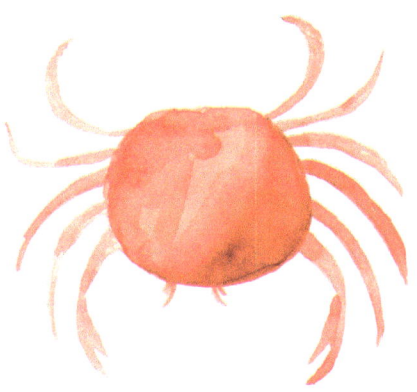

PLACE the water, Old Bay, salt, and hot sauce in an 8-quart saucepan. Bring to a rolling boil. Add the potatoes and bring to another boil. Boil for 10 minutes. Add the corn and sausage and bring to another boil. Boil for 10 minutes. Add the shrimp and continue to boil anywhere from 1–3 minutes, just until your shrimp turn pink; no more.

PLACE a very large colander over a very large bowl. Drain the meat and vegetables. Reserve the broth in the bowl, if desired (you'll probably end up with around 8 cups, which is enough for a few extra soup recipes, or you may simply discard the broth). Place all the meat and vegetables on a large platter. Garnish, if desired, and serve with sauces. Cover and refrigerate the leftovers. Makes 4 servings.

Chapter Nine: The Fourth of July

Shrimp Sauce

Start to finish: 7 minutes

½ cup ketchup
½ cup chili sauce (such as Heinz)
4 teaspoons lemon juice
4 teaspoons prepared horseradish

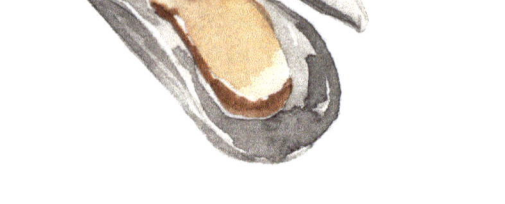

Whisk all the ingredients in a medium bowl. Cover and refrigerate the leftovers. Makes 1 cup.

Sausage Sauce

Start to finish: 7 minutes

½ cup stone ground mustard
¼ cup packed light brown sugar
2 tablespoons mayonnaise
1 teaspoon prepared horseradish

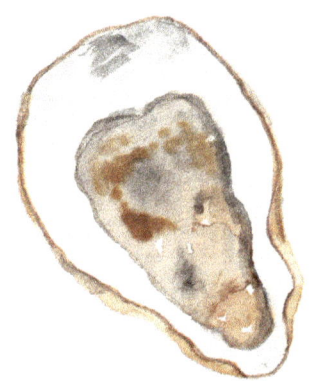

Whisk all the ingredients in a small bowl. Cover and refrigerate the leftovers. Makes about ¾ cup.

Corn Sauce

Start to finish: 5 minutes

½ cup salted butter, very soft
1 teaspoon Old Bay Seasoning
½ teaspoon cayenne pepper

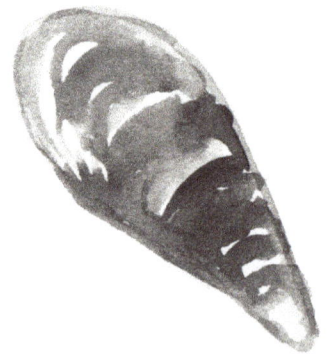

Whisk all the ingredients in a small bowl. Cover and refrigerate the leftovers; bring to a spreadable room temperature before serving. Makes ½ cup.

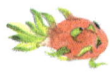

Potato Sauce

Prep: 8–10 minutes

½ cup salted butter, very soft
1 teaspoon onion powder
1 teaspoon salt
½ teaspoon garlic powder
½ teaspoon black pepper
1 cup sour cream, room temperature (light is okay)
¼ cup chives, minced

Whisk the butter and the 4 seasonings in a medium bowl. Add the sour cream and chives and mix well. Cover and refrigerate the leftovers; bring to a spreadable room temperature before serving. Makes about 1½ cups.

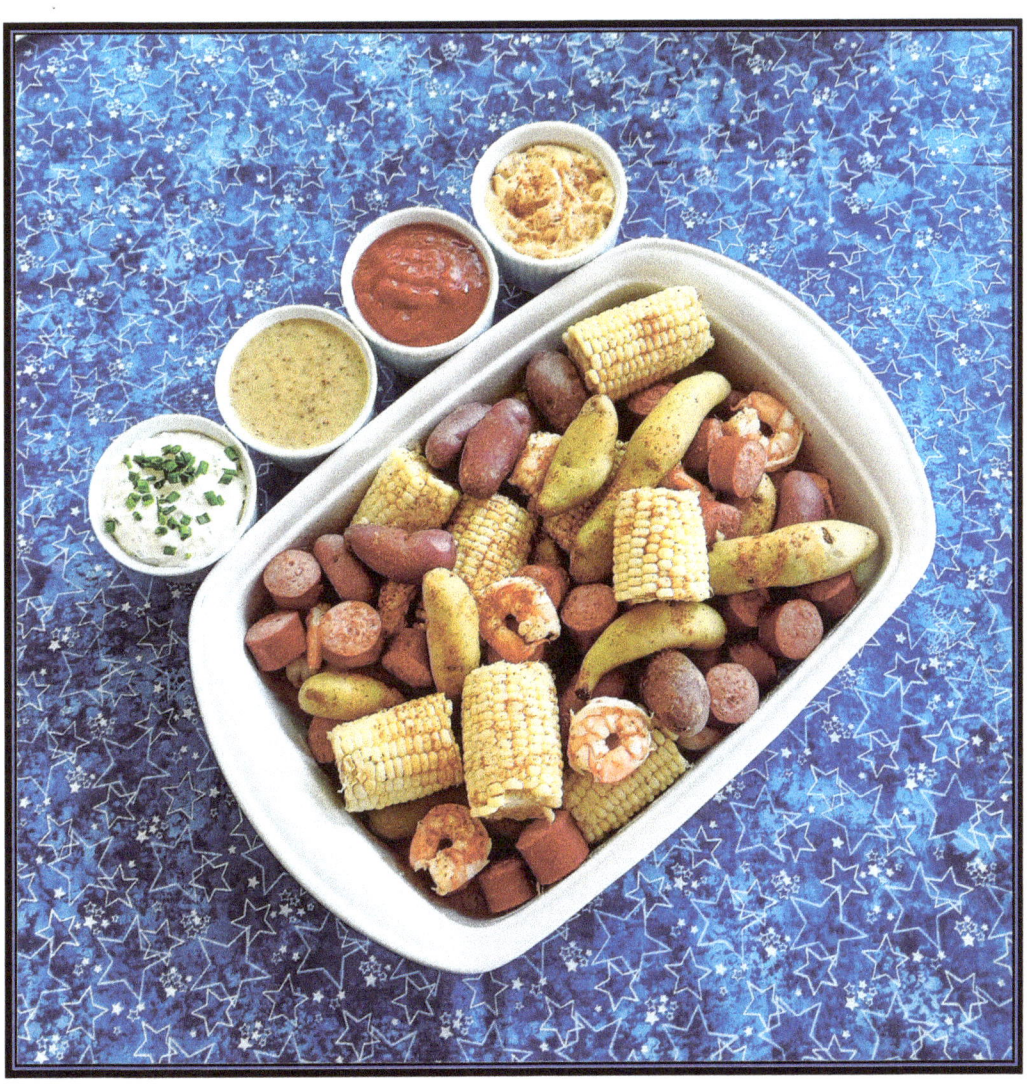

Boil Bonus Soup

START TO FINISH: ABOUT 40 MINUTES

You will probably end up with about eight cups of **strongly** seasoned broth from the previous recipe. You can discard this or use it judiciously in your favorite gumbo recipe or something like the following recipe. If you decide to reserve all your boil broth, you could make four batches of a soup like this one; freeze it in 2-cup portions for future use. You'll have to watch your seasoning for this soup, depending on what leftovers you end up utilizing.

If you only have about four cups of boil leftovers, feel free to add other vegetables or meats, all chopped coarsely. Items such as frozen peas, chopped carrot, or diced chicken will work out fine.

2–3 tablespoons Corn Sauce (page 140, or just use plain salted butter)
1 cup onion, coarsely chopped
6 cups assorted boil leftovers (cut corn off cobs; chop everything else coarsely)
2 cups boil broth (from the previous recipe, or use low-sodium
    chicken broth or clam juice)
4½ cups water, divided
⅓ cup all-purpose flour
⅓ cup Shrimp Sauce (page 140)
⅓ cup Sausage Sauce (page 140)
¾ cup Potato Sauce (page 141)

GARNISH: additional boil sauces, Old Bay Seasoning, and/or hot sauce

use a 4-cup glass measuring cup to measure most everything for the recipe; don't bother to rinse it out. Melt the Corn Sauce in a 6-quart saucepan. Sauté the onion 5 minutes over rather high heat. Add the boil leftovers, broth, and 4 cups water. Bring to a boil. Cook over medium heat, uncovered, 10 minutes. Stir a few times. Whisk the remaining water and flour together and add to the pot. Cook a few more minutes on medium heat. Add Shrimp Sauce and Sausage Sauce. Lower the heat and mix in the Potato Sauce. Season, though, as I mentioned above, **watch it!** Cover and refrigerate any leftovers; don't freeze. Makes 6–8 servings.

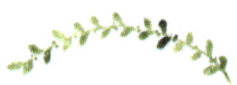

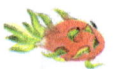

Cranberry Spinach Salad

IN ADVANCE: TOASTING NUTS AND COOLING
PREP: 15 MINUTES

Try not to assemble this until right before you serve it, because your spinach will wilt. Make it more of a main dish for a different occasion with the addition of some shredded chicken and/or a little cheese like feta or blue.

2 ounces slivered almonds, lightly toasted and cooled
    (sliced almonds will also work)
5–6 ounces fresh baby spinach
2 ounces dried cranberries
¼ cup almond oil
1 tablespoon sugar
2 tablespoons white wine vinegar
1 teaspoon lemon juice
2 teaspoons honey mustard
½ teaspoon salt
½ teaspoon white pepper
½ teaspoon poppy seed

TOSS the prepared almonds, spinach, and cranberries in a very large bowl. Combine the remaining ingredients in a shaker bottle. Season, if desired. Shake well and pour over greens. Toss well and serve immediately. Not recommended as leftovers. Makes 4–6 servings.

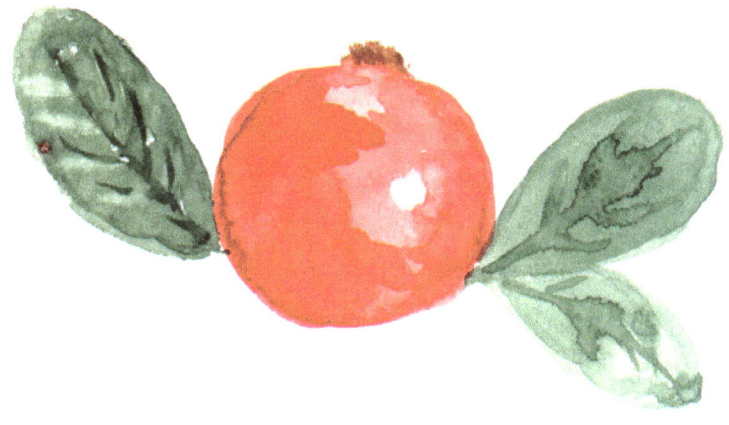

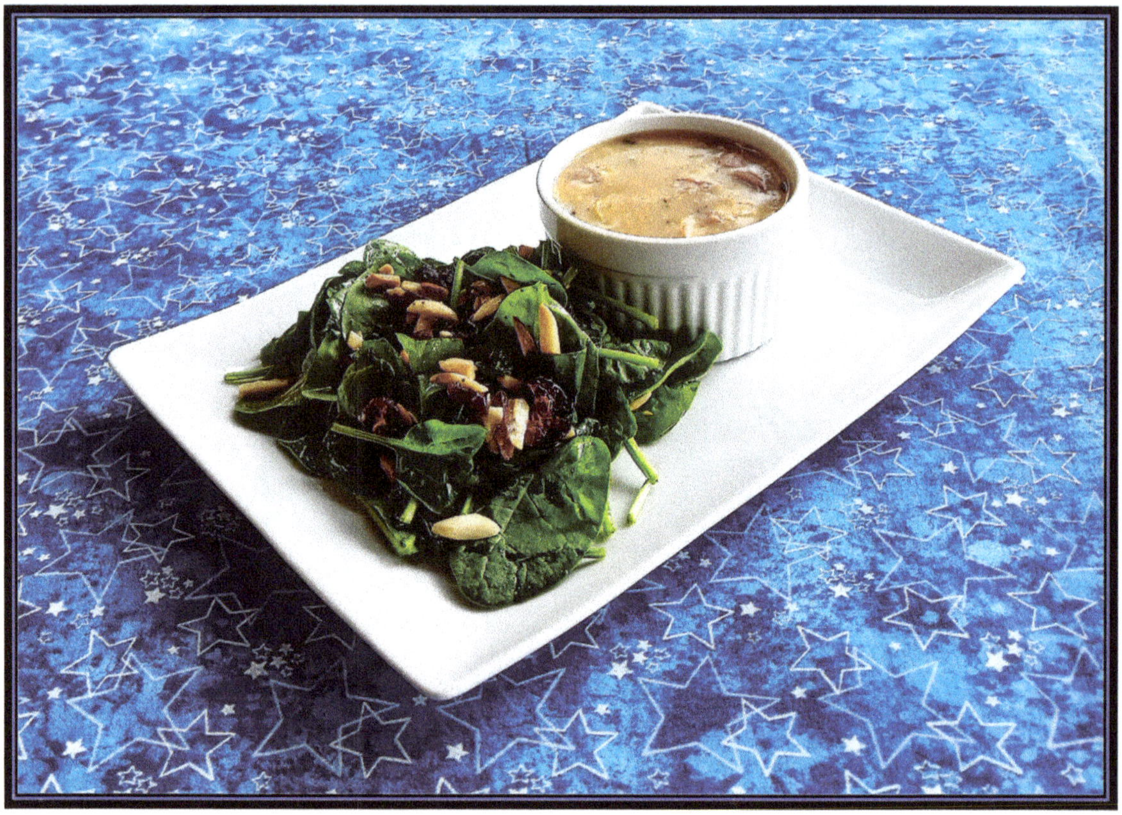

Left:
Cranberry Spinach Salad, page 143

Right:
Boil Bonus Soup, page 142

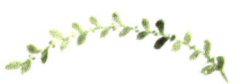

 144   Celebrating Comfy, Cozy Foods from North America: CH&M, Volume 3

Uncle Donny's Tropical Apple Cider Punch

ACTIVE PREP: ABOUT 15 MINUTES
FREEZE: OVERNIGHT
STAND: ABOUT 90 MINUTES

My uncle Donny was a solitary lifelong bachelor. He lived with his parents until they died, sold the 12-room family mansion on Long Island, New York, lived in an apartment for a few years, then finally moved out here to Albuquerque at the end of 2007 to spend more time with his brother, my father. Tragically, less than three months later, my dad suddenly died.

Donny attended all our family events, including my children's and grandchildren's birthday parties, throughout the years, though he usually ended up sitting in the living room by himself watching something like golf, which was strange since he never played the game. He was a generous man who always brought a greeting card with a modest cash gift. His sense of humor could be as dry as the New Mexican desert after a couple of weeks without any rain. He always arrived at an event about 45 minutes early, which meant more time for awkward conversations while I was doing my best to get a meal going. (I'll admit I sometimes fibbed about the time of an event to prevent him from coming so early, because carrying on conversations while rushing around my kitchen was sometimes difficult.) Inevitably, he would bring two bottles of room-temperature Martinelli's sparkling apple cider. I'd always be sure to have a bottle that he had previously brought already chilled; then, new ones would end up on a pantry shelf, waiting for the next event. We usually only consumed one bottle; you know, not everyone wants to have a glass of Martinelli's all the time.

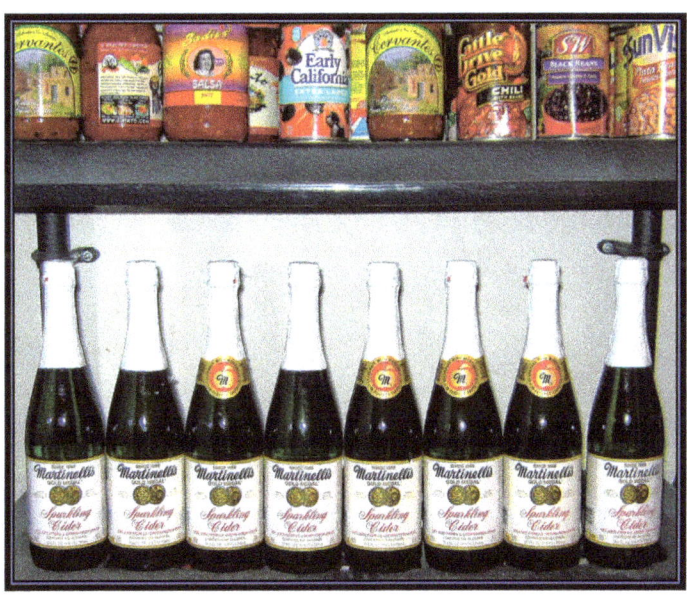

Unfortunately, the pandemic was especially tough on him as an introverted senior living alone in a rather small retirement apartment community. He never contracted COVID-19, but he passed away in September 2020 from other maladies. He was a veteran of the Korean War, and he worked for the New York parks department for 40 years. He loved country music, wrestling (WWE), and birdwatching. Ironically, I only actually got to know him well in the last four months of his life, when I went to visit him daily. Between COVID-19 lockdowns, a general lack of nursing/hospice personnel, and a patient who was particularly particular about medical staff, I became his part-time nurse. This spared him from being transferred to a nursing home. I learned much about my family history, which was surprisingly heartbreaking at times, but overall, this experience helped me understand him better. Our time at the end was often frustrating and sad, but I feel honored I was able to be there for him.

Start this recipe the night before serving.

1 pound frozen mixed fruit mix (preferably with mango
    and pineapple, but other fruits and mixes are fine)
1½ cups unsweetened pineapple juice, chilled (12 ounces)
1½ cups ginger ale, chilled (12 ounces, regular or diet)
750 ml. bottle sparkling apple cider, chilled
    (any flavor variety is fine)
1 cup lime juice, chilled
1 cup simple syrup, chilled (see the recipe on page 22,
    if you would like to make your own)

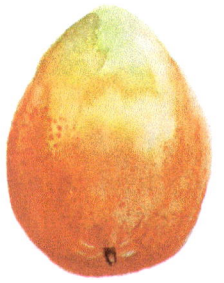

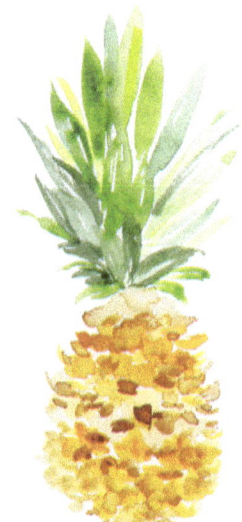

THE NIGHT BEFORE SERVING: Place fruit mix in a blender and let it stand for an hour or so. Add pineapple juice and blend thoroughly. Spoon into ice cube trays and freeze overnight.

ABOUT THIRTY MINUTES BEFORE SERVING: Place ice cube trays on your counter and let stand.

POUR the ginger ale, cider, lime juice, and simple syrup into a medium-sized punch bowl and combine. Add the ice cubes and stir to mix. Each serving should have a few of the prepared ice cubes. Cover and refrigerate the leftovers. Makes about 7 cups.

> **HERE ARE A FEW ALTERNATIVES TO THE INGREDIENTS LISTED ABOVE:**
>
> You can use different frozen fruit mixes. You may substitute a lemon/lime soft drink. You may substitute a bottle of your preferred variety of sparkling wine for the cider. And the last option would be to make the original recipe and add a cup (or two... or three?) of a clear hard liquor, such as vodka (various flavors are okay, such as citrusy ones or vanilla), rum (coconut would be good), or tequila. How much you add depends on how strong you like your punch; start with one cup and see how it goes.

Snickers Salad

START TO FINISH: ABOUT 20 MINUTES

So, there I was a few years ago, playing that *Quiz RPG: World of Mystic Wiz* game (see my Post-Watergate Chicken Salad on page 56). The question was: "From what part of America does 'Snickers Salad' originate?" The available answers were New England, Deep South, Midwest, and Northwest. I chose Deep South—I was wrong (again; no wonder I gave up this game!); it was the Midwest. After conducting some vigorous research (the kind that would lend itself to inserting a "winking emoticon" here), I discovered this is another one of those perfect potluck dishes that will practically guarantee an empty bowl by the end of the event.

As I wrote previously, I still usually picture a "salad" as having some fresh foods such as vegetables, fruits, and maybe some type of protein somewhere in the mix. Snickers Salad does require an apple as an ingredient, so I guess that qualifies it as a salad. Right. Your basic salad here consists of Snickers candy, Granny Smith apples, and Cool Whip. I mentioned this to Bob and I could see his eyes light up. I'll admit it—mine did too—Snickers is my favorite basic candy bar, although I do feel that a toffee-crunch Symphony bar could be a contender for first place. Many of Tony's Chocolonely bars are fast becoming favorites, but I digress.

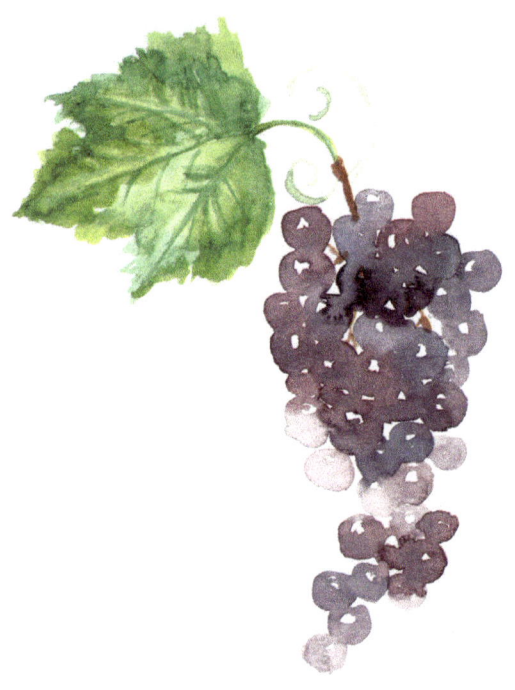

Those simple ingredients produce a pile of white fluff in a bowl; visually, it looks pretty bland. The Snickers Salad has many variations. You can add relatively crunchable items such as candy sprinkles, peanuts, chocolate chips, crushed pretzels, grapes, bananas, or crushed pineapple. Or you can mix various items in with the Cool Whip before you add your mix-ins: vanilla pudding mix, buttermilk (why would you add this?), lemon juice, sour cream, softened cream cheese, marshmallow creme, or mayonnaise (no! not mayo!!!). You can then pour some dessert sauce over this, such as caramel or fudge. From all these ingredients, I've come up with a really snazzy version.

Be sure to use a tart variety of apple; you need to offset the sweetness, and Granny Smith is the perfect choice. I'm sure many other types of candies would work well for this salad—Butterfinger bars, Heath bars, or Twix bars would make nice substitutes for the Snickers bars. All these candies can become rather hard after a time in the refrigerator, so serve this immediately or bring it to room temperature for about an hour before serving, if you have refrigerated it.

8-ounce container Cool Whip
3 ounces semi-sweet miniature chocolate chips
3 ounces cocktail peanuts, finely chopped
30 large red seedless grapes
2 medium-sized Granny Smith apples, unpeeled
6 (1.86-ounce) Snickers bars, unwrapped

Garnish: purchased caramel ice cream sauce, purchased fudge or chocolate sauce, additional miniature chocolate chips, and/or additional chopped cocktail peanuts

In a very large bowl, combine the Cool Whip, chocolate chips, and peanuts well. Cut the grapes in half and mix in. Core the apples, then cut into small chunks and mix in. Cut the Snickers bars into thirds, lengthwise. Cut into ¼" slices and mix in well. Serve immediately with desired garnishes. Cover and refrigerate the leftovers; let them stand out for about an hour before serving again so the candy can soften up a bit. Makes 8–10 servings.

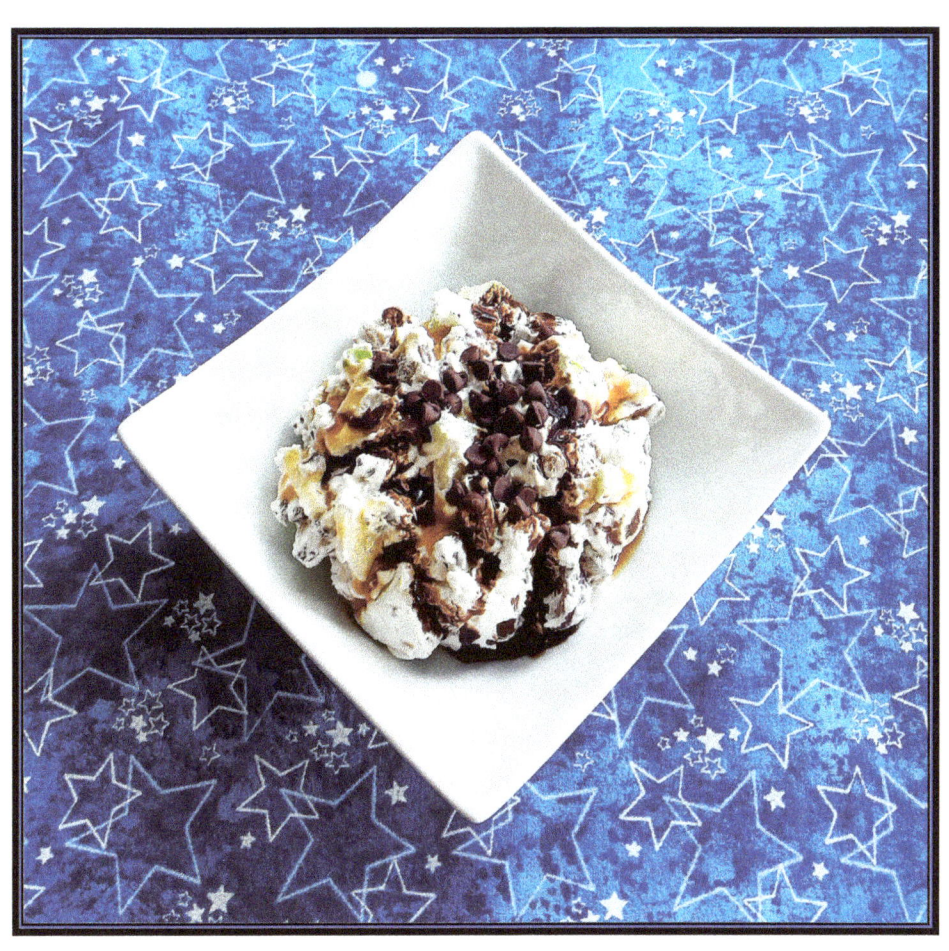

CHAPTER TEN

MAIN EVENTS

- Beefy Enchiladas
- "Perhaps This Chicken Needs Paprika?"
- Hidden Treasure Meatloaf
- Partial to Panko Fish
- Bodacious Brisket
- Savory Seasoning Pork Chops
- Taco Rice Casserole
- Truth or Consequences Stuffed Peppers
- Marcella's Flat Enchiladas
- The Whole Enchilada
- Taco Tuesday Tacos
- Vader's Killer Taters
- Callista's Birthday Pizza

Main Events

HERE'S AN ASSORTMENT of meaty main dishes, many of which will pair nicely with hot or cold sides from previous or upcoming chapters.

Beefy Enchiladas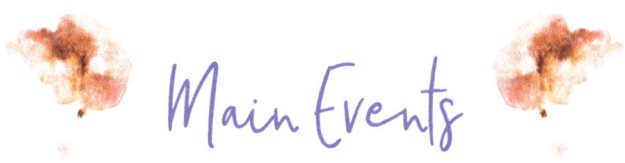

PREP: ABOUT 45 MINUTES
BAKE: 50 MINUTES
STAND: 10–15 MINUTES
OVEN: 375°

You might think that enchiladas are generally corn tortillas rolled up around some sort of filling, but they are also served flat around Albuquerque. Perhaps the word merely means "with chile"? New Mexican enchiladas are usually cheesier (and less healthy, oh, well...) than their Mexican counterparts. You can substitute other ground meats here, or even switch to a vegetarian version by chopping up something like a pound or so of summer squashes (bell peppers, corn, and additional onion would also combine well with the squash) and giving them a sauté. Use my Calabacitas recipe (page 104) for a delicious vegetarian filling.

1 pound ground beef sirloin
1 tablespoon chili powder
1 teaspoon salt, divided
1 teaspoon black pepper, divided
14.5-ounce can stewed tomatoes, drained and cut into ½″ chunks
¼ cup salted butter
2 tablespoons minced garlic
1 cup onion, coarsely chopped
½ cup all-purpose flour
2 teaspoons dried oregano (2–3 tablespoons fresh, minced)
1½ cups 1% milk
14.5-ounce can low-sodium chicken broth
8 ounces sharp cheddar cheese, shredded and divided
8 ounces roasted and chopped green chile, drained
12 corn tortillas, about 6–7″ in diameter

GARNISH:

You can top this dish with anything you like on the **NICE NEW MEXICAN & MEXICAN GARNISHES** list.

COAT a 3-quart deep skillet with cooking spray. Fry the beef over rather high heat until the pink is gone, breaking it up. Cook until it is almost dry. Add the chili powder, ½ teaspoon salt, ½ teaspoon pepper, and the tomatoes and combine well. Let it stand in the pan.

PLACE the butter in a 3-quart saucepan and melt over moderately high heat. Add the garlic and onion and sauté 3 minutes. Whisk in the flour, oregano, and the remaining salt and pepper well. Whisk in the milk and chicken broth and cook over moderately high heat until the sauce starts thickening somewhat. Add 4 ounces of cheddar and whisk to melt. Add the green chile, mix, and turn off the heat.

PREHEAT the oven to 375°. Coat a 13" by 9" baking dish with cooking spray or grease lightly; set aside. Add ½ cup of the sauce into the meat mixture; combine well. Pour 1½ cups of the sauce into the prepared dish and spread to cover the bottom of the dish. Spread 4 tortillas on a dinner plate and microwave 20–30 seconds on HIGH to soften them (if it seems necessary; some corn tortillas are already soft enough to fold easily). Spoon about ¼ cup of the beef mixture down the middle of one tortilla. Enclose loosely and place seam side down in the prepared pan. Repeat this process with the remaining tortillas, arranging 8 in a row, then the final 4 crosswise, 2 by 2. Mix any stray meat filling into the sauce. Pour the remaining sauce all over; spread to cover all the tortillas. Cover with foil and bake 30 minutes. Remove the foil and sprinkle the remaining cheese all over. Bake another 20 minutes. Let stand 10–15 minutes before serving. Cover and refrigerate the leftovers; enchiladas freeze well. Makes 4–6 servings.

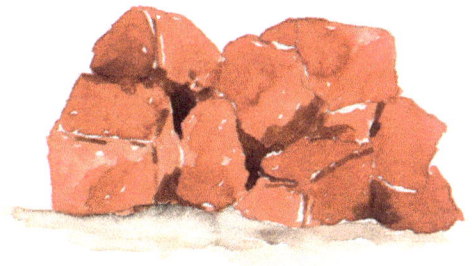

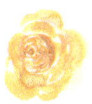

Chapter Ten: Main Events

"Perhaps This Chicken Needs Paprika?"

START TO FINISH: ABOUT 1 HOUR

This was an official question asked by my daughter Chloë, and the correct answer was "yes." Serve this over your favorite carbs, such as rice, egg noodles, or mashed potatoes. Or skip the chicken preparation completely and just start with the pork gravy. Bake up some plump biscuits and pour this gravy over them for a deluxe breakfast.

8–10 boneless, skinless chicken thighs
    (around 2½ pounds)
Salt, black pepper, and smoked paprika
2 tablespoons salted butter
8 ounces bulk pork sausage (any flavor is fine)
¾ cup shallots, finely chopped
¼ cup all-purpose flour
½ teaspoon poultry seasoning
¼ teaspoon black pepper
¼ teaspoon smoked paprika
14.5-ounce can low-sodium chicken broth
⅓ cup heavy cream
4 ounces roasted and chopped green chile,
    with juice

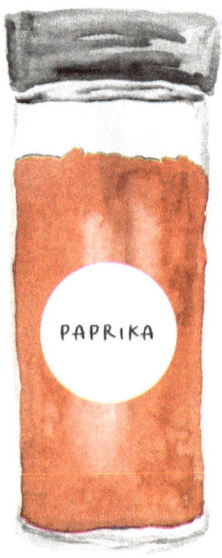

COAT a 5-quart deep skillet with cooking spray. Place the chicken on a cutting board and spread out each thigh. Pull off any large and easily removable portions of fat and discard them. Sprinkle each thigh moderately with salt, pepper, and paprika. Place butter in the skillet and melt over rather high heat. Place the seasoned sides of the chicken down in the pan; fry 3–4 minutes, shaking the pan occasionally to keep them from sticking. Sprinkle the same 3 seasonings on the top sides of all the chicken moderately. Turn all over and brown the other side, about 3–4 minutes. Remove to a plate and set aside. Reuse the pan with all the drippings.

ADD the sausage and shallots to the pan and fry over rather high heat until the pink is gone, breaking up the meat. Add the flour, poultry seasoning, ¼ teaspoon pepper, and ¼ teaspoon paprika to the skillet and mix in. Add the remaining ingredients and bring to a boil. Add the chicken back to the pan, with any accumulated juices. Cover and cook on the lowest heat 30 minutes. Turn the chicken over, raise the heat one notch and cook, uncovered, 10–15 minutes, until the chicken is very tender. Spoon sauce over the chicken a couple of times. Season the sauce, if desired. Serve with a carbohydrate of your choice. Cover and refrigerate the leftovers. Makes 6 servings.

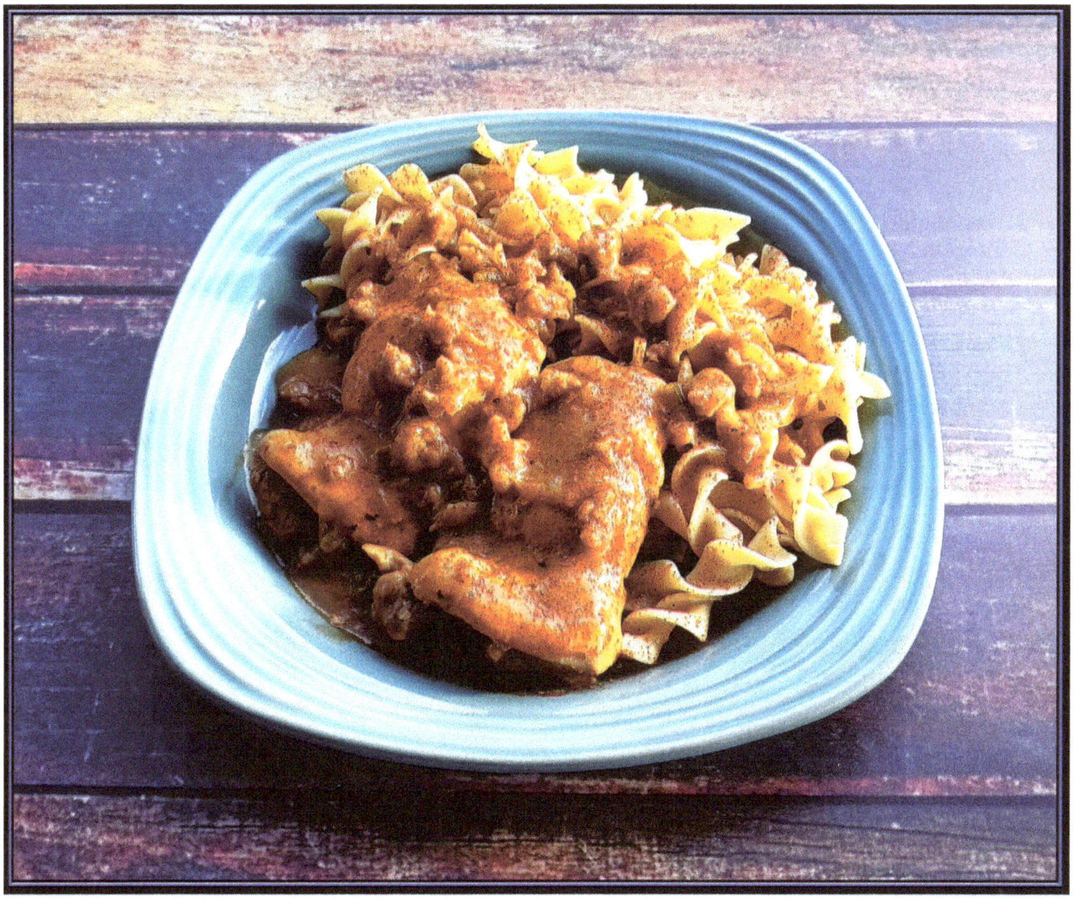

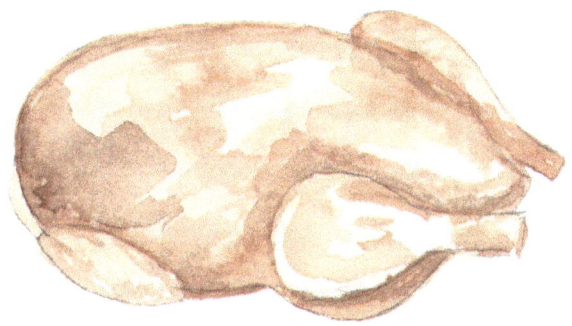

Hidden Treasure Meatloaf

Prep: about 35 minutes
Bake: 90 minutes
Stand: 5 minutes
Oven: 375°

What is hidden within? A whole bunch of healthy vegetables that picky little halflings generally prefer not to eat in their original forms. This makes two large meatloaves, so it's great for a crowd, or you can freeze one for later consumption.

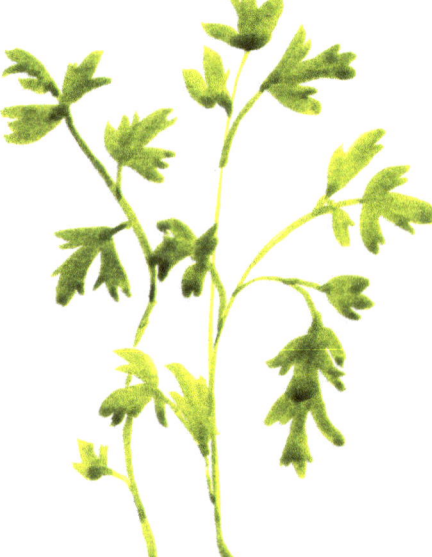

8 ounces onion
8 ounces carrot
8 ounces celery
A large red bell pepper
6 large garlic cloves
1 cup fresh parsley (loosely packed; not too stemmy)
2 cups old-fashioned oats, divided
4 teaspoons salt
2 teaspoons black pepper
2 teaspoons rubbed sage (3 tablespoons fresh)
2 teaspoons dried thyme (3 tablespoons fresh)
1 cup half-and-half
2 large eggs
1 pound lean ground beef
1 pound ground pork
1 pound ground chicken
About 1 cup prepared barbecue sauce (any variety)

Garnish:

You could offer more barbecue sauce, ketchup, salsa, chile sauces, Sriracha sauce, hot sauces, or whatever items you like on meatloaf.

PREHEAT the oven to 375°. Coat (2) 9" by 5" loaf pans with cooking spray or grease lightly. Cut off stems, peel, and core the first 4 vegetables. Cut them into 1" chunks and place them in a large food processor. Add the garlic cloves and process well. Scrape down the sides and process again. Add the parsley, 1 cup oats, and the 4 seasonings and process well. Scrape the sides and process again. Set aside.

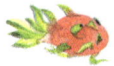

COMBINE the half-and-half and eggs in a 2-cup glass measuring cup and whisk well; set aside. Place the 3 meats in a very large bowl and combine well with your hands. Mix in the prepared vegetables, then mix in the egg mixture. Add the remaining 1 cup of oats and mix well with your hands. Divide into the prepared pans evenly; smooth the tops. Bake 1 hour. Spread barbecue sauce on each loaf, about ½ cup on each one. Bake another 30 minutes (they should reach 160° in the center). Let them stand in the pans 5 minutes. Slice and serve with your preferred garnishes, if desired. Cover and refrigerate the leftovers; they freeze well. Makes 16–20 slices.

> **HERE'S AN EVEN MORE HALFLING-FRIENDLY TREATMENT:**
>
> Coat 24 regular-sized muffin cups well with cooking spray. Divide the meat mixture between all. Bake 30 minutes. Spoon about a scant tablespoon of barbecue sauce on top of each. Bake another 15 minutes. Let stand in the pans 2–3 minutes before serving. Makes 24.

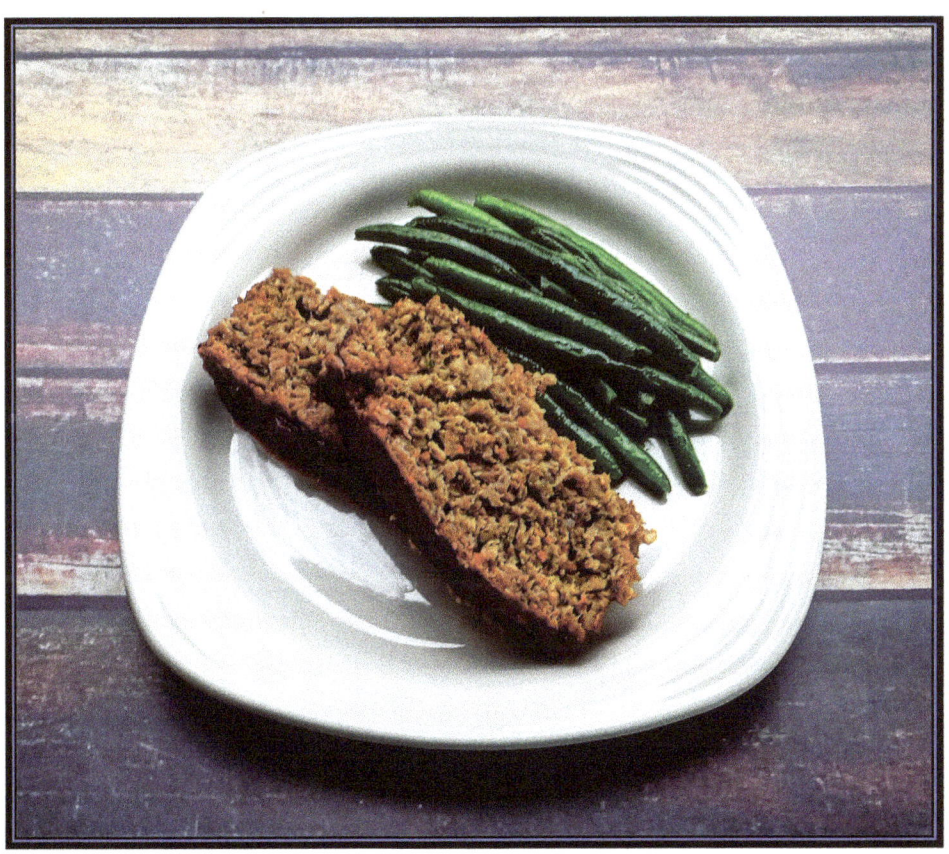

Partial to Panko Fish

START TO FINISH: ABOUT 30 MINUTES
OVEN: 450°

I have tested a few different fish fillets for this recipe, and they have all worked well. Mahi-mahi, cod, tilapia, and salmon are all fine.

1 large egg
2 tablespoons half-and-half
1 teaspoon salt, divided
¼ cup panko breadcrumbs
2 tablespoons dry Parmesan and/or Romano cheese
1 tablespoon all-purpose flour
1½ teaspoons coarse lemon pepper
½ teaspoon cayenne pepper
4 boneless, skinless fish fillets (thaw as directed
      if frozen; each can weigh around 5–7 ounces)
2 tablespoons olive oil
2 tablespoons salted butter

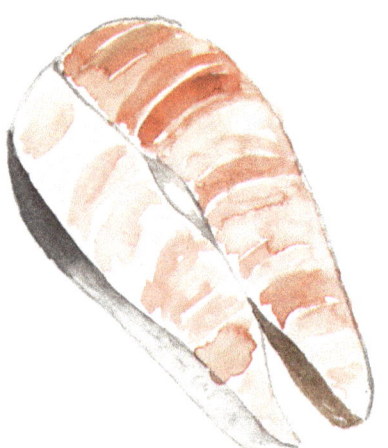

PREHEAT the oven to 450°. Coat a medium baking sheet with cooking spray and set aside. Combine the egg, half-and-half, and ½ teaspoon salt in a shallow bowl with a whisk; set aside. Combine the panko, cheese, flour, lemon pepper, remaining ½ teaspoon salt, and cayenne in another shallow bowl and set aside. Set the fish on a plate and pat dry with paper towels. Place the oil in a large skillet and set the heat to rather high.

DIP one fillet in the egg mixture, then the panko mixture to coat well all over. Place in the skillet. Repeat with all the fillets. Sprinkle any remaining crumbs to fill in any empty spaces (discard the egg mixture). Fry 2–3 minutes. Carefully turn them over; fry another 2–3 minutes. They should all be golden brown on both sides. Place on the prepared sheet. Cut the butter into 4 slices and place one on each fillet. Bake 8–12 minutes, until the center flakes with a fork but it is still moist within (total baking time will depend on the relative thickness of each fillet). Cover and refrigerate the leftovers. Makes 4 servings.

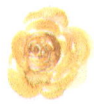

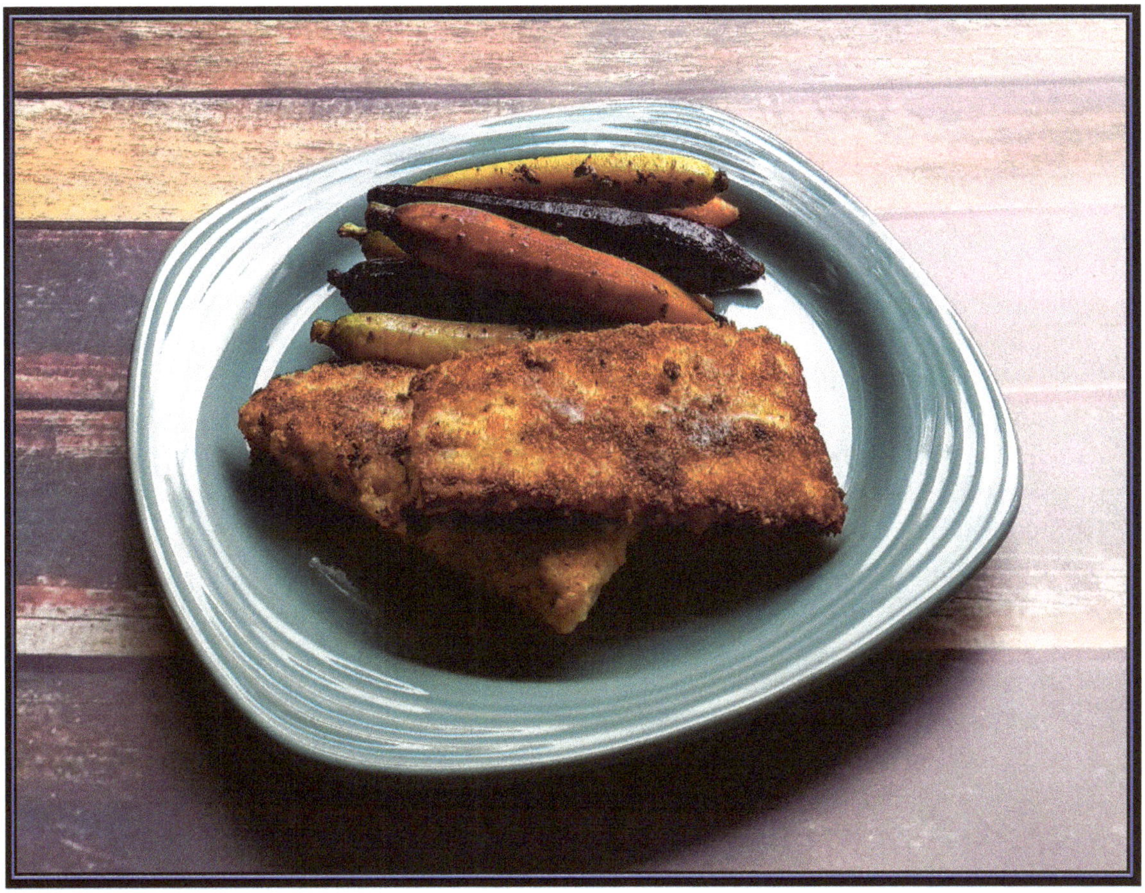

Chapter Ten: Main Events 159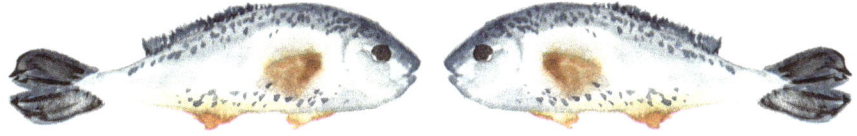

Bodacious Brisket

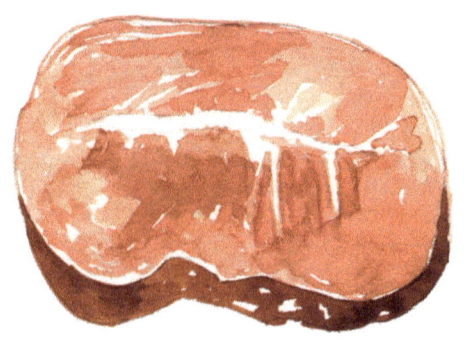

Prep: about 30 minutes
Bake: 6½ hours
Stand: 15 minutes
Oven: 275°

My second cookbook has a Bodacious Brisket Soup, so I figured I better just stick with that adjective for this rather boldly flavored brisket. This special occasion dish cries out for mashed potatoes and some sort of green vegetable to keep it company. Why is this a special occasion dish? Because you need to take out a loan to pay for a five-pound brisket. The last time I made this, I went to Costco to begin my quest for the perfect five-pound brisket. My choices were either two-and-a-half-pound miniatures or ten-pound behemoths. You can imagine I was thrilled to get a miniature (which fit perfectly in an 11" by 7" dish); I don't know where I would even begin to bake such a behemoth. What pan would it fit in? I don't own one big enough…

Start your preparation SEVEN hours before serving.

1 tablespoon smoked paprika
1 tablespoon ground coriander
1 tablespoon five-spice powder
2 teaspoons black pepper
1 teaspoon salt
1 teaspoon cayenne pepper
A 5-pound beef brisket
¼ cup packed light brown sugar
¼ cup ketchup
¼ cup Dijon mustard
2 tablespoons soy sauce
1 teaspoon liquid smoke
½ cup water
¼ cup cornstarch (all-purpose flour will also work)

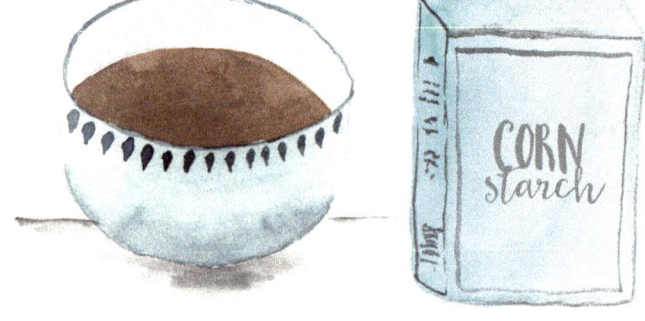

SEVEN HOURS BEFORE SERVING: Preheat the oven to 275°. Coat a 13" by 9" baking dish with cooking spray. Combine the first 6 seasonings in a 4-cup glass measuring cup with a whisk and set aside. Place the brisket in the pan, with the fat side up. Sprinkle 1 tablespoon spice mix all over and press it in. Turn the meat over. Sprinkle the remaining spice mix all over evenly.

PLACE the brown sugar, ketchup, mustard, soy sauce, and liquid smoke in the 4-cup glass measuring cup and whisk well. Pour and spread all over the meat (rinse out the measuring cup and use again later). Cover the pan with heavy-duty aluminum foil and bake 6 hours. Remove the foil and set it aside for later use. Bake the brisket another 30 minutes. Put the brisket on a cutting board and cover with the foil. Let it rest 15 minutes.

MEANWHILE, set a rather small colander on top of the glass measuring cup. Carefully pour the pan juices into the cup. Add water to measure a total of 3 cups. Pour into a 2-quart saucepan. Bring to a boil. Combine the ½ cup water and cornstarch in the 4-cup glass measuring cup well with a whisk. Whisk this into the pot and cook on medium heat to thicken, whisking often. You can season the gravy, but judiciously; it probably won't need anything extra, especially salt. Slice the meat thinly on a diagonal, or just pull it apart with forks. Discard the bottom layer of fat. Serve with gravy. Cover and refrigerate the leftovers; they freeze well. Makes 10–12 servings.

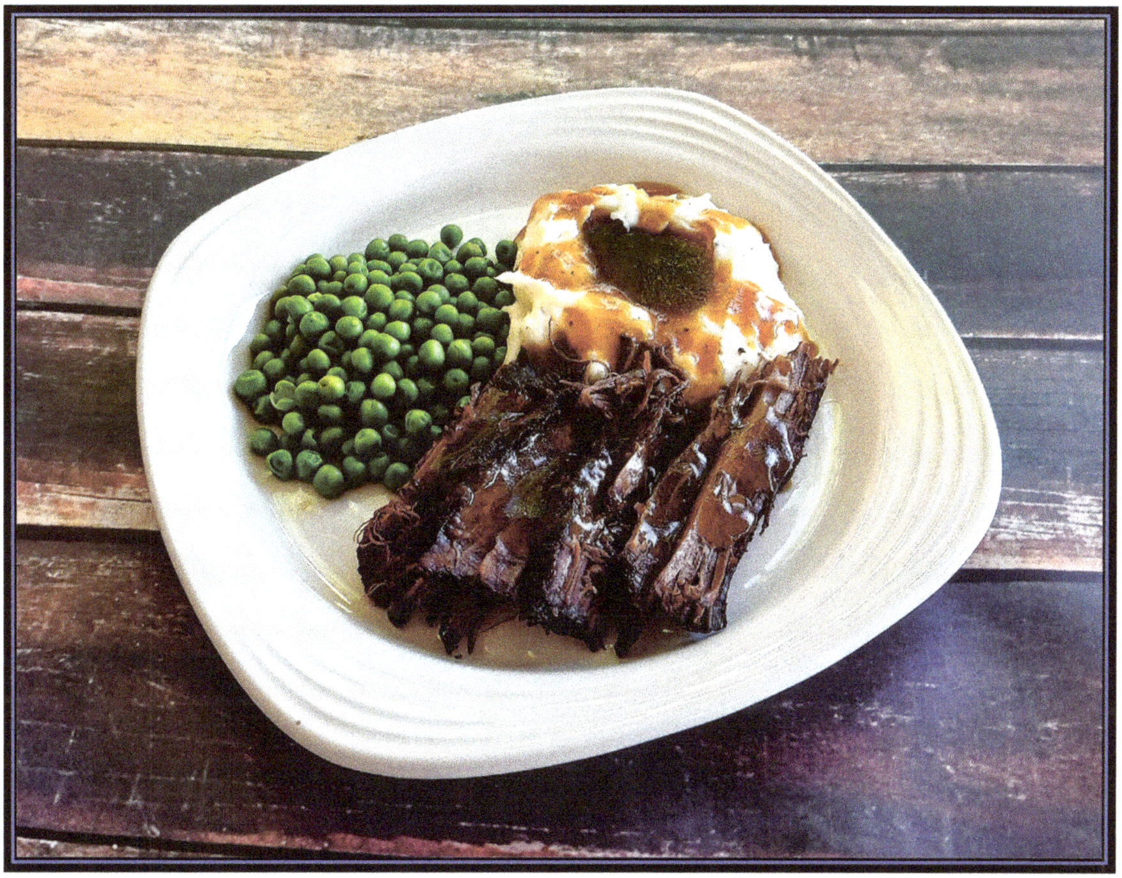

Chapter Ten: Main Events   161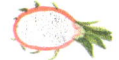

Savory Seasoning Pork Chops

START TO FINISH: ABOUT 25 MINUTES

Here's a speedy protein perfect for a hectic weeknight.

4 pork loin center cut chops, bone-in, about ¾" thick
    (stay close to 1¾–2 pounds)
1½ teaspoons Savory Seasoning (page xi)
3 tablespoons plain dry breadcrumbs
1 ounce fresh Parmesan and/or Romano cheese, finely shredded
2 tablespoons olive oil

LET the chops stand at room temperature for 30 minutes or so. Combine the Savory Seasoning, breadcrumbs, and cheese in a shallow bowl. Coat a 5-quart deep skillet with cooking spray. Place the oil in the skillet and turn the heat to rather high. Swirl the oil in the pan to coat the entire surface. Press one side of a chop into the prepared cheese mixture. Press it down to make sure that the side is coated well. Place this side down in the pan. Repeat with the other chops. Sprinkle the remaining crumb mixture over all of them evenly; press it in and try to fill in any bare spots. Fry 3 minutes, until golden brown. Carefully turn all of them over. Fry another 3 minutes, until golden brown. Turn the heat to the lowest setting. Cover and cook 3–4 minutes, until desired doneness. Turn off the heat and let them rest in the covered pan about 3 minutes. Cover and refrigerate the leftovers. Makes 4 servings.

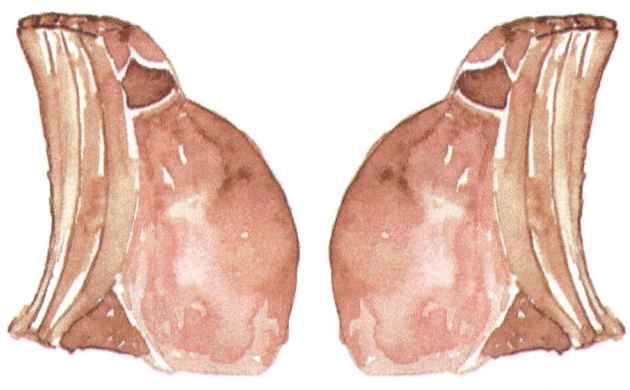

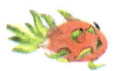

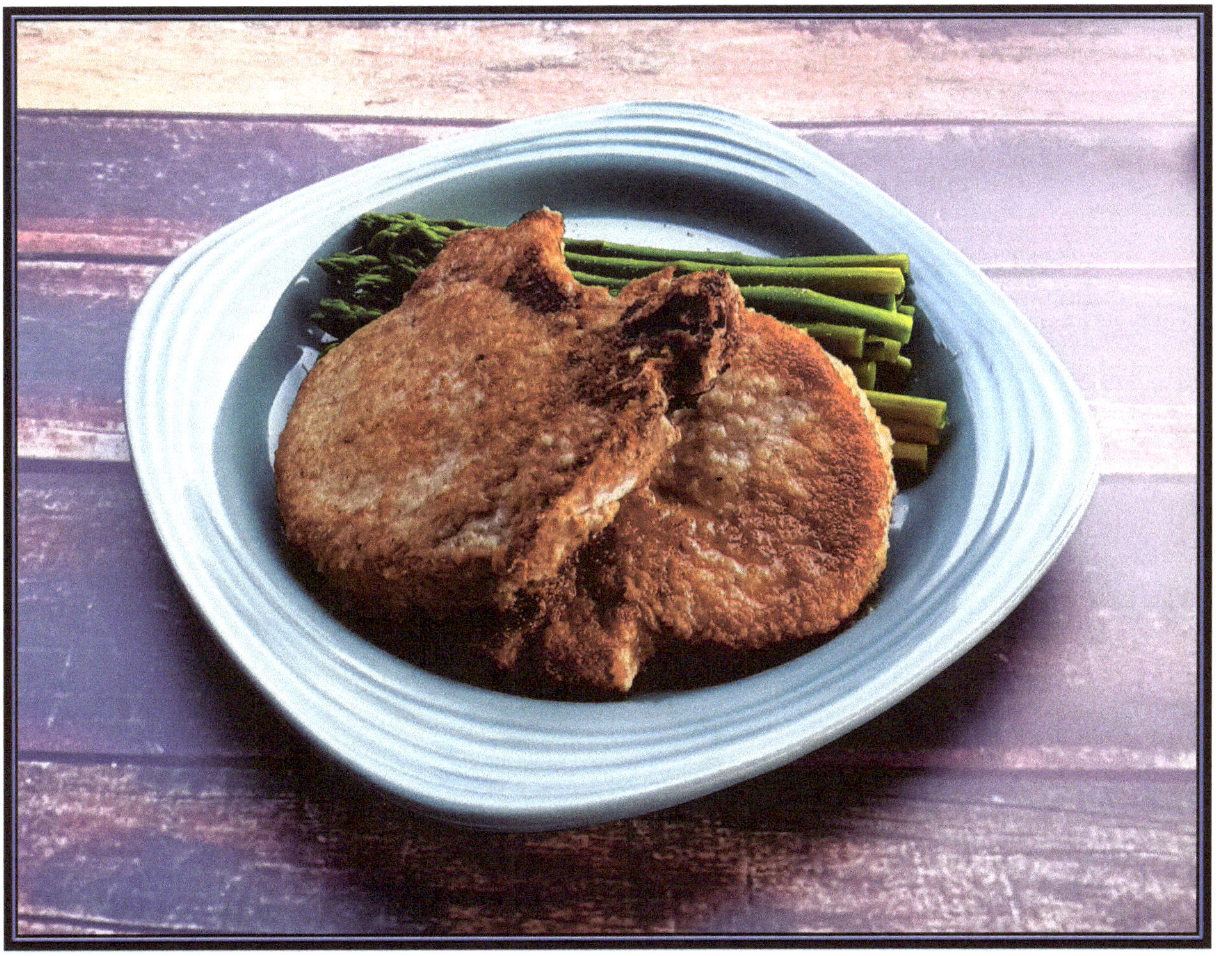

Chapter Ten: Main Events 163

Taco Rice Casserole

START TO FINISH: ABOUT 1 HOUR AND 20 MINUTES

This is an easy stovetop skillet meal. Repurpose any leftovers in a burrito or next to some scrambled eggs for a hearty brunch option.

1 pound ground beef sirloin
1 large bell pepper, any color, cored and chopped coarsely
1 cup onion, coarsely chopped
1 cup long-grain rice
14.5-ounce can diced tomatoes, with juice
8 ounces roasted and chopped green chile, with juice
1 tablespoon chili powder
1½ teaspoons salt
1 teaspoon ground cumin
1 teaspoon dried oregano (2–3 tablespoons fresh, minced)
1 teaspoon black pepper
1 teaspoon garlic powder
1½ cups mild olives, pitted, drained, and sliced (green or black)
½ cup water
14.5-ounce can low-sodium chicken broth
½ cup minced fresh cilantro (optional)
8 ounces fiesta blend cheese, finely shredded

GARNISH:

> Have a look at the **NICE NEW MEXICAN & MEXICAN GARNISHES** list and choose your favorites.

COAT a 5-quart deep skillet with cooking spray. Place the beef, bell pepper, and onion in the pan and fry over very high heat until the pink is gone, breaking up the meat. Add the rice, tomatoes, chile, the 6 seasonings, olives, water, and broth. Stir to combine, then bring to a boil. Cover and cook on the lowest heat 40–45 minutes, until the rice is tender. Stir a couple of times. Season, if needed. Mix in the cilantro, if using. Sprinkle the cheese all over, turn off the heat, cover, and let stand 10 minutes. Garnish, if desired. Cover and refrigerate the leftovers; they freeze well. Makes 6–8 servings.

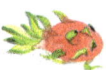

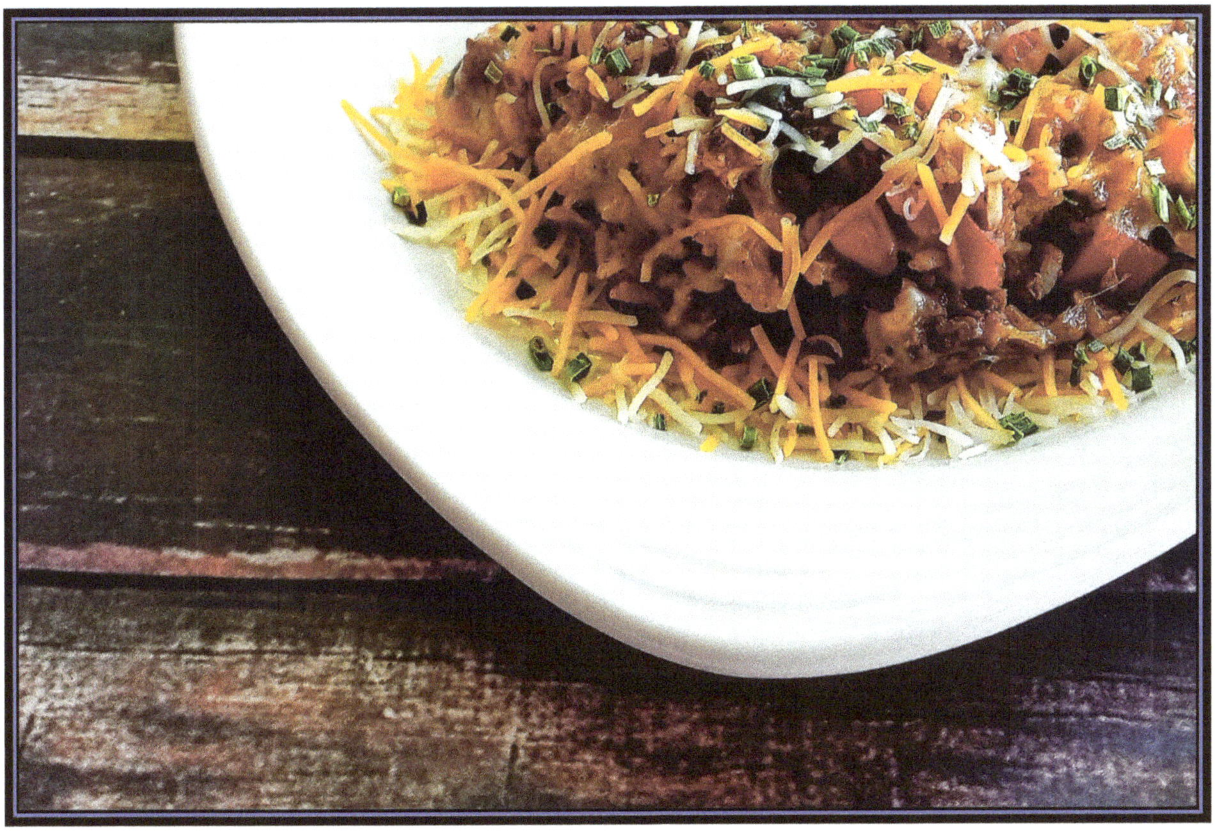

Truth or Consequences Stuffed Peppers

IN ADVANCE: TOASTING NUTS, COOLING, AND CHOPPING
PREP: ABOUT 35 MINUTES
BAKE: 70 MINUTES
OVEN: 375°

Once upon a time (in 1950, to be exact), a town named Hot Springs in central New Mexico voted to change its name because a popular radio/television show called *Truth or Consequences* held a contest. Ralph Edwards, the host of the show, said he would broadcast from any town willing to do this legally. Edwards kept his word, and thus, history was made. Why would the citizens of this town do this? Besides the fun factor, I'm not sure why, though it's probably good for tourism. The show might be gone, but the town is still called Truth or Consequences. It's usually called T or C, for short.

Chapter Ten: Main Events   165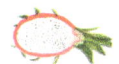

If you find that you have run out of sauce (at the leftover stage), you can pour red chile or salsa over these. You could even omit the tomato sauce preparation and start with two cups of red chile for smoky, spicy goodness.

4 ounces walnuts, lightly toasted, cooled, then chopped finely in advance
4 large bell peppers (any color, though I usually use red, yellow,
      and orange ones; as symmetrical as possible)
1½ teaspoons salt, divided, plus some additional salt for sprinkling in the peppers
1 cup low-sodium chicken broth
8-ounce can tomato sauce
1 pound ground turkey
½ cup onion, finely chopped
½ cup frozen corn
2 tablespoons cornmeal
1 large egg
2 tablespoons chili powder
½ cup half-and-half
1 teaspoon black pepper
1 teaspoon dried oregano (2–3 tablespoons fresh, minced)
1 teaspoon garlic powder
8 ounces pepper jack cheese, shredded
Cooked rice (about 1½ cups of uncooked rice should be plenty)

CUT the stem of each bell pepper down to 1" (if necessary). Cut each in half from stem to bottom. Use a small sharp knife to cut away the inner core and seeds, leaving the stems intact. Sprinkle the pepper interiors lightly with salt; set aside.

PREHEAT the oven to 375°. Coat a 13" by 9" baking dish with cooking spray or grease lightly. Combine ½ teaspoon salt, broth, and tomato sauce in a 2-cup glass measuring cup with a whisk. Pour into the prepared dish and set aside.

PLACE the prepared nuts in a large bowl. Add the turkey, onion, corn, cornmeal, egg, chili powder, half-and-half, 1 teaspoon salt, pepper, oregano, and garlic powder and mix well with your hands. Divide the meat mixture evenly and press the meat into each pepper half. Lay the peppers in the prepared pan, with the meat facing up. Cover with foil. Bake 50 minutes.

REMOVE the foil. Sprinkle the cheese over each evenly. Bake another 20 minutes, uncovered. Gently pull out the stems. To serve: place a portion of cooked rice on a plate (or in a bowl), place pepper on top, then spoon tomato sauce from the pan over all of them, as desired. Cover and refrigerate the leftovers; they freeze well. Makes 8.

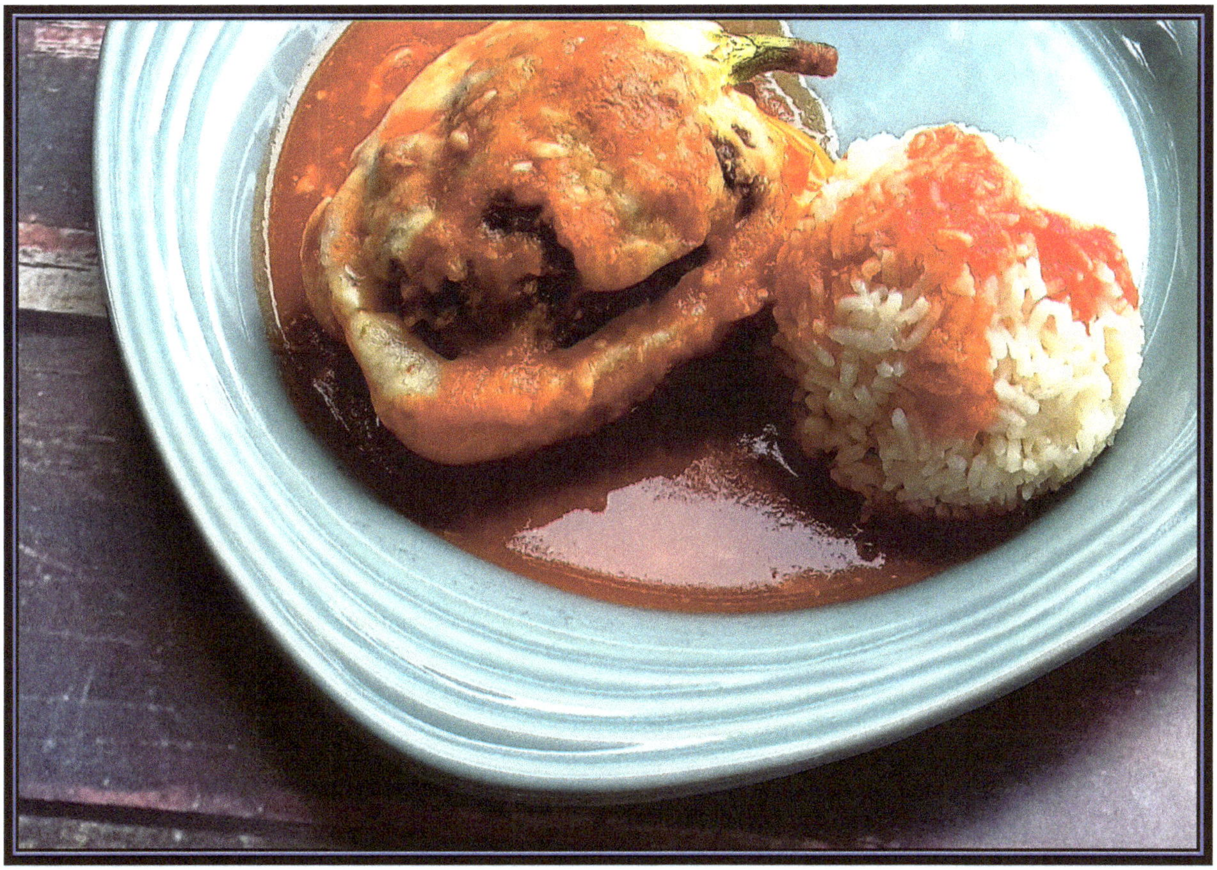

Marcella's Flat Enchiladas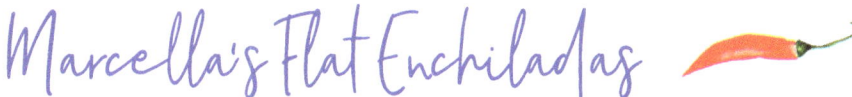

START TO FINISH: ABOUT 35 MINUTES

I was lucky enough to have a really kind, loving mother-in-law named Marcella. A couple of times a year during the '90s, she would announce she was making her special enchiladas. This occasion would produce a veritable feeding frenzy in her tiny North Valley kitchen. This kitchen also had a three-foot-square table in the center. It was always there, and ended up being the place for plates and garnishes. Everyone assembled their own plate, and you definitely needed a knife and fork for this meal. She would make large quantities of the ingredients listed below, and some people (meaning my husband and his brother) would often end up getting THREE helpings.

Chapter Ten: Main Events   167

For such basic items and such a deceptively basic dish, there might appear to be a lot of preparation involved, yet the recipe really only takes a little while to put together. I am scaling this down to feed four people and I have listed previously prepared ingredients, if you find all of this to be daunting and you don't want to prepare the chile sauce and beans by yourself. A cast iron skillet is a requirement if you want to stick with Marcella's tried-and-true technique. If you do end up making everything from scratch and you end up with leftovers, don't worry; everything can be used in future dishes.

½ cup vegetable oil
8 corn tortillas, 6–7" in diameter
4 cups red chile sauce (see page xxviii to make your own in advance)
15.5-ounce can pinto beans, with juice (you need about 2 cups;
    see page 92 to make your own in advance)
1 pound ground beef chuck (no substitute, if you want the
    authentic Marcella experience)
1 teaspoon salt
½ cup water
8 ounces sharp cheddar cheese, finely shredded (fiesta blend is fine)

MANDATORY GARNISH:

You must set out a bowl of shredded iceberg lettuce, as well as a bowl of chopped white onions, and another of chopped tomatoes. A couple of cups of each item should suffice, maybe 3 cups of the lettuce.

OPTIONAL GARNISH:

Occasionally, someone would fry an egg over medium in another skillet (use a bit of tub margarine for an authentic Marcella experience) to serve on top, so you would need 1 egg for each serving. A bowl of roasted and chopped green chile was usually around, too. My daughters remember there being a bowl of sliced black olives (canned) on the table, though Bob and I don't remember that particular item. However, it would be a welcome addition.

PLACE the oil in a 10" cast iron skillet. Heat to sizzling over rather high heat. Using tongs as your cooking utensil, fry each tortilla about 20 seconds on each side, then remove to paper towels. Repeat with each tortilla and keep a double layer of paper towels between each one. Reserve 1 tablespoon oil and set aside (you can use any remaining oil for other items; be sure to use a heat-proof container to pour the hot oil in, if you plan to save it). You may complete this step in advance.

HEAT the red chile sauce in a 2-quart saucepan to a simmer. Heat the beans in a 1½-quart saucepan to a simmer. Place the reserved oil in the skillet and fry the chuck over rather high heat until all the pink is gone, breaking up the meat. Add the salt and water and bring to a boil. Cook on lowest heat 10 minutes, uncovered. Stir a few times.

TO ASSEMBLE: Get out 4 dinner plates. With tongs, dip a tortilla in the red chile sauce and place on a plate. Repeat with 3 more tortillas. Divide meat evenly over all 4 plates. Use a slotted spoon to do this (Marcella never drained the meat, and this also adds a bit of savory, salty broth to the dish). Using a slotted spoon, place beans evenly over each plate, about ½-cup per person. Sprinkle about ⅓ cup of cheese over each. Pour about ⅓ cup of red chile sauce over each. Dip the remaining tortillas in the sauce and place on top. Divide the remaining cheese over all 4 plates. Then place lettuce, onions, and tomatoes on top of each. Pour the desired amount of extra sauce all over each one. Place a prepared egg and any other garnishes you choose on top of each, if desired. Cover and refrigerate the leftovers separately. Makes 4 servings.

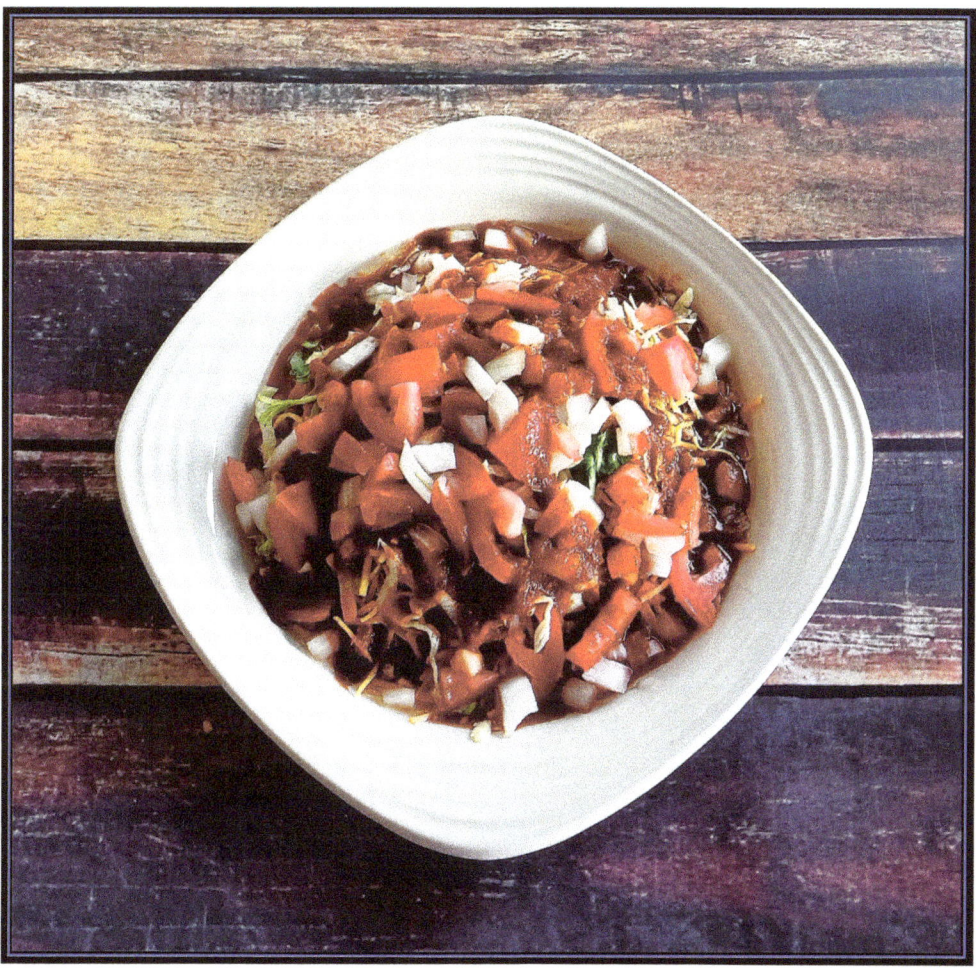

The Whole Enchilada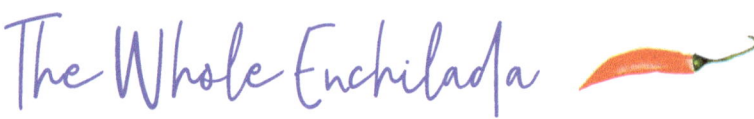

Prep: about 39 minutes
Bake: 50 minutes
Stand: 10 minutes
Oven: 375°

This is a mellow casserole that is easy to customize with different proteins, or you can omit the meat for a meatless option. You could also use ground meats; just precook a pound of your choice in a medium skillet, drain, and add to the beans. Too mellow? Double the green chile.

10-ounce can of diced tomatoes with green chiles (such as Ro*Tel)
3 tablespoons salted butter
1 cup onion, coarsely chopped
1 tablespoon minced garlic
¼ cup all-purpose flour
½ teaspoon salt
½ teaspoon garlic salt
14.5-ounce can low-sodium chicken broth
4 ounces roasted and chopped green chile, with juice
1 cup sour cream, room temperature (light is okay)
12 corn tortillas, 6–7" in diameter
16-ounce can refried beans
1 pound cooked chicken, coarsely chopped
8 ounces sharp cheddar cheese, shredded and divided

Garnish:

> This is another great place to use some of those
> **Nice New Mexican & Mexican Garnishes.**

PLACE the tomatoes with green chile in a strainer and set aside to drain well. Place the butter in a 2-quart saucepan. Melt over rather high heat. Add the onion and garlic and sauté 2 minutes. Add the flour, salt, and garlic salt and whisk well. Add the broth and green chile and cook over medium heat until it thickens somewhat. Whisk in the sour cream and cook on a low simmer 1 minute; don't boil. Set aside.

PREHEAT the oven to 375°. Coat a 13" by 9" baking dish with cooking spray or grease lightly. Pour 1 cup of the prepared sauce into the pan. Cut each tortilla into 8 wedges. Place half of these in the pan rather evenly. Place the refried beans in a large glass bowl and microwave on HIGH 1 minute to soften them. Mix 1 cup of the sauce into the beans well. Mix the chicken and half of the cheese into the beans. Place in the pan and spread to coat all the tortillas. Place the remaining tortilla wedges all over evenly. Pour the remaining sauce all over, covering all the tortillas. Sprinkle the reserved tomatoes and green chiles all over. Cover with foil and bake 30 minutes.

REMOVE the foil and sprinkle the remaining cheese all over. Bake another 20 minutes, uncovered. Let stand 10 minutes before serving. Garnish, if desired. Cover and refrigerate the leftovers; they freeze well. Makes 6–8 servings.

Taco Tuesday Tacos

START TO FINISH: ABOUT 45 MINUTES

Tacos can really be interpreted in a million different ways, but here is the filling we use at home when it is taco night (inevitably held on a Friday night, which is not as charmingly alliterative as Tuesday). We use the regular-sized corn tortilla crispy shells. Definitely not the large ones, because they are way too big. You can use this filling in any sort of taco container you want. You can make your own corn tortillas and fry them up as you would like. You can use miniature flour tortillas, if you like your tacos to be a bit on the doughier side. Let's say you want to get those giant shells and make a "healthy" salad option out of your taco meat. Then, this recipe might make four or six of those.

Occasionally, I will order something like a vegetarian taco plate at various restaurants, or I will convince myself to try the healthier version of a taco and get the fish ones. Usually, I'm disappointed in what I get. I think part of this is because the small, non-crispy corn tortillas that are served with these types of fillings are never strong enough to support the filling and the tortillas fall apart. I've even seen places supply two corn tortillas for each taco, but even those can fall apart. Then I wish I had just ordered a burger. Oh, well.

I've also seen the regular tacos offered at many Mexican/New Mexican restaurants around town. These are usually rather bland offerings: crispy corn tortillas filled with salted ground beef (not much of any other seasonings), iceberg lettuce, a few chopped tomatoes, and a bit of cheddar cheese on top. Then, they often don't automatically supply you with any salsa to pour over it before you crunch it. You can splurge and get something like a Navajo taco, which is a decadent, open-faced, knife-and-fork kind of taco served on top of a divine piece of fry bread (look it up, yum).

Regardless of how you prefer to eat your tacos, here is a beefy, cheesy, pleasantly spicy filling to help you get there. You can choose whatever type of carrying case you want to set this meat in. The spice mix will certainly work on other ground meats, such as turkey, and it will also work on a vegetable sauté. The recipe will make 12 regular-sized tacos, or probably eight larger tacos, or four to six salads.

These are officially also known as White Person Tacos, but they are better than your average version.

1 tablespoon chili powder
2 teaspoons all-purpose flour
1 teaspoon salt
1 teaspoon black pepper
1 teaspoon onion powder
1 teaspoon garlic powder
1 teaspoon dried oregano
1 teaspoon ground cumin
1 teaspoon smoked paprika
1 pound ground beef sirloin
1 cup onion, coarsely chopped
¾ cup water
6 ounces fiesta blend cheese, finely shredded
12 regular-sized crispy corn taco shells (or whatever container you prefer)

Garnish:

You can start with your typical shredded iceberg lettuce (the most boring kind of lettuce ever invented, perhaps), a few chopped tomatoes, and some salsa or taco sauce, any variety. But you could also consult the **Nice New Mexican & Mexican Garnishes** list and broaden your horizons with some items there. Olives, onions, radishes, etc., can be fun to add.

COMBINE the first 9 ingredients in a small bowl with a whisk. Set aside. Coat a 3-quart deep skillet with cooking spray. Place the beef and onion in the pan and fry over very high heat until all the pink is gone, breaking up the meat. Drain this only if it seems to need it; otherwise, fry it until it is just about dry. Sprinkle the seasoning mix all over and add the water. Bring to a boil, then cook on a gentle boil, uncovered, about 15 minutes or so. Stir a few times, especially near the end of cooking. Your sauce will reduce and thicken, but you still want your beef to be a bit saucy. Sprinkle the cheese all over. Reduce the heat to the lowest setting, cover, and cook until the cheese has melted, about 2 minutes.

MEANWHILE, heat your chosen taco shells as directed on the package. Divide the meat for each. Garnish, as you like. Cover and refrigerate the leftovers. Makes 12 regular-sized tacos. This might serve 4–6, depending on the appetite of your diners. I usually eat 2 (I used to eat 3); Bob usually eats 5, but this also depends on whether I have made some salad to go with them (like my Black Bean Salad on page 58, then I might only eat one taco with the salad).

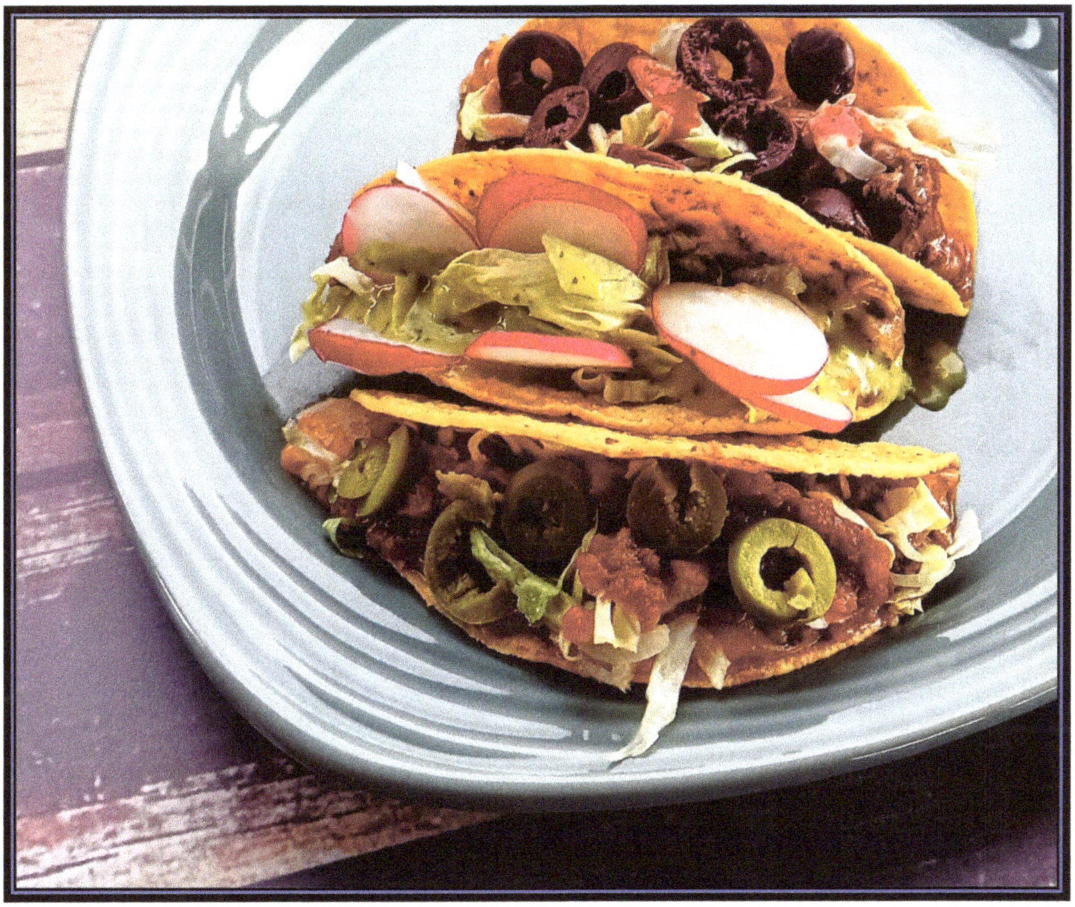

Chapter Ten: Main Events

Vader's Killer Taters

Prep: about 45 minutes
Bake (simultaneous): depending on your taters, around 25-30 minutes
Oven: 450°

> Just in time for the next Boonta Eve Classic (or maybe the next Super Bowl), I present to you an epic Empire dish to serve while cheering on your favorite team. The Empire would certainly appreciate the "bread and circuses" aspect of our own galaxy's ancient and modern cultures, wouldn't it? It keeps the masses in line. I don't know if Darth Vader would appreciate the spice inherent in this dish—hold on—we never see Lord Vader eat anything, do we? He must have been fed intravenously through his suit. That's quite a tragic change from the carefree young Anakin Skywalker, who seemed to enjoy dining. Be careful, Anakin! This Southwestern poutine might set your taste buds on fire! Oh, dear...

1 pound chorizo (or hot Italian sausage), casings removed
1 cup red onion, coarsely chopped
2 pounds seasoned frozen potatoes (your choice—skinny, curly, or steak fries, tater tots or crowns, etc.)
6 tablespoons salted butter
½ cup all-purpose flour
½ teaspoon pepper
½ teaspoon crushed red pepper flakes
1 quart low-sodium chicken broth
4 ounces roasted and chopped green chile, with juice
12 ounces cheese curds (if these aren't available, use queso panela or fresco; fresh mozzarella or paneer will also work in a pinch)

GARNISH:

If you really want an oozy, cholesterol-rich treat, fry up a few eggs and serve them on top. If you want to get some more vegetables in here, chop up some scallions and sprinkle all over the top.

PREHEAT the oven to 450°. Coat a 5-quart deep skillet with cooking spray. Fry the sausage and onion over rather high heat until the pink is gone, breaking up the meat. Drain and set aside; re-use the pan. Coat a large baking sheet with cooking spray. Pour the potatoes on the sheet, then coat them all over with cooking spray. Bake as directed on the package, but add 5 minutes to the total time. Stir potatoes 3 times. You want them to be very crispy, but not burnt.

MEANWHILE, melt the butter in the skillet over rather high heat. Whisk in the flour and the 2 seasonings until thicker and smooth. Add about half of the broth and whisk well to make a smooth gravy. Whisk in the remaining broth and chile and boil 2 minutes. Add the meat and onion back to the pan. Lower the heat to medium/low and cook, uncovered, on a gentle boil, 15 minutes. Stir a few times.

WHILE the gravy is cooking, break or chop up the cheese curds into more manageable chunks, around ½" or so, and set aside.

TO SERVE: You can serve this as a sort of casserole by placing all the potatoes in a 13" by 9" baking dish (or even a 15" by 11" dish, depending on whether you want to spread it all out a bit more), topping them with all the cheese, then pouring all the gravy over them. This is the perfect treatment for a party. Or you can also serve this individually by dividing the potatoes on each plate, topping them with cheese, and pouring gravy over all. You might even prefer to place the cheese on top of the gravy. Either way will be fine. Regardless, you will want to serve it immediately, garnished, or not. The hot gravy and potatoes will sort of melt the cheese, but not completely—which is just how you want to serve it. Cover and refrigerate the leftovers separately; the gravy can be frozen, and you can cook up fresh potatoes at a future date. Makes 6–8 servings.

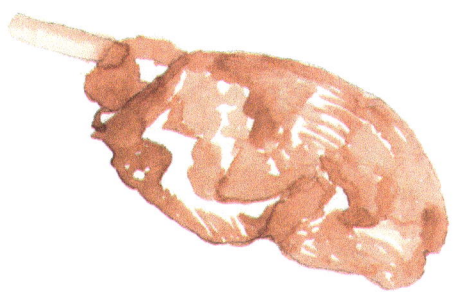

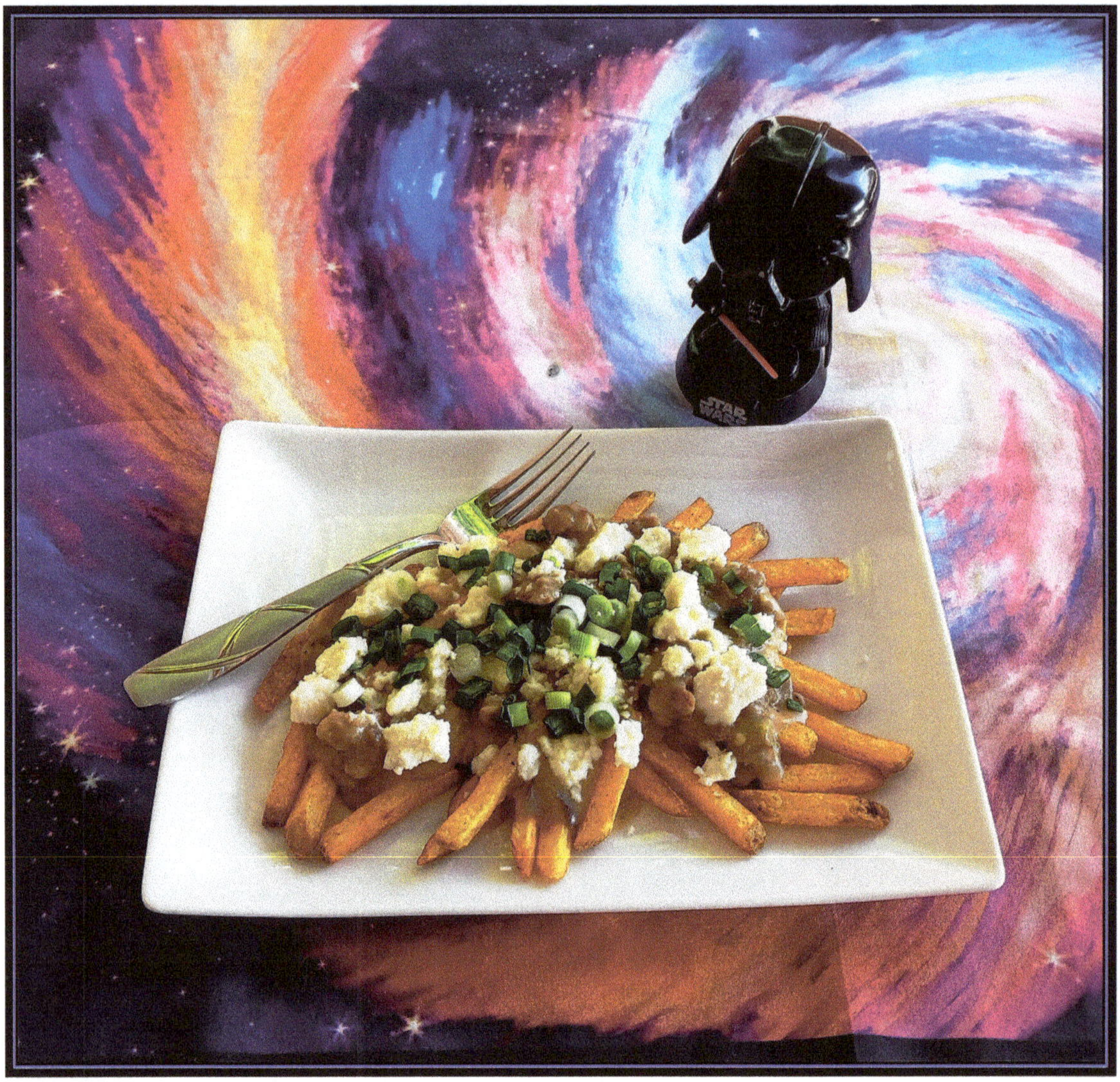

DARTH VADER SAYS:

"Give yourself to the cheese curds. It is the only way you can
please your friends. Yes, your thoughts betray you...
You may alter the recipe...
Pray don't alter it too much."

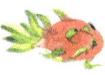

Callista's Birthday Pizza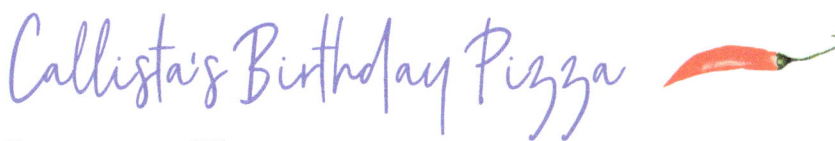

Prep: about 35 minutes
Bake: 16 minutes, per pizza
Stand: 3 minutes, per pizza
Oven: 450°

Well, I guess the title gives it away! Yes, this is my younger daughter's favorite birthday treat. But please don't limit yourself to serving this only on birthdays. There's the Super Bowl, or baby showers, or just any Friday night to celebrate the end of a work week. It's best to bake these loaded pizzas one at a time, right in the middle of your oven. Be sure to use a substantial pizza crust for these.

1 tablespoon vegetable oil
2 tablespoons minced garlic
¾ cup shallots, finely chopped
1 tablespoon chili powder
½ teaspoon salt
½ teaspoon black pepper
1 pound ground beef sirloin
16-ounce can refried beans
½ cup salsa, any variety
2 packaged full-sized (12") pizza crusts, preferably thicker ones
    (I use Boboli original crusts)
16-ounce jar sliced and tamed jalapeños, drained well
    (or use regular, spicy ones)
10 ounces queso panela, crumbled into rather small chunks
4 ounces sharp cheddar cheese, finely shredded

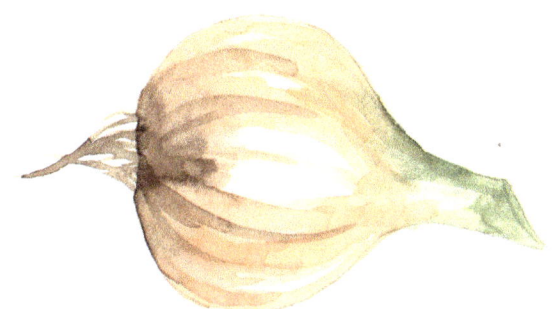

Garnish:

> Many of the **Nice New Mexican & Mexican Garnishes** will complement this recipe.

COAT a 3-quart deep skillet with cooking spray. Place the oil in the pan and turn the heat to rather high. Fry the garlic, shallots, the 3 seasonings, and the beef over rather high heat until the pink is gone and it is almost dry, breaking up the meat. Season, as desired. Set aside.

Chapter Ten: Main Events

PREHEAT the oven to 450°. Place the beans in a medium glass bowl and microwave on HIGH for about a minute to soften them. Mix the salsa in well and set aside.

PLACE the pizza crusts on 2 pans or pizza stones. Spread the bean mixture evenly on both, leaving a ½" border all around. Divide the meat evenly and spread on both. Divide the jalapeños evenly and place on both. Sprinkle the queso panela evenly over both. Sprinkle the cheddar over both. Bake 1 pizza 16 minutes. Let stand 3 minutes before cutting. Repeat baking and standing for the other pizza. Garnish, as desired. Cover and refrigerate the leftovers. Makes 6–12 servings.

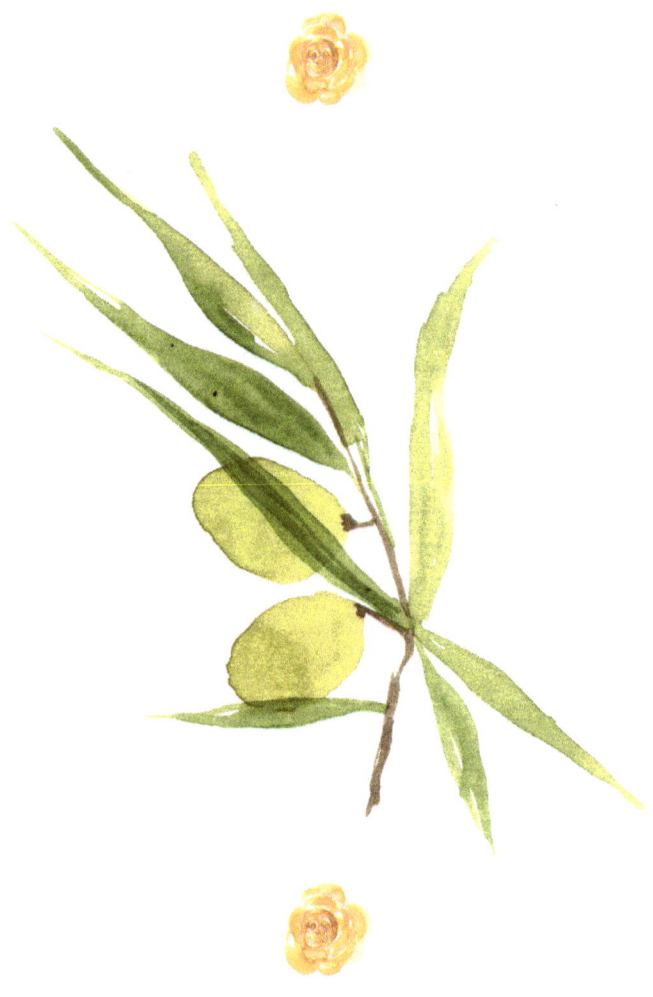

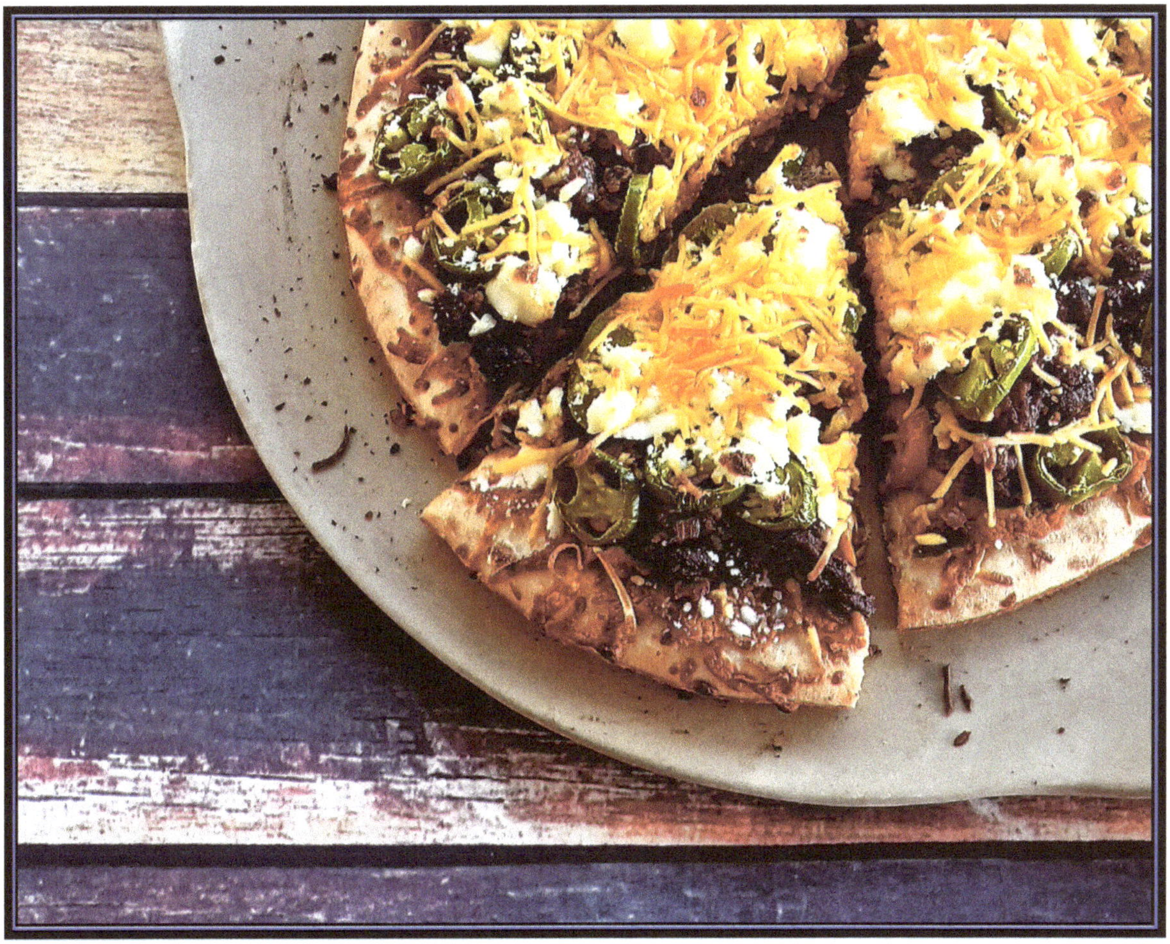

Chapter Eleven

Thanks-giving

Sam's Fairly Large Crowd Po-ta-toes

Roasted Baby Carrots

Caulisprouts

Spinach au Gratin

Chloë's Grits Dressing

Walter's Favorite Cranberry Relish

The One-Bowl Thanksgiving Leftover Casserole

Thank Goodness for Enchilada Casseroles

Cranberry Cheesecake

The Half-Pound Cake

Cran-Apple Streusel Pie

The Little Halflings' Pumpkin Patch

Warren's Pumpkin Cheesecake

Cyrus's No-Bake Pumpkin Tarts

Pumpkin Sparkle Pie

William's Chili Pumpkin Bread
with Pepitas Honey Butter

Isabella's Pumpkin Pie Ice Cream

Pumpkin Pancakes

Thanksgiving

THANKSGIVING IS PROBABLY the most traditional holiday around our house, though I am no longer roasting whole turkeys. A boneless, skinless turkey breast suits us all just fine. And isn't the modern Thanksgiving meal all about the sides and desserts? I've included an assortment of suitable recipes from which I rotate year to year. Plus, I have a few items that utilize your leftovers. I decided to split my pumpkin recipes into their own subsection, where I named a few recipes for my grandchildren. You'll see you can mix and match recipes depending on whether you end up with leftover canned pumpkin or if you have carved a giant pumpkin and need a few places to put some. See page xvi for a homemade pumpkin spice recipe.

Most everything in this chapter feeds six to eight, or eight to ten. Various savory items are baked at 350°, which allows you some wiggle room if you have other recipes that require higher or lower temperatures; you can increase or decrease a few minutes either way for these casual items (when I say casual, I mean they are not items such as cakes or breads which would require more specific settings for success). The desserts will serve more people. Some items are easy to reduce by half; many items can be increased according to your needs.

Make it a memorable Southwestern event by cooking up a pot of my Red Chile Sauce (page xxviii) to serve as a gravy alternative, especially on your mashed potatoes. Does turkey benefit from a red chile blanket? Try it and see.

Do you need a big pan of macaroni and cheese to accompany your Thanksgiving spread? Taters and dressing are generally the favorite carbohydrate choices around our table, but you can find a few good mac & cheese options in Chapter Twelve. Many could easily be doubled and placed in a 13" by 9" baking dish.

Sam's Fairly Large Crowd Po-ta-toes

START TO FINISH: ABOUT 55 MINUTES

Sam is a rather common name and it technically does not belong to any sort of specific fantasy world, but this is definitely a recipe that someone like the hobbit Samwise Gamgee could have made for his large family (13 children!).

The garlic powder is optional, or you can use a double recipe of my Magical, Mythical Garlic: Regular Roast (page xvii). Prepare the garlic in advance, mash it, then add it to the finished taters. Add two or three cups of finely shredded Parmesan cheese to the finished product for variety. Cheddar works well, too.

10 cups water
1 tablespoon salt, divided
5 pounds russet potatoes, peeled, and cut into 1" chunks
½ cup salted butter
1 cup half-and-half
2 teaspoons black pepper
1 tablespoon garlic powder (optional; use more if you love garlic, say, 2 tablespoons)

Garnish: extra pats of butter and some finely chopped fresh chives

PLACE the water, 1 teaspoon salt, and the potatoes in an 8-quart saucepan. Bring to a boil. Cook over medium heat, partially covered, 20–25 minutes, until the potatoes are fork tender. Stir a couple of times. Reserve 1 cup of the cooking liquid and set aside. Drain in a large colander and set aside.

ADD the reserved water back to the pot, as well as the remaining 2 teaspoons salt, butter, half-and-half, pepper, and garlic (in whatever form you are using, if you are). Heat on a rather high setting until the butter has melted. Add the potatoes and mash by hand or use a hand mixer. Season, as needed. Garnish, if you like. Cover and refrigerate the leftovers. Makes 10–12 servings.

Roasted Baby Carrots

Prep: 10 minutes
Roast: about 2 hours
Oven: 350°

Don't use skinny carrots for this dish; try to get the plumpest baby carrots you can. I usually throw these in the oven at right about 11 a.m. to serve them at 1 p.m., which is our traditional time to eat Thanksgiving dinner.

2 tablespoons salted butter
2 tablespoons packed light brown sugar
2 tablespoons olive oil
1 tablespoon crushed ginger
1 teaspoon salt
1 teaspoon black pepper
1 teaspoon crushed rosemary (2–3 tablespoons fresh, minced)
2 pounds baby carrots

PREHEAT the oven to 350°. Coat a 13″ by 9″ baking dish with cooking spray or grease lightly. Place the butter in a very large glass bowl. Microwave on HIGH in 20-second intervals to melt, for a total of 40–60 seconds. Add the brown sugar, oil, and the 4 seasonings and whisk well. Add the carrots and mix well. Place the carrots in the prepared dish. Roast 1½ to 2 hours. Stir a couple of times. They will start to caramelize nicely near the end of roasting. Season. Cover and refrigerate the leftovers. Makes 6–8 servings.

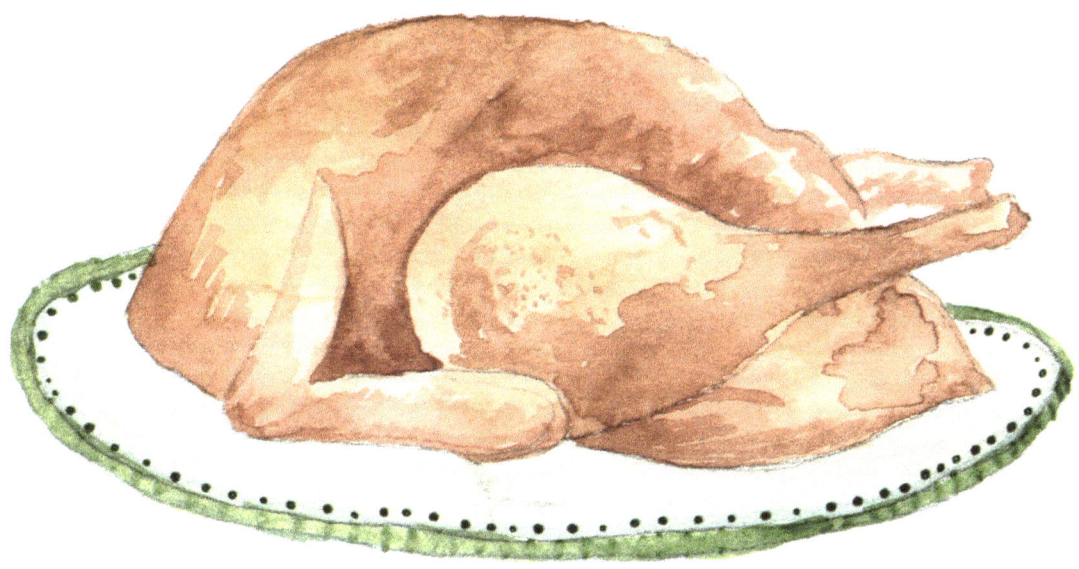

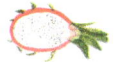

Caulisprouts

PREP: 15 MINUTES
ROAST: 1 HOUR
OVEN: 350°

This recipe is perfect for anyone who loves stinky cruciferous vegetables. Such as myself. Not my husband, however.

2 tablespoons salted butter
2 tablespoons olive oil
1 teaspoon fine sea salt
½ teaspoon black pepper
½ teaspoon garlic powder
½ teaspoon dried thyme (2–3 tablespoons fresh, minced)
½ teaspoon sugar
12 ounces fresh cauliflower florets, around 1½" or so
12 ounces fresh Brussels sprouts, cut in half
A medium-sized red onion (around 8 ounces);
    peel, cut off stems, and cut into 8 wedges
2 ounces Parmesan and/or Romano cheese, finely shredded

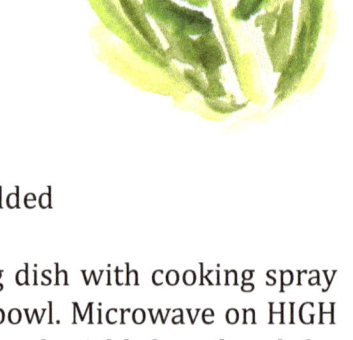

PREHEAT the oven to 350°. Coat a 13" by 9" baking dish with cooking spray or grease lightly. Place the butter in a very large glass bowl. Microwave on HIGH in 20-second intervals to melt, for a total of 40–60 seconds. Add the oil and the 5 seasonings and whisk well. Add the 3 vegetables and toss to coat. Pour into the prepared pan. Roast 45 minutes. Stir a couple of times. Sprinkle the cheese over all. Roast another 15 minutes. Cover and refrigerate the leftovers. Makes 6–8 servings.

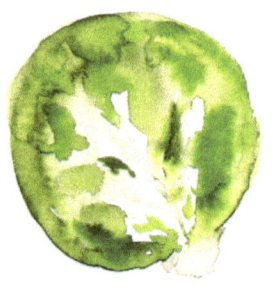 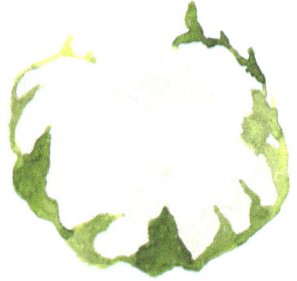 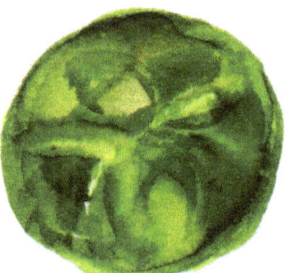

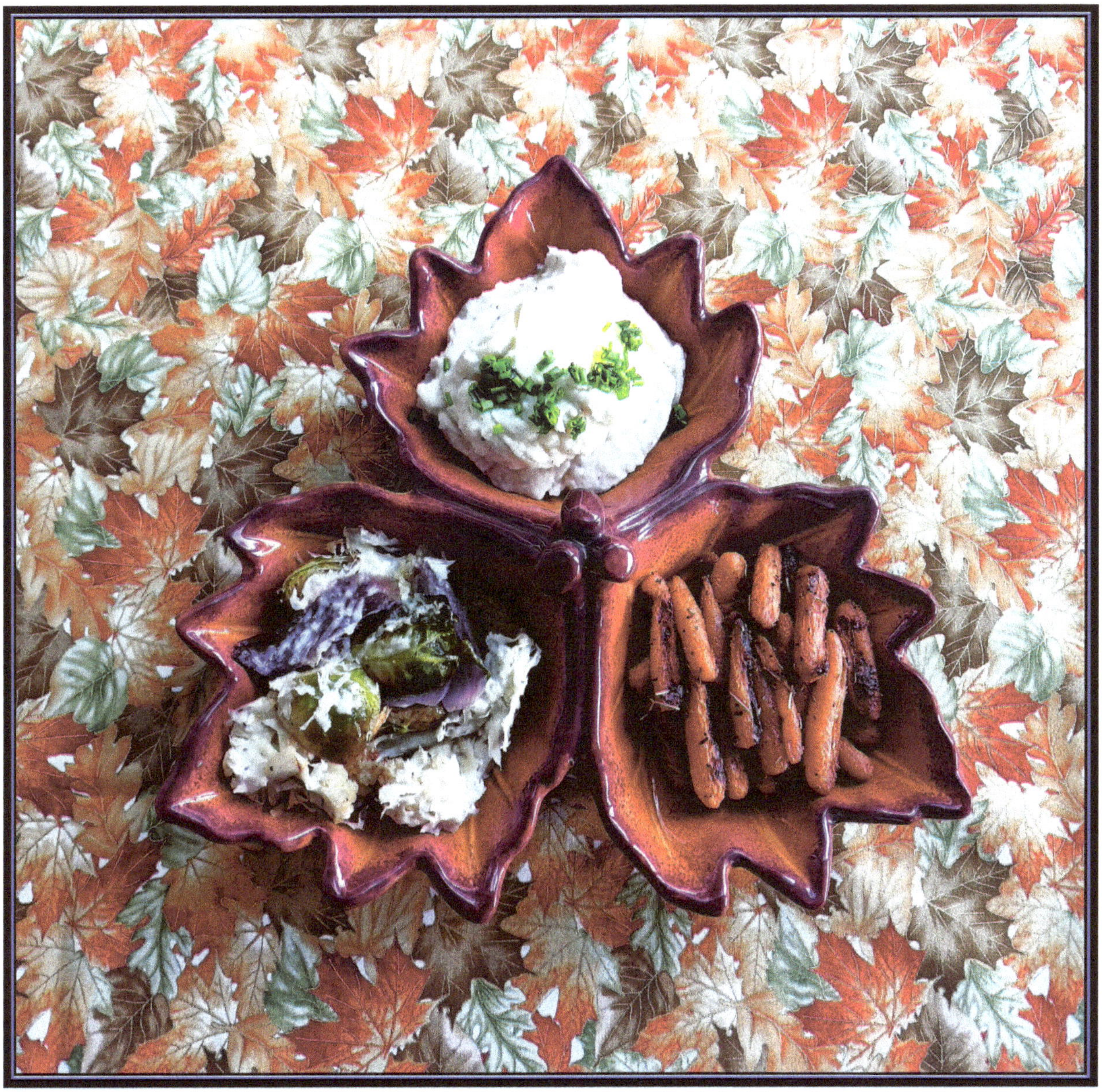

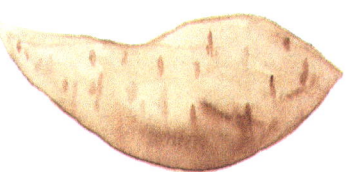

CLOCKWISE, FROM TOP:
Sam's Fairly Large Crowd Po—ta—toes, page 183
Roasted Baby Carrots, page 184
Caulisprouts, page 186

Chapter Eleven: Thanksgiving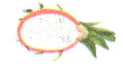

Spinach au Gratin

PREP: ABOUT 35 MINUTES
BAKE: 30 MINUTES
STAND: 5 MINUTES
OVEN: 350°

I think I saw something like this among the billion recipes on the internet and the concept sounded good. I've brought it down to manageable proportions, because one can eat only so much cheesy spinach at a time.

Leftover fatigue? Combine some of this dish with some chicken or vegetable broth for an impromptu soup, whisk well, and heat. Add a little cooked bacon if you are so inclined. Pour some over various types of carbs, such as rice or potatoes.

6 cups water
2 pounds frozen chopped spinach
½ cup salted butter
1 cup onion, coarsely chopped
8 ounces light cream cheese (Neufchâtel), softened
½ cup half-and-half
1 teaspoon salt
1 teaspoon black pepper
1 teaspoon hot sauce
4 ounces buttery crackers (such as Ritz), broken up coarsely
4 ounces Gruyère cheese, shredded
Paprika

BRING water to boil in a 6-quart saucepan. Add the spinach and bring to another boil. Cook on medium heat 5 minutes. Drain and let the spinach stand in the colander. Don't squeeze the spinach. Rinse and reuse the pan.

PREHEAT the oven to 350°. Coat an 11" by 7" baking dish with cooking spray or grease lightly. Melt the butter in the saucepan. Add the onion and sauté 5 minutes over rather high heat. Add the cream cheese, half-and-half, salt, pepper, and hot sauce and cook over medium/low heat, whisking until the cheese melts. Take off the heat. Add the crackers and mix in. Add the spinach and mix in. Pour into the prepared pan. Sprinkle the Gruyère all over. Sprinkle moderately with paprika, as desired. Bake 30 minutes. Let stand 5 minutes before serving. Cover and refrigerate the leftovers (it can be frozen). Makes 10–12 servings.

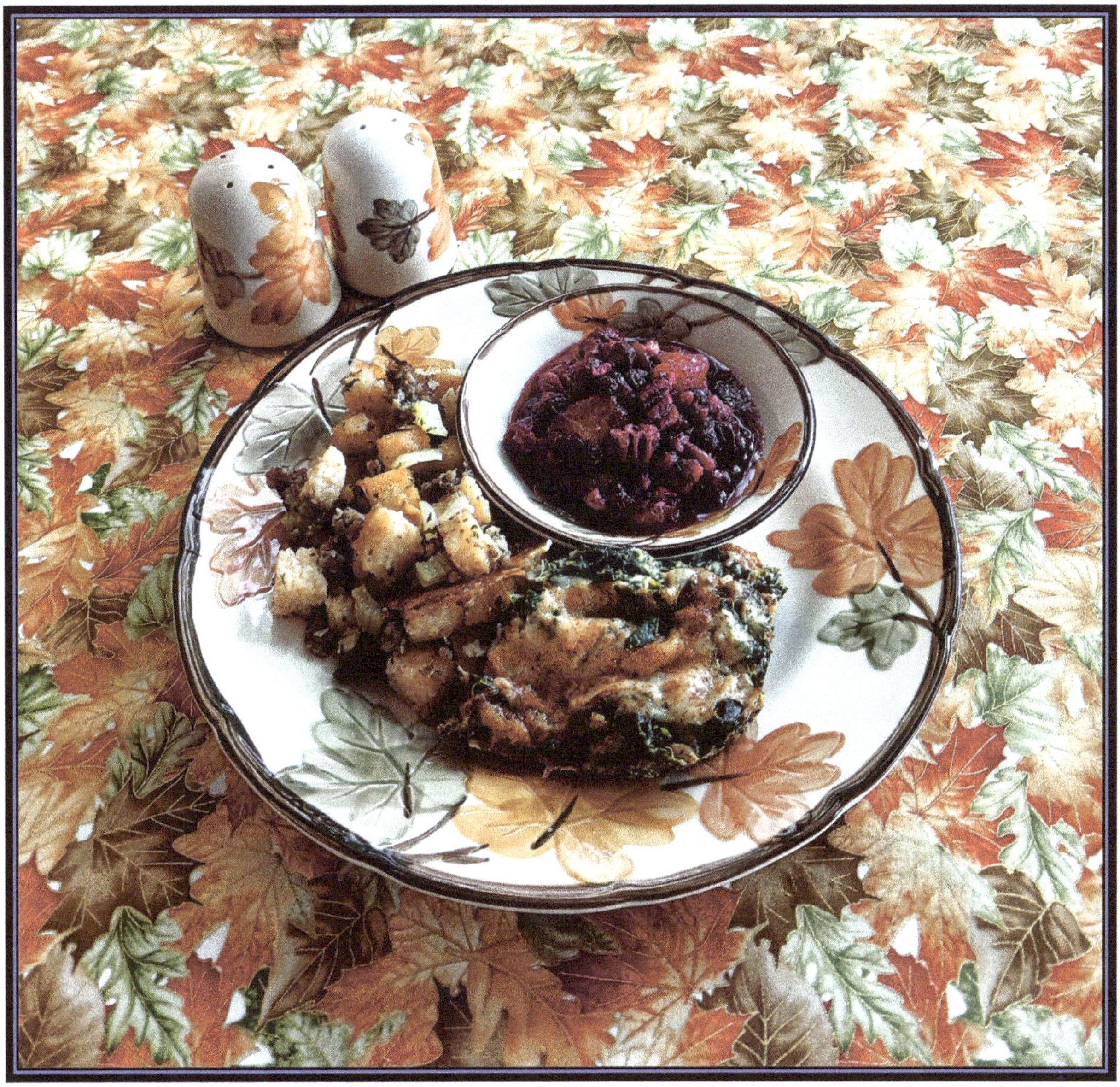

CLOCKWISE, FROM TOP:
Walter's Favorite Cranberry Relish, page 192
Spinach au Gratin, page 188
Chloë's Grits Dressing, page 190

Chapter Eleven: Thanksgiving   189

Chloë's Grits Dressing

ACTIVE PREP: ABOUT 50 MINUTES
COOL: 1 HOUR
CHILL: OVERNIGHT
BAKE: 40 MINUTES AND 45 MINUTES
STAND: 1 HOUR
OVEN: 450° AND 350°

For a few years, my mom used to give my sister and me a copy of the latest *Southern Living* Christmas cookbook. These books have dozens of craft ideas (some of which I have made), tons of sweet recipes, and plenty of savory holiday recipes as well. My mom's version of stuffing/dressing was basically the recipe on the back of a big bag of Pepperidge Farm herb-seasoned cubes, cooked with bacon, butter, celery, and onion. She made enough to stuff a moderate bird, with an extra bowl on the side. But after some experimenting with various dressing/stuffing recipes in these books, pretty much everyone concluded that the book's grits dressing was the favorite, especially of my daughter Chloë.

However, I discovered that I had to change the *Southern Living* recipe quite a bit to make it more specific and easier to prepare. You really need to refrigerate those grits overnight, or you will not be able to cut them into cubes. As a rule, I don't include recipes in my cookbooks that are heavily influenced by other cookbooks, but I'm going to make an exception for just this one.

Start this recipe (at least) the night before you want to serve it. If you plan to make it a little more in advance, you can certainly assemble the dish two or even three days before you need it. I start my grits preparation the night before Thanksgiving; then, I bake the grits croutons first thing on Thanksgiving morning. But my boneless, skinless turkey breast usually doesn't enter the oven until around 10 a.m., and I have plenty of time to deal with assembling the whole dish. If you are roasting a large bird, however, you'd probably want to go ahead and prepare the entire recipe a couple of days before the holiday. Then, you can just take out the dish about 30 minutes before you need to bake it along with anything else you might be baking.

1 quart low-sodium chicken broth
1¼ cups quick-cooking grits
2 ounces Parmesan and/or Romano cheese, finely shredded

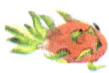

1 pound hot bulk pork sausage
⅓ cup salted butter
2 cups celery, coarsely chopped (leaves are okay to use, too)
2 cups onion, coarsely chopped
1 tablespoon minced garlic
2 tablespoons dried parsley (or ½ cup fresh, minced)
1 large egg
1 tablespoon water

THE NIGHT (OR TWO NIGHTS) BEFORE ASSEMBLING: Place the broth in a 3-quart saucepan and bring to a boil. Slowly whisk in the grits. Cover and cook on moderately low heat 7 minutes. Whisk a couple of times. Whisk in the cheese well. Coat a 13″ by 9″ baking dish with cooking spray or grease lightly. Place the dish on a cooling rack. Pour the grits into the prepared dish, smooth the top, and let them cool 1 hour. Cover and refrigerate overnight.

TO PREPARE THE GRITS CROUTONS: Preheat the oven to 450°. Coat 2 large baking sheets with cooking spray or grease lightly. Flip the grits over onto a cutting board. Cut into ¾″ cubes (I use a pizza slicer to do this). Use a spatula to transfer the cubes onto one baking sheet. Make sure all the cubes are separated. Bake 20 minutes.

USE a spatula to loosen all the cubes. Place the other pan on top. Using 2 potholders, hold the pans together and carefully flip the pans over. Shake the pan gently to redistribute and separate the cubes into 1 layer. Bake 20 minutes. Shake the pan to loosen the cubes. Let stand on the pan for at least 1 hour before the next steps.

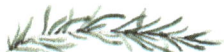

TO ASSEMBLE: Preheat the oven to 350°. Coat an 11″ by 7″ baking dish with cooking spray or grease lightly. Coat a 5-quart deep skillet with cooking spray. Fry the sausage over rather high heat until the pink is gone, breaking it up. Drain; reuse the skillet.

MELT the butter in the skillet over rather high heat. Add the celery, onion, and garlic and sauté over rather high heat 5 minutes, scraping up any brown bits. Add the parsley and sausage to the pan and mix. Separate any conjoined croutons and add them to the pan; mix in gently. Pour all into the prepared dish. Whisk the egg and water in a 1-cup glass measuring cup. Drizzle over all (cover and refrigerate if making in advance; let the pan sit at room temperature for about 30 minutes before the final baking). Bake 45 minutes. Cover and refrigerate the leftovers. Makes 8–10 servings.

Chapter Eleven: Thanksgiving   191

Walter's Favorite Cranberry Relish

IN ADVANCE: LIGHTLY TOASTING NUTS, COOLING, AND CHOPPING
PREP: 25 MINUTES
STAND: 1 HOUR
CHILL: OVERNIGHT

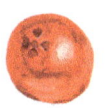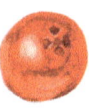

Nobody around my house is keen on the can of cranberry jelly. **Prepare this the night before you want to serve it (two or three nights in advance is also fine);** then, you can cross one thing off your list. After the relish has been refrigerated overnight, you could reserve one cup to make The Half-Pound Cake on page 198, if you like, or one and a half cups to make the Cranberry Cheesecake on page 195.

4 ounces pecan halves, lightly toasted, cooled, and chopped coarsely in advance
11-ounce can mandarin oranges, in light syrup
¾ cup orange juice
¾ cup sugar
1 tablespoon ground cinnamon
½ cup seedless raspberry jam (red plum or red currant are also fine)
1 pound fresh cranberries, thawed if frozen
5 ounces raisins

THE NIGHT BEFORE SERVING: Drain the oranges over a 3-quart saucepan. Set the oranges aside. Add the juice, sugar, cinnamon, and jam to the pot and mix well with a whisk over medium heat until the jam melts. Add the cranberries and raisins and bring to a boil. Cook over medium/low heat (a rolling simmer, but don't let it boil over) 10 minutes, uncovered. Stir a few times. Mix in the prepared pecans and oranges. Let stand 1 hour, uncovered. Pour into a 6-cup glass container. Cover and refrigerate overnight. Cover and refrigerate the leftovers; they can be frozen. Makes 6 cups.

The One-Bowl Thanksgiving Leftover Casserole

PREP: ABOUT 20 MINUTES
BAKE: 50 MINUTES
STAND: 10–15 MINUTES
OVEN: 375°

This is for that inevitable time after Turkey Day when you have become absolutely tired of placing all of your leftovers on a plate and microwaving them.

You can change this around and cook it at other times, of course. Roast beef would be a nice substitute, or obviously chicken would work. This is a full dish, so you need to use a pan underneath, just in case it dribbles over. Letting it stand for 10 minutes will reduce the liquid content of the casserole, which can vary according to your vegetable choices. For the green vegetables, you can use items such as peas, lima beans, green beans, or Brussels sprouts (cut in half). For the orange or yellow vegetables, use items such as carrot, corn, or summer squash. You can even use vegetables that have been part of their own casseroles. Add fresh or frozen items to total three cups of vegetables.

2 cups cold, leftover, seasoned mashed potatoes
¼ cup 1% milk
1½ cups leftover cooked green vegetables
1½ cups leftover cooked orange and/or yellow vegetables
8 ounces cooked turkey, coarsely chopped or diced
1½ cups leftover turkey gravy (preferably not too thick; a 12-ounce jar is okay to use)
¾ cup all-purpose flour
½ teaspoon salt
½ teaspoon black pepper
4 ounces sharp cheddar cheese, finely shredded
⅓ cup soft salted butter

PREHEAT the oven to 375°. Coat an 11″ by 7″ baking dish with cooking spray or grease lightly. Place the dish on a large baking sheet. Combine the potatoes well with the milk in a large bowl. Season, if necessary. Spread evenly into the prepared dish; reuse the bowl. Cut any larger vegetables into more manageable bite sizes. Place the vegetables in the bowl. Add the turkey and gravy and combine well. Pour over the potatoes and spread evenly. Rinse and dry the bowl.

COMBINE the flour, salt, pepper, and cheese in the bowl. Add the butter and mix in with a wooden spoon and/or your hands to make a clumpy mixture. Sprinkle evenly over the turkey mixture. Bake 50 minutes. Let stand 10–15 minutes before serving. Cover and refrigerate any leftovers. Makes 6 servings.

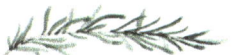

Thank Goodness for Enchilada Casseroles

Prep: about 40 minutes
Bake: 55 minutes
Stand: 10–15 minutes
Oven: 375°

Repurpose your turkey in this delicious enchilada casserole dish. Chicken will also work, as will various other precooked proteins, such as beef or shrimp.

3 tablespoons salted butter
¼ cup all-purpose flour
½ teaspoon black pepper
½ teaspoon garlic salt
½ teaspoon onion salt
½ teaspoon jalapeño powder
14.5-ounce can low-sodium chicken broth
¾ cup half-and-half
¾ cup salsa verde (see page 48 for a recipe)
1 cup sour cream, room temperature (light is okay)
2 tablespoons vegetable oil
1 cup onion, coarsely chopped
3 large jalapeños, cut off stems, scrape out seeds with a spoon, and chop finely
1 pound cooked turkey, diced or shredded
10 ounces queso fresco, crumbled and divided
12 corn tortillas (6–7" diameter)
2 ounces sharp cheddar cheese, finely shredded
Chipotle powder (or chili powder)

Garnish:

> Take a look at the **Nice New Mexican & Mexican Garnishes** list for suggestions.

MELT the butter in a 3-quart saucepan over rather high heat. Add the flour and the 4 seasonings and whisk together until fully combined and smooth. Add the broth and half-and-half and whisk over medium/high heat until thicker. Take off the heat and mix in the salsa verde and sour cream. Set aside.

HEAT the oil in a 5-quart deep skillet. Sauté the onion and jalapeños 5 minutes over rather high heat. Add the turkey, 6 ounces queso fresco, and ½ cup of the prepared sauce to the skillet and mix in. Set aside.

PREHEAT the oven to 375°. Coat a 13" by 9" baking dish with cooking spray or grease lightly. Pour 1½ cups of the sauce into the prepared dish and spread to cover the bottom of the dish. Spread 4 tortillas on a dinner plate and microwave 20–30 seconds on HIGH to soften them (if it seems necessary; some corn tortillas are already soft enough to fold easily). Spoon about ¼ cup of the turkey mixture down the middle of one tortilla. Enclose loosely and place the seam side down in the prepared pan. Repeat this process with the remaining tortillas, arranging 8 in a row, then the final 4 crosswise, 2 by 2. Any stray filling can be mixed into the sauce. Pour the remaining sauce all over them; spread to cover all the tortillas. Cover with foil and bake 30 minutes.

REMOVE the foil. Sprinkle the remaining queso fresco all over. Sprinkle the cheddar all over evenly. Sprinkle moderately with chipotle powder. Bake, uncovered, 25 minutes. Let stand 10-15 minutes before serving. Garnish, if you like. Cover and refrigerate the leftovers; enchiladas freeze well. Makes 4–6 servings.

Cranberry Cheesecake

IN ADVANCE: TOASTING NUTS AND COOLING
PREP: 25 MINUTES
BAKE: 70 MINUTES, PLUS 1 HOUR IN OVEN (HEAT OFF)
COOL: 1 HOUR
CHILL: OVERNIGHT
OVEN: 350°

This cheesecake was designed to utilize some of Walter's Favorite Cranberry Relish. However, you can use a 14-ounce can of whole berry cranberry relish, or one and a half cups of any other relish recipe. **Prepare this the night before you want to serve it.**

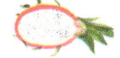

4 ounces pecan halves, lightly toasted and cooled in advance
4 ounces graham crackers
½ cup all-purpose flour
1¼ cups sugar, divided
½ teaspoon salt, divided
6 tablespoons salted butter, melted
1½ pounds light cream cheese (Neufchâtel), softened
3 large eggs
¼ cup Cointreau (other orange-flavored liqueurs or orange juice will be fine)
1 teaspoon vanilla extract
1½ cups prepared Walter's Favorite Cranberry Relish
    (page 192, or other; see recipe introduction)

Garnish: whipped cream

The night before serving: Preheat the oven to 350°. Coat a 9" springform pan with cooking spray or grease lightly. Wrap a 12" piece of foil around the outside bottom of the pan; set aside. Place the prepared pecans, graham crackers, flour, ¼ cup sugar, and ¼ teaspoon salt in a large processor. Process well. Add the butter and process. Scrape the sides and bottom of the bowl and process again. Pour into the prepared pan. Press up the pan sides about 1½", then press onto the bottom of the pan evenly. Reuse the processor; don't bother to wash it.

Place the cream cheese, eggs, 1 cup sugar, ¼ teaspoon salt, Cointreau, and vanilla in the processor and process well. Scrape the sides and bottom of the bowl and process again. Pour into the prepared pan. Place the cranberry relish in a medium bowl and stir it up to soften it, if it has been refrigerated (or if it has been in a can). Drop the relish in generous tablespoons all over the cheese. Use a butter knife to swirl it gently. Try not to disturb the crust underneath. Bake 70 minutes. Turn off the heat and leave the cake in the oven 1 hour. Place on a rack for 1 hour. Refrigerate overnight. Release the pan sides, using a sharp knife to assist you if necessary, and slice. Garnish, if you like. Cover and refrigerate the leftovers. Makes 12–16 servings.

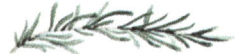

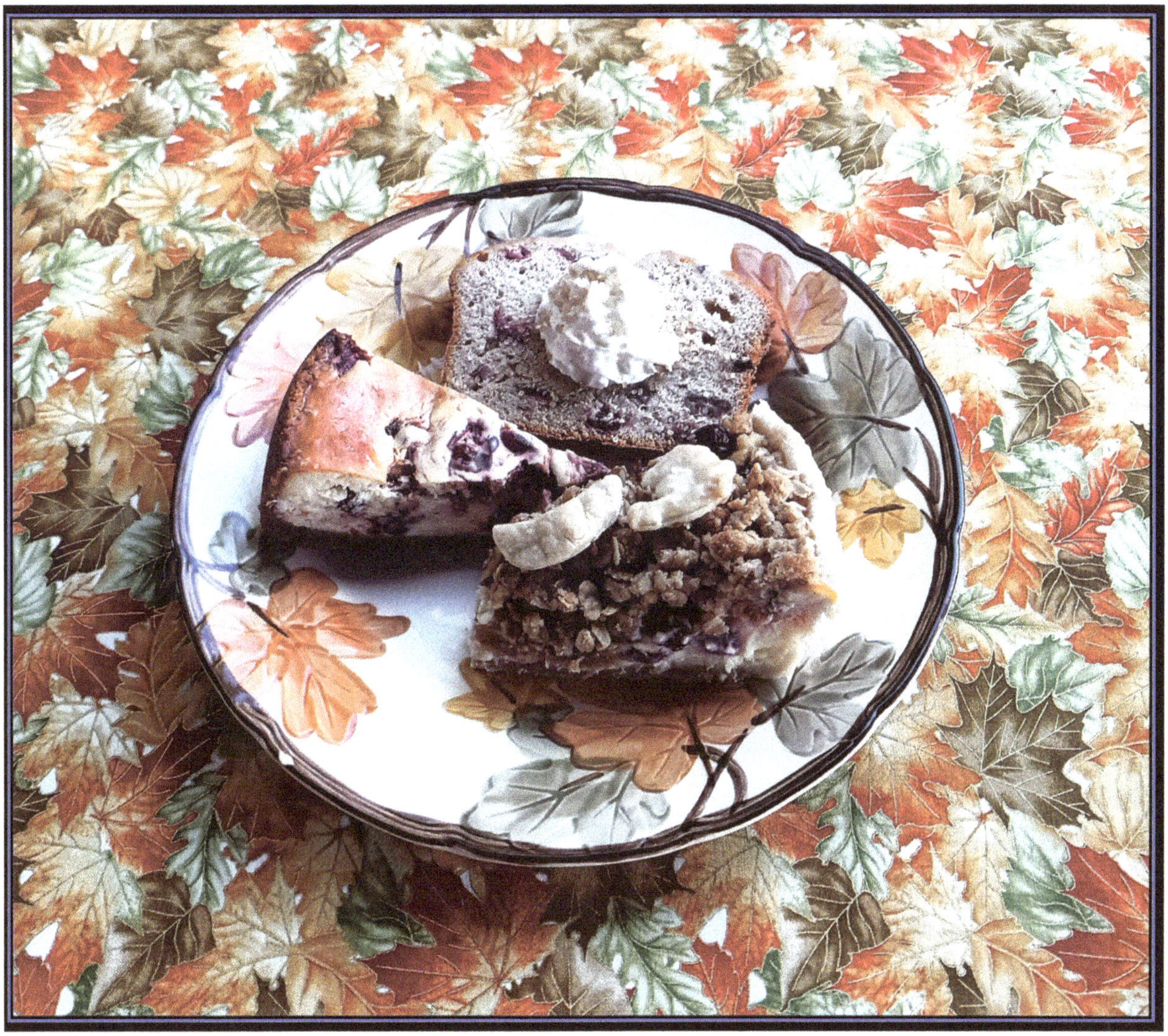

CLOCKWISE, FROM TOP:
The Half-Pound Cake, page 198
Cran-Apple Streusel Pie, page 199
Cranberry Cheesecake, page 195

Chapter Eleven: Thanksgiving 197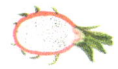

The Half-Pound Cake

Prep: about 15 minutes
Bake: 1 hour 25 minutes
Cool: 2½ hours
Oven: 325°

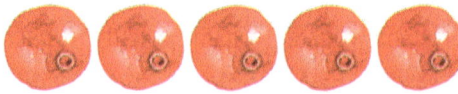

This is so titled because the primary ingredients all measure just about a half pound each. As with the previous recipe, you may substitute your own cranberry relish. I usually set aside a cup of Walter's Favorite Cranberry Relish and make this a couple of weeks after the holiday.

1 cup salted butter, softened
1¼ cups sugar
5 large eggs, room temperature
1 tablespoon vanilla extract
1¾ cups all-purpose flour (plus extra for dusting the pan)
2 teaspoons ground cinnamon
1 teaspoon salt
½ teaspoon baking powder
1 cup sour cream, room temperature (light is okay)
1 cup Walter's Favorite Cranberry Relish
    (page 192, or other recipe), room temperature

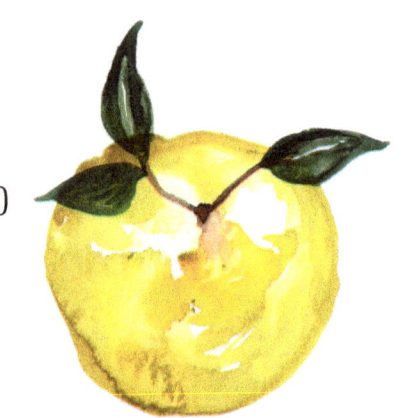

PLACE THE OVEN RACK ONE LEVEL BELOW THE CENTER POSITION. Preheat the oven to 325°. Coat a 9" by 5" loaf pan with cooking spray or grease lightly. Sprinkle some flour in the pan and shake to coat the bottom and sides; shake out any excess. Place the butter and sugar in a very large bowl and beat on medium speed for 2 minutes, using a stand mixer or a hand mixer. Add the eggs, one at a time, beating on medium 30 seconds after each addition. Add the vanilla with the final egg. Scrape down the sides; don't worry if the batter happens to appear curdled. Add the flour, cinnamon, salt, and baking powder and mix on medium another minute. Scrape down the sides and mix another minute. Add the sour cream and mix on medium 1 minute.

    ADD the cranberry relish and mix on the lowest speed, just until incorporated. Pour into the prepared pan. Smooth the top. Bake 1 hour and 25 minutes, until the center tests with slightly moist crumbs. Place on a rack for 30 minutes. Use a knife at the edges to facilitate removal from the pan, if necessary,

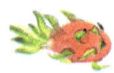

and place on the rack to cool at least 2 hours before cutting. Cover and keep at room temperature or refrigerate. Makes 10–12 servings.

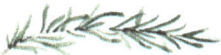

Cran-Apple Streusel Pie

IN ADVANCE: PIE CRUST PREPARATION, CRANBERRY PREPARATION
IN ADVANCE: TOASTING NUTS, COOLING, AND CHOPPING
PREP: ABOUT 20 MINUTES
BAKE: 53 MINUTES
COOL: 2 HOURS
CHILL: OVERNIGHT
OVEN: 375°

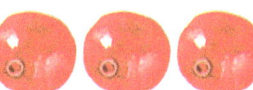 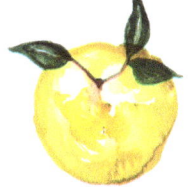

You can use a homemade pie crust or a purchased one for this pie, though homemade is preferred. Isn't it always? **Be sure to make this the night before you want to serve it.**

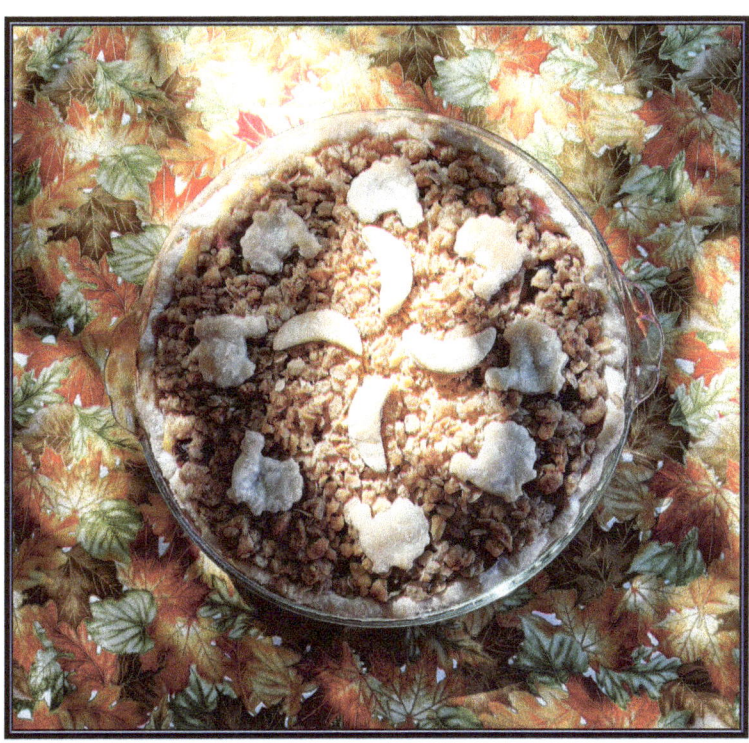

A single pie crust (homemade is preferred; see page xix)
4 ounces fresh cranberries, cut in half (thaw, if using frozen)
3 ounces walnuts, lightly toasted, cooled, and chopped finely in advance
6 ounces light cream cheese (Neufchâtel)
⅓ cup sugar
1 teaspoon salt, divided
2 large eggs
¾ cup old-fashioned oats
¼ cup all-purpose flour
⅓ cup packed light brown sugar
½ teaspoon ground cinnamon
6 tablespoons salted butter, softened
21-ounce can apple pie filling
3 ounces dried cranberries

GARNISH:

As usual, you can't go wrong with whipped cream or vanilla ice cream.

THE NIGHT BEFORE SERVING: Prepare your pie crust as necessary. When it is ready to go, preheat the oven to 375°. Roll out the crust and place it in a 9½" (glass) pie dish. Crimp or flute the edge generously (easier to do with a homemade crust). If using a homemade crust, you can cut small decorations out of the scraps if you like. Place the cream cheese in a large glass bowl and microwave on HIGH in 20-second intervals just until it is very soft, but not liquefied; about a minute total. Whisk in the sugar, ½ teaspoon salt, and eggs. Mix in the fresh cranberries. Pour into the prepared crust. Bake 25 minutes. Rinse out the bowl and dry it.

MEANWHILE in the bowl, combine the oats, flour, brown sugar, cinnamon, ½ teaspoon salt, and the prepared walnuts. Mix in the butter with your hands until crumbly. Set aside.

REMOVE the pie from the oven; maintain the heat. Carefully spread the apple pie filling evenly over the cheese mixture. Sprinkle the dried cranberries all over. Pour the oat mixture all over evenly and spread to the edges. Decorate, if desired. Bake 28 minutes. Cool on a rack 2 hours. Refrigerate overnight. Let stand at room temperature 1–2 hours before serving. Garnish, as desired. Cover and refrigerate the leftovers. Makes 8 servings.

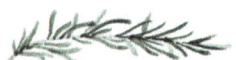

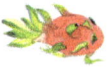

The Little Halflings' Pumpkin Patch

I ended up with quite a few pumpkin recipes and my four grandkids are all pumpkin fanatics, so I sectioned them off into their own little garden. You are welcome to use a purchased pumpkin pie spice, but I do have a recipe for my own on page xvi. I really don't like to fuss with fresh pumpkins; there's too much carving involved, and then there are all the seeds and membranes, so I use canned. A typical 15-ounce can of pumpkin yields about one and three-quarters cups, maybe a smidge more. These recipes can be mixed and matched to utilize the whole can. Pumpkin can be frozen, though it might get a bit watery, but that's not a big deal, and I have found that frozen pumpkin does not badly affect the final product.

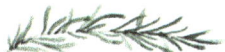

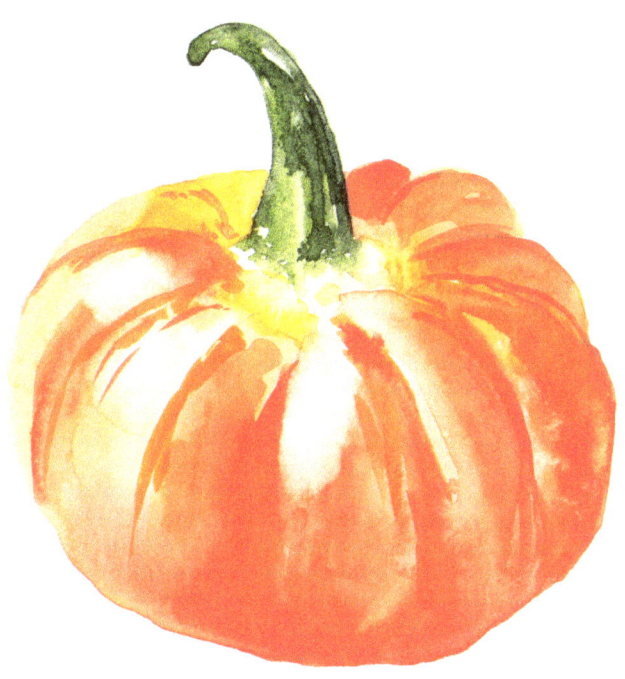

Warren's Pumpkin Cheesecake

IN ADVANCE: TOASTING NUTS AND COOLING
PREP: ABOUT 35 MINUTES
BAKE: 70 MINUTES, PLUS 1 HOUR IN OVEN (HEAT OFF)
COOL: 1 HOUR
CHILL: OVERNIGHT
OVEN: 350°

Here's another decadent cheesecake, perfect for any late autumn or winter holiday. **Be sure to prepare this the night before serving.**

6 ounces pecan halves, lightly toasted and cooled in advance, divided
8 ounces purchased crispy gingersnap cookies
8 ounces graham crackers
¼ cup all-purpose flour
1¼ cups sugar, divided
6 tablespoons salted butter, melted
½ cup packed light brown sugar
4 teaspoons pumpkin pie spice, divided (see page xvi for a recipe)
½ teaspoon salt, divided
¼ cup half-and-half
1½ pounds light cream cheese (Neufchâtel), softened
3 large eggs
¾ cup plain pumpkin
¼ cup bourbon (or whiskey or orange juice)
1 teaspoon vanilla extract

GARNISH: whipped cream and a drizzle of caramel sauce

THE NIGHT BEFORE SERVING: Preheat the oven to 350°. Coat a 9" springform pan with cooking spray or grease lightly. Wrap a 12" square of aluminum foil around the outside bottom of the pan; set aside. Place the gingersnaps and graham crackers in a large food processor. Process to crumbs. Remove 1 cup of the crumbs and place in a medium bowl; set aside. Add the flour, ¼ cup sugar, and 2 ounces of the prepared pecans to the processor and process well. Add the butter and process well. Scrape the sides and bottom and process again. Pour into the prepared pan. Press the mixture 2" up the sides, then press evenly on the bottom. Reuse the processor; don't bother to wash it.

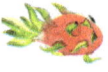

FINELY chop the remaining pecans and add to the reserved crumb mixture. Add the brown sugar, 1 tablespoon pumpkin pie spice, ¼ teaspoon salt, and the half-and-half to the bowl and mix well. Set aside.

PLACE the cream cheese, eggs, 1 cup sugar, pumpkin, bourbon, remaining 1 teaspoon pumpkin pie spice and ¼ teaspoon salt, and vanilla in the processor and process well. Scrape the sides and bottom of the bowl and process again. Pour into the prepared pan. Dollop the reserved crumb mixture all over in generous tablespoons. Gently press most of the crumbs into the cheese mixture while leaving some of it exposed on the top. Bake 70 minutes. Turn off the heat and leave in the oven 1 hour. Place on a rack for 1 hour. Refrigerate overnight. Release the pan sides, using a sharp knife to assist you if necessary, and slice. Garnish, if you like. Cover and refrigerate the leftovers. Makes 12–16 servings.

Cyrus's No-Bake Pumpkin Tarts

PREP: ABOUT 30 MINUTES
CHILL: AT LEAST 5 HOURS (OVERNIGHT IS BEST)

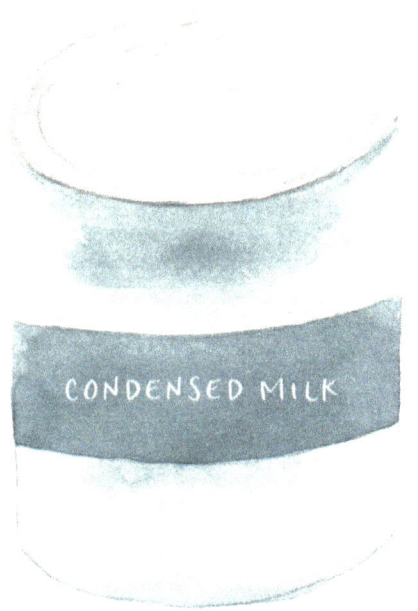

These little tarts can be made the night before you need them or first thing in the morning, since they need about 5–6 hours to set up in the refrigerator. They are perfect to serve to children, who will be happy to get a whole pie for themselves!

You could also make two regular-sized pies with this filling. If you choose this option, you will need to assemble them the night before serving so the pumpkin mixture will have adequate time to firm up. You can certainly make your own graham cracker crust, if you are inclined to do so.

Chapter Eleven: Thanksgiving 203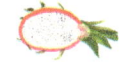

- 18 mini graham cracker pie crusts (such as Keebler)
- 15-ounce can plain pumpkin
- 1 pound mascarpone cheese, softened
- 14-ounce can sweetened condensed milk (fat-free or light varieties are fine to use)
- ¼ cup packed light brown sugar
- 1 tablespoon pumpkin pie spice (see page xvi for a recipe)
- ½ teaspoon salt
- 1½ tablespoons raw sugar (turbinado; cinnamon sugar would also work)

GARNISH:

A dollop or squirt of whipped cream is all you need.

AT LEAST FIVE OR SIX HOURS BEFORE SERVING (OVERNIGHT IS OPTIMAL): Set all the pie crusts on baking sheets just for easier transportation. Place the pumpkin, cheese, condensed milk, brown sugar, pumpkin pie spice, and salt in a very large bowl. Beat with a hand mixer until well blended. Spoon into each pie crust evenly. Sprinkle each with some raw sugar. Refrigerate until fairly firm, at least 5–6 hours. Garnish, if you like. Refrigerate the leftovers, but don't freeze them. You can cover them loosely with plastic wrap for longer storage. They will last for quite a few days in the fridge. Makes 18.

Pumpkin Sparkle Pie

IN ADVANCE: PIE CRUST PREPARATION
IN ADVANCE: TOASTING NUTS, COOLING, AND CHOPPING
PREP: ABOUT 20 MINUTES
BAKE: 50 MINUTES
COOL: 2 HOURS
CHILL: OVERNIGHT
OVEN: 375°

In the right light, the top of this pie will sparkle, at least in theory. **Make this the night before serving.**

A single pie crust (homemade is preferred; see page xix)
4 ounces pecans, lightly toasted, cooled, and chopped coarsely in advance
15-ounce can plain pumpkin
2 large eggs
¾ cup packed light brown sugar
½ cup half-and-half
1 teaspoon ground cinnamon
½ teaspoon salt
½ teaspoon ground allspice
½ teaspoon ground cloves
½ teaspoon ground nutmeg
½ teaspoon ground mace
4 ounces sweetened coconut flakes
2 ounces crystallized ginger, finely chopped
2 tablespoons caramel sauce (purchased or homemade)
¼ cup raw sugar (turbinado)

Garnish: whipped cream

The night before serving: Prepare your pie crust as necessary. When it is ready to go, preheat the oven to 375°. Roll out the crust and place it in a 9½" (glass) pie dish. Crimp or flute the edge generously (easier to do with a homemade crust). If using a homemade crust, you can cut small decorations out of the scraps if you like.

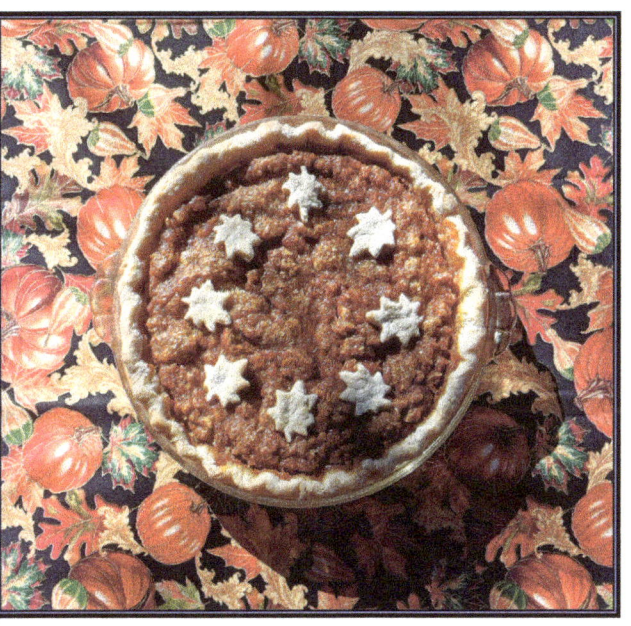

Place the pumpkin, eggs, brown sugar, half-and-half, and the 6 seasonings in a large bowl. Whisk well. Add the pecans, coconut, and ginger and mix well. Pour into the prepared crust. Drizzle the caramel sauce all over. Sprinkle the raw sugar all over. Decorate, if desired. Bake 50 minutes. Place on a rack and cool for 2 hours. Refrigerate overnight. Let stand at room temperature for 2–3 hours before serving. Garnish, as desired. Cover and refrigerate the leftovers. Makes 8 servings.

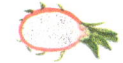

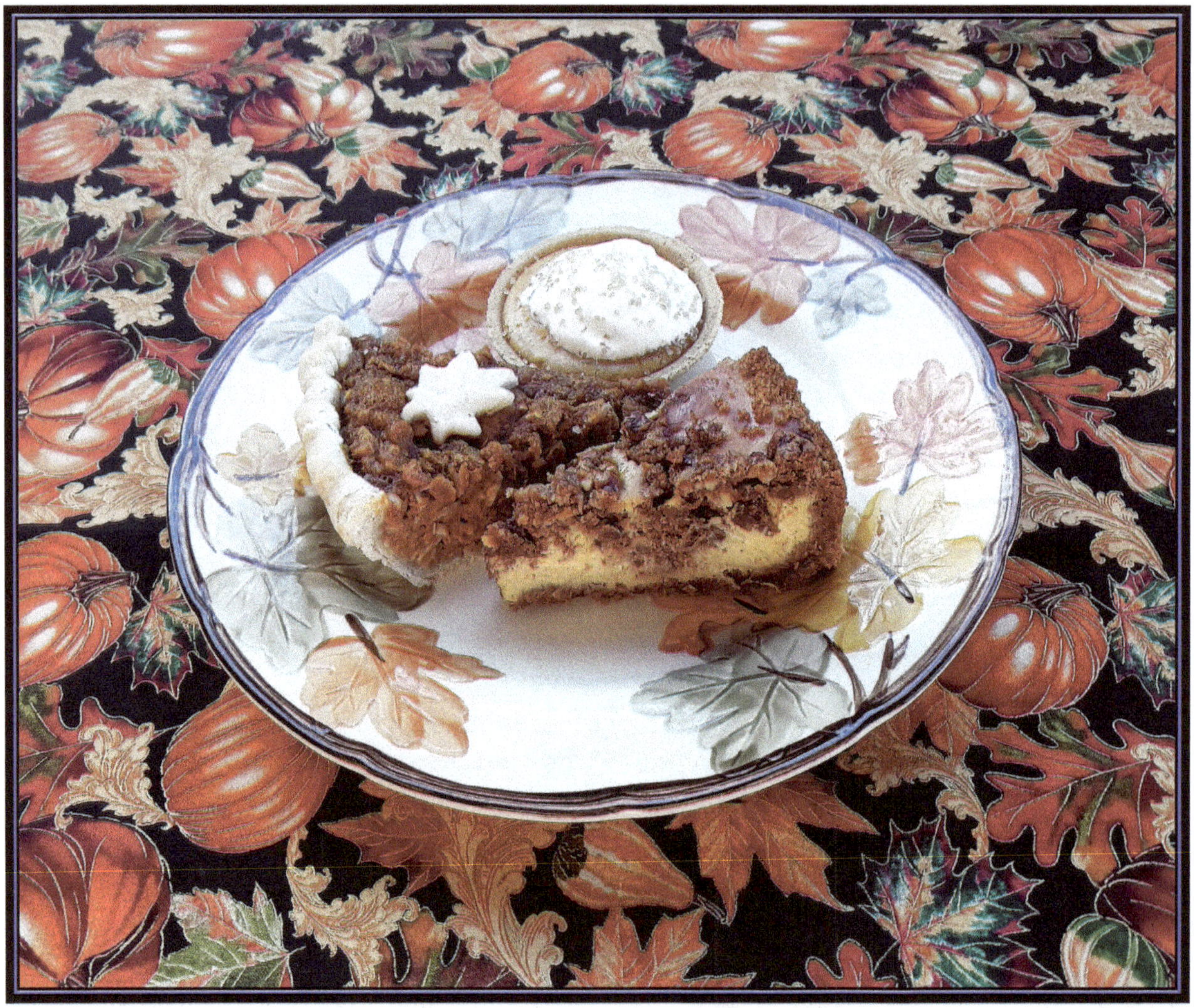

CLOCKWISE, FROM TOP:
Cyrus's No-Bake Pumpkin Tarts, page 203
Warren's Pumpkin Cheesecake, page 202
Pumpkin Sparkle Pie, page 204

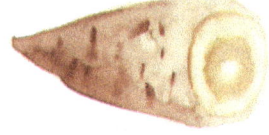

William's Chili Pumpkin Bread with Pepitas Honey Butter

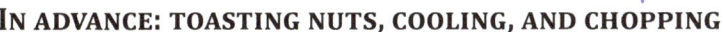

IN ADVANCE: TOASTING NUTS, COOLING, AND CHOPPING
PREP: 15 MINUTES
BAKE: 1 HOUR
COOL: 1½ HOURS
OVEN: 350°

This is a hearty quick bread, perfect for dessert or even breakfast.

3 ounces pecans, lightly toasted, cooled, and chopped finely in advance
1 cup sugar
½ cup packed light brown sugar
1 cup plain pumpkin
2 large eggs
½ cup vegetable oil
⅓ cup water
2 cups all-purpose flour
1 tablespoon pumpkin pie spice (see page xvi for a recipe)
1 tablespoon chili powder
1 teaspoon baking soda
1 teaspoon salt
½ teaspoon baking powder

PEPITAS HONEY BUTTER, RECIPE BELOW

PREHEAT the oven to 350°. Coat a 9" by 5" loaf pan with cooking spray or grease lightly. Place the sugar, brown sugar, pumpkin, eggs, oil, and water in a large bowl and whisk until well combined. Combine the prepared pecans and the remaining ingredients well in a medium bowl. Add to the sugar mixture and mix well (wipe this bowl out and use for the butter below). Pour into the prepared pan. Bake 1 hour. Place on a rack and cool 30 minutes. Remove from the pan and cool on the rack 1 hour before cutting. Slice and serve with softened honey butter. Cover and store at room temperature. Makes 10–12 servings.

Pepitas Honey Butter

Prep: 5 minutes

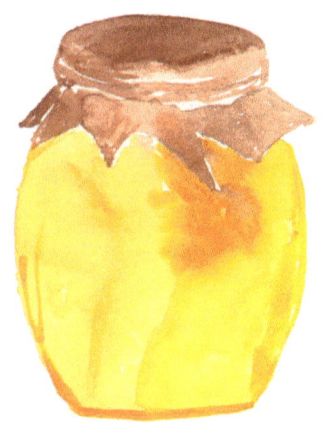

½ cup salted butter, very soft
2 tablespoons honey
½ teaspoon vanilla extract
1 ounce roasted and salted pepitas (pumpkin seeds)

PLACE the butter, honey, and vanilla in a medium bowl and combine well. Add the pepitas and mix in well. Cover and refrigerate the leftovers, but bring them to a spreadable room temperature to serve. Makes ¾ cup.

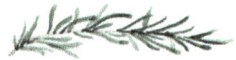

Isabella's Pumpkin Pie Ice Cream

Active prep: about 19 minutes
Mix: 35 minutes
Freeze: 3–4 hours

This is my daughter Chloë's favorite ice cream. She loved it even more when she was pregnant with her daughter. Then her daughter also ended up loving it, so I named it after her—seeing that she enjoyed it both *in utero* and *ex*.

¾ cup half-and-half
¼ cup heavy cream
½ cup liquid egg substitute
1 cup plain pumpkin
½ cup packed light brown sugar
¼ cup plus 2 tablespoons sugar
1 tablespoon pumpkin pie spice (see page xvi for a recipe)
½ teaspoon salt, divided
3 tablespoons salted butter
2 ounces pecans, coarsely chopped
2 ounces graham crackers, broken into ½" pieces

PLACE the half-and-half, cream, egg substitute, pumpkin, brown sugar, ¼ cup sugar, pumpkin pie spice, and ¼ teaspoon salt in a 4-cup glass measuring cup. Whisk until well combined. Pour into a 6-cup automatic ice cream maker and mix 30 minutes.

MEANWHILE, melt the butter in a medium skillet over rather high heat. Add the 2 tablespoons sugar and ¼ teaspoon salt and stir to dissolve. Add the pecans and graham crackers and sauté 1 minute, stirring constantly. Take off the heat and let it stand.

WHEN the ice cream is almost finished mixing, gently break up the nut mixture with a spatula or wooden spoon and add it to the machine. Mix another 5 minutes. Place into a 6-cup container. Cover and freeze anywhere from 3–4 hours, depending on how firm you like your ice cream. Stir a few times. Cover and freeze the leftovers; when it has become very firm, let it stand on your counter for about 15 minutes before serving again. Makes about 5 cups.

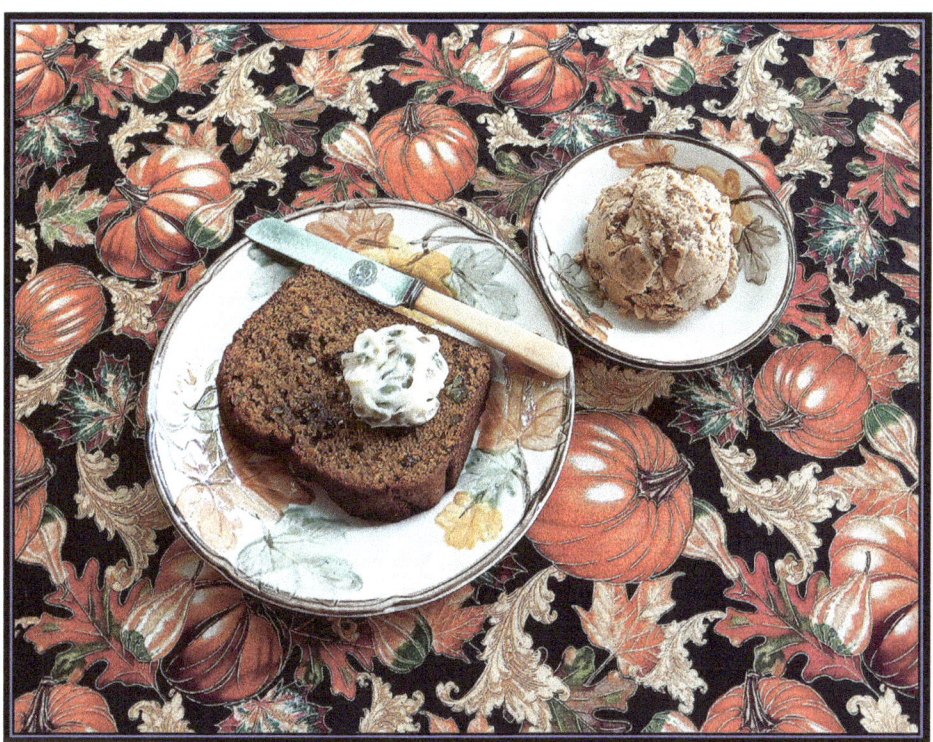

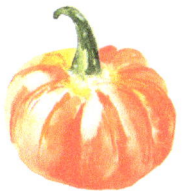

LEFT:
William's Chili Pumpkin Bread with Pepitas Honey Butter, page 207

RIGHT:
Isabella's Pumpkin Pie Ice Cream, page 208

Pumpkin Pancakes

IN ADVANCE: TOASTING NUTS, COOLING, AND CHOPPING
START TO FINISH: ABOUT 30 MINUTES

Just in case having pumpkin for dessert isn't enough, here is a breakfast recipe. Maybe this is still dessert.

2 ounces pecans, lightly toasted, cooled, and chopped finely in advance
1 cup all-purpose flour
¼ cup cake flour
2 tablespoons sugar
1 tablespoon baking powder
¾ teaspoon salt
4 teaspoons pumpkin pie spice (see page xvi for a recipe)
4 ounces white chocolate chips (you may use a 4-ounce bar of white chocolate instead, chopped into whatever size bits/chunks you feel are appropriate)
1 cup buttermilk
½ cup 1% milk
1 large egg
2 tablespoons vegetable oil
1 teaspoon vanilla extract
1 teaspoon maple extract
¾ cup plain pumpkin

GARNISH: spreadable or melted butter and maple syrup

In a large bowl, combine the 2 flours, sugar, baking powder, salt, pumpkin pie spice, white chocolate chips, and the prepared pecans. Set aside. Place the buttermilk, milk, egg, oil, and the 2 extracts in a 4-cup glass measuring cup. Whisk well, then add the pumpkin and whisk again. Add all to the flour mixture and whisk until combined well. Let it stand while you heat the griddle.

COAT a griddle or a very large skillet with cooking spray. Heat to moderately high. When ready, pour the batter in about ¼-cup portions. Cook until a few bubbles appear on top. Carefully flip over. Modulate heat to prevent burning. Repeat with the remaining batter, spraying the griddle again. Serve with butter and maple syrup, if desired. Cover and refrigerate the leftovers. Makes 15–16.

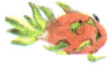

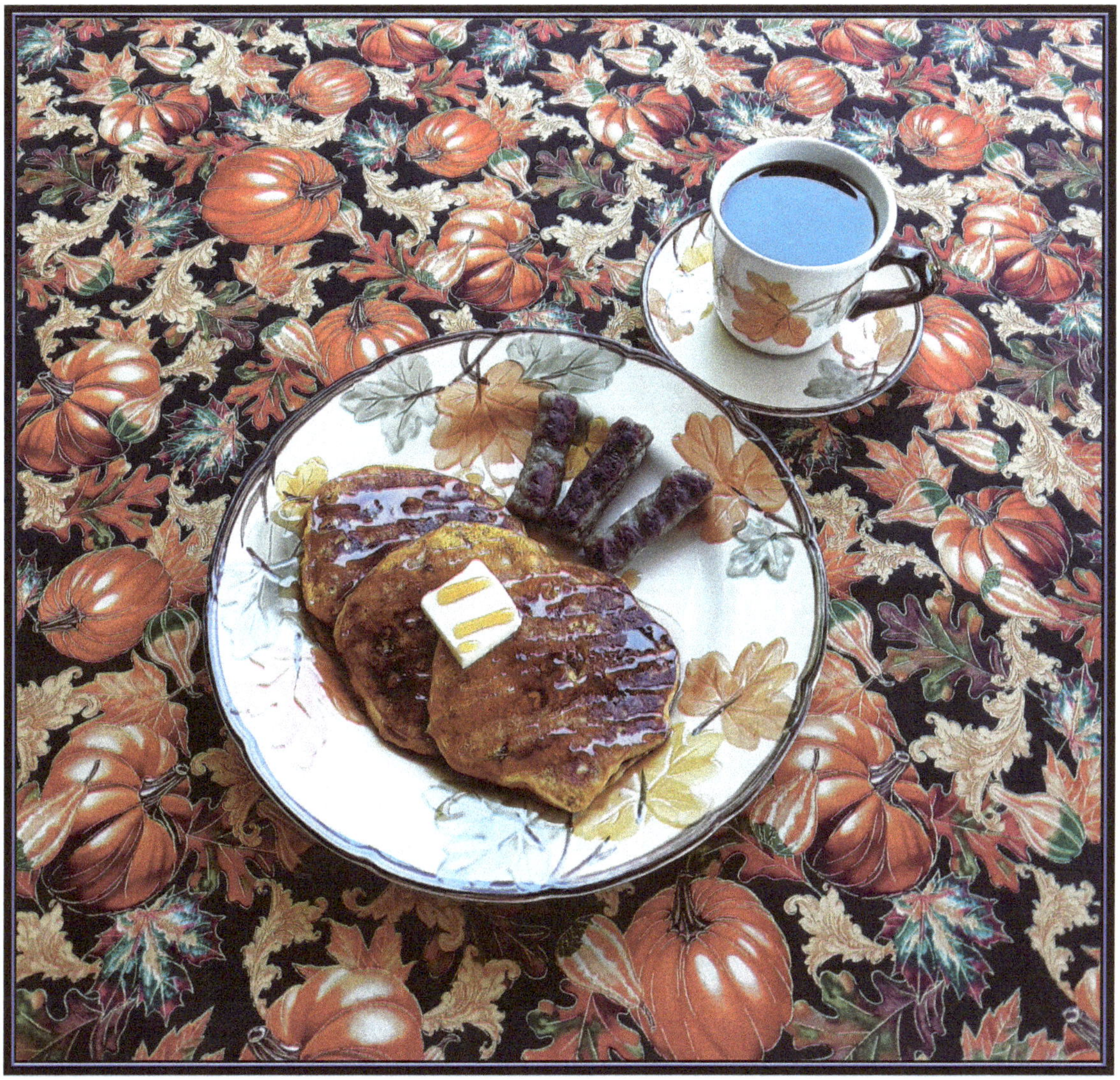

CHAPTER TWELVE

PASTA

- Spaghetti Western
- Saucy Soupy Mac & Cheese
- Cajun-Style Fettuccine
- Upscale Mac & Cheese
- Vodka Penne
- Hearty Bacony Mac & Cheese
- Santa Fe Fettuccine
- Creamy Dreamy Mac & Cheese
- Frankenstein's Bowties
- Sheldon's Spaghetti
- Tony's Tuna Casserole
- Halfling/Monster Mac & Cheese

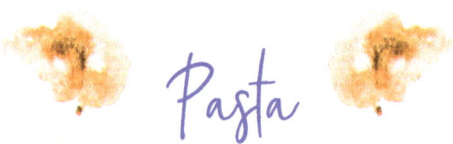

Pasta

So, MAYBE THERE are a million varieties of pasta shapes? Maybe. And cooks and chefs are always debating about which kinds are best for holding sauces or which kinds have the best chewability. Don't even start on what *al dente* means because we all have our preferences as to how soft we want our pasta (though if it's falling apart on you, it's probably way too soft).

In the following recipes, I have listed particular types of pasta as guidelines, but you are free to substitute various items if you need to do so. If I say spaghetti, you can substitute fettuccine or linguine or long fusilli. If I say elbow macaroni, you can substitute ditalini or orecchiette. If I say (short) fusilli, you can substitute bowties, campanelle, rotini, wagon wheels, etc. How about some pasta shaped like Darth Vader? Or some tri-color dinosaur shapes? Do you want to make your own pasta? Go for it if you have the time. You can use anything you like, though obviously, your cooking times might change according to your chosen pasta shape. I love to pick out exotic pastas when I get the chance.

Green chile is a welcome addition to any of the recipes that don't already have some in this chapter; use anywhere from four to eight ounces, roasted, chopped, and drained.

Portion sizes are suggestive and are based on a strangely elaborate rubric that I invented just for these types of recipes. I remember an old *Bon Appétit* recipe that made a 13" by 9" pan of lasagna that they said served six people, but when I make a pan like that, I cut it into 12 or 15 portions. Then people can take two if they need to. I also have a cookbook by Giada de Laurentiis that contains various recipes requiring a pound of pasta, with meats and vegetables, serving four people. Yes, FOUR people. So, I guess it depends on whether you want a Cheesecake Factory-sized bowl of pasta for dinner or a more moderately-portioned Lean Cuisine-sized bowl for lunch—then, you never know whether somebody will want seconds or leftovers for another meal. All the recipes in this chapter are based on eight or twelve ounces of pasta. Some have meats and/or vegetables as well. Everything can be doubled easily or cut in half; plus, pasta dishes generally keep well and can be frozen. Just add a dash of an appropriate liquid to compensate for any dryness that might occur when you reheat, such as milk, cream, water, or broth.

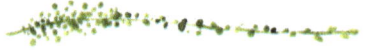

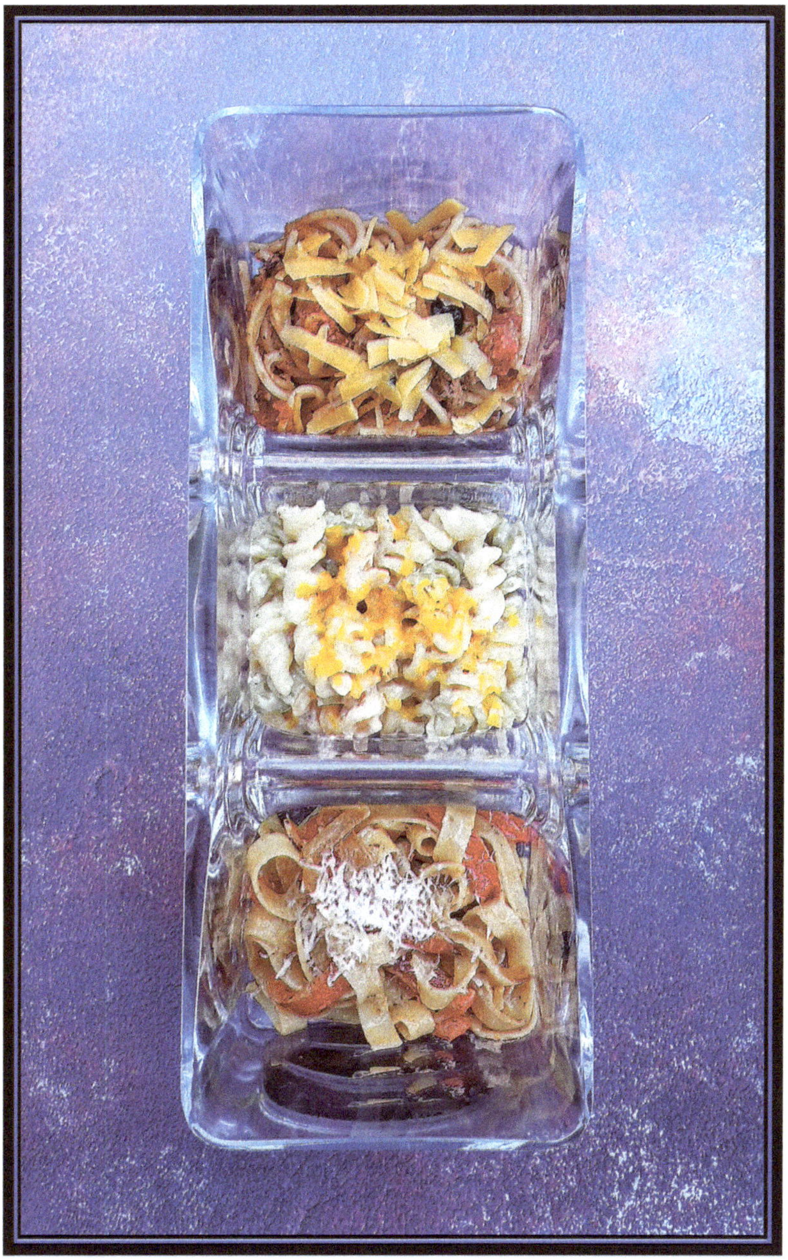

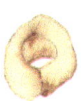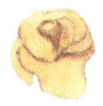

TOP TO BOTTOM:
Spaghetti Western, page 216
Saucy Soupy Mac & Cheese, page 218
Cajun-Style Fettuccine, page 219

Chapter Twelve: Pasta   215

Spaghetti Western

PREP: ABOUT 45 MINUTES
BAKE: 30 MINUTES
STAND: 15 MINUTES
OVEN: 350°

Perhaps not a dish served in the Wild West, but you can certainly crank up an old movie to set the mood, say, something by Sergio Leone. For serious Westerns, I tend to gravitate toward things like *Unforgiven* or *Deadwood,* but for funny Westerns, you can't beat *Blazing Saddles.* None of those really qualify as true spaghetti Westerns. Check out my bean-centered recipes to accompany a viewing of *Blazing Saddles.* This casserole ends up with some deliciously crispy noodles on top.

1½ cups mild olives, pitted, drained, and sliced (green or black)
14.5-ounce can diced tomatoes
3 quarts water
1½ teaspoons salt, divided
8 ounces spaghetti, broken into thirds
1 pound ground beef sirloin
1 tablespoon minced garlic
1 cup onion, coarsely chopped
¾ cup half-and-half
¼ cup heavy cream
¼ cup tomato paste
4 ounces roasted and chopped green chile, with juice
1 teaspoon dried oregano (2–3 tablespoons fresh, minced)
¾ teaspoon black pepper
¾ teaspoon garlic salt
¾ teaspoon onion salt
6 ounces sharp cheddar cheese, shredded; divided

PLACE the prepared olives in a medium bowl. Drain the tomatoes well in a large colander; add to the olives. Set aside; reuse the colander.

BRING water and 1 teaspoon salt to a boil in a 6-quart saucepan. Cook the spaghetti as directed on the package. Reserve ½ cup cooking liquid, then drain in the same colander. Set aside; reuse the pot.

PREHEAT the oven to 350°. Coat an 11″ by 7″ baking dish with cooking spray and set aside. Coat the pot with cooking spray. Fry the beef, garlic, onion, and the remaining ½ teaspoon salt over very high heat, breaking up the meat until the pink is gone. Pour over the pasta in the colander. Reuse the pot.

WHISK the reserved pasta water, half-and-half, cream, tomato paste, green chile, and the 4 seasonings in the pot and cook over medium heat until well combined. Turn off the heat; add the olives and tomatoes. Add the pasta and meat and combine. Add 4 ounces of shredded cheddar and mix. Season, if necessary. Pour into the prepared pan. Bake 30 minutes.

REMOVE the dish from the oven and turn off the heat. Sprinkle the remaining cheese over evenly. Return to the oven and leave there 15 minutes. Cover and refrigerate the leftovers. Makes 4–6 main-dish servings; 8–12 side-dish servings.

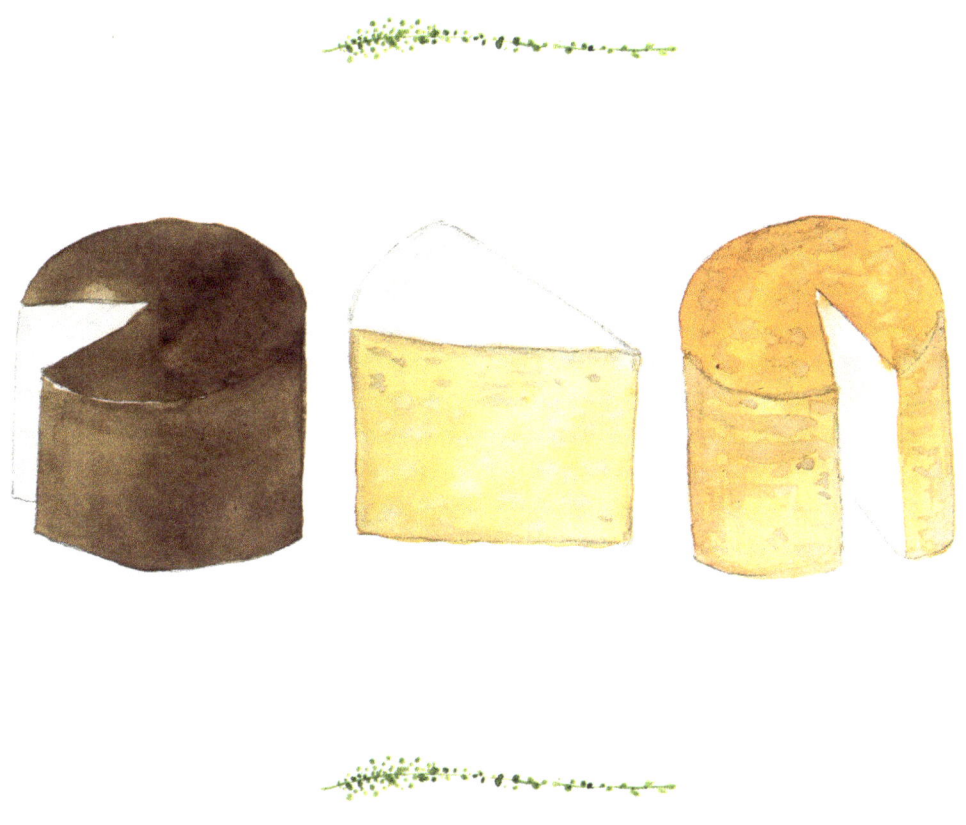

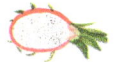

Chapter Twelve: Pasta   217

Saucy Soupy Mac & Cheese

START TO FINISH: ABOUT 42 MINUTES

We used to have a fun noodle restaurant in town, and a few of my recipes were developed to mimic their menu items. This one was my daughter Callista's favorite. If fontina cheese is hard to find, good substitutes are Havarti or Muenster.

This is meant to be kind of soupy in your bowl. If you would prefer it to be a little less so, cover the pot and let it stand for a minute or so; keep in mind that your cheese choice will affect the thickness of your sauce.

8 ounces fusilli or rotini
1 tablespoon salted butter
1 tablespoon all-purpose flour
½ teaspoon salt
½ teaspoon black pepper
12-ounce can evaporated milk (low-fat and fat-free are fine)
¼ cup heavy cream
4 ounces colby jack cheese, shredded
4 ounces fontina cheese, shredded

GARNISH: more colby jack cheese, finely shredded

COOK the fusilli as directed on the package in a 4-quart saucepan. Drain and set aside; reuse the pot. Melt the butter over rather high heat, then whisk in the flour, salt, and pepper. Slowly add the evaporated milk and cream and whisk over medium/high heat until it thickens slightly. Add the 2 cheeses and whisk until melted. Mix in the pasta. Season, as desired. Serve in bowls and garnish generously with more colby jack, if desired. Cover and refrigerate the leftovers. Makes 3–4 main-dish servings; 6–8 side-dish servings.

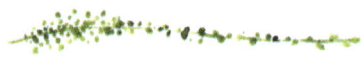

Cajun-Style Fettuccine

START TO FINISH: ABOUT 45 MINUTES

This is rather spicy (as it should be!), but of course you may increase the cayenne and hot sauce if you need to. I usually start heating my pasta water first, then I start the vegetable sauté, but I do have some high-altitude concerns where I live.

¼ cup salted butter
1 tablespoon minced garlic
2 cups onion, cut into ¼" slivers
2 large red bell peppers, cored and cut into ¼" slivers
½ cup dry white wine, such as chardonnay
1½ teaspoons salt
1 teaspoon black pepper
1 teaspoon cayenne pepper
1 teaspoon dried thyme (or 2–3 tablespoons fresh, minced)
1 teaspoon smoked paprika
1 teaspoon hot sauce
1 cup heavy cream
12 ounces fettuccine

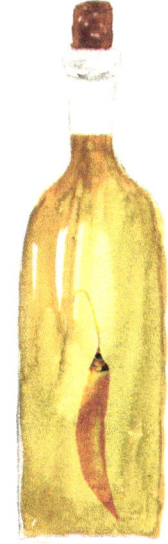

GARNISH: fresh Parmesan and/or Romano cheese, finely shredded

MELT the butter over very high heat in a 5-quart deep skillet. Add the garlic, onion, and bell pepper and sauté 5 minutes. Add the wine and boil 3 minutes. Add the 5 seasonings, hot sauce, and cream and bring to a boil. Cook, covered, on the lowest heat 10 minutes. Stir twice. Raise the heat to a low simmer and cook, uncovered, 7–8 minutes or so. Stir a few times.

MEANWHILE, cook the fettuccine as directed on the package in a 6-quart saucepan. Reserve ½ cup of the cooking liquid, then drain. Combine the pasta with the sauce in the pot or the skillet; either one is fine. Add some or all the reserved cooking liquid only if it seems to need it. Season, as desired. Garnish, if you like. Cover and refrigerate the leftovers. Makes 6–8 main-dish servings; 12–16 side-dish servings.

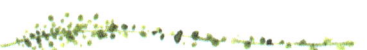

Upscale Mac & Cheese

PREP: ABOUT 35 MINUTES
BAKE: 30 MINUTES
STAND: 5 MINUTES
OVEN: 350°

This is only considered upscale because you get to use European cheeses, shallots, and panko.

8 ounces small macaroni (such as elbows or ditalini)
3 tablespoons salted butter, divided
¾ cup shallots, finely chopped
1 tablespoon all-purpose flour
¾ teaspoon salt
¾ teaspoon white pepper
¾ teaspoon dry mustard
1½ cups 1% milk
½ cup heavy cream
5.2-ounce package of Boursin cheese (or about ⅔ cup
    of any soft garlic/herb-type of cheese)
4 ounces Gorgonzola cheese, crumbled
4 ounces Gruyère cheese, shredded (Swiss or Jarlsberg would also be fine)
½ cup panko breadcrumbs (plain or seasoned)

COOK pasta as directed on the package in a 4-quart saucepan. Drain and set aside; reuse the pot.
   PREHEAT the oven to 350°. Coat a 2-quart casserole dish with cooking spray. Place 1 tablespoon butter in the saucepan and melt over rather high heat. Sauté the shallots 2 minutes. Add the flour and the 3 seasonings and whisk until combined. Add the milk and cream. Whisk over medium/high heat until bubbly and thicker. Add the 3 cheeses and whisk in until melted. Season, if necessary. Mix in the pasta and pour all into the prepared dish. Sprinkle the breadcrumbs evenly over all the pasta. Melt the remaining butter in a small glass bowl in the microwave on HIGH (about 20–30 seconds total); drizzle over all. Bake 30 minutes. Remove and let stand 5 minutes before serving. Cover and refrigerate the leftovers. Makes 4–6 main-dish servings; 8–12 side-dish servings.

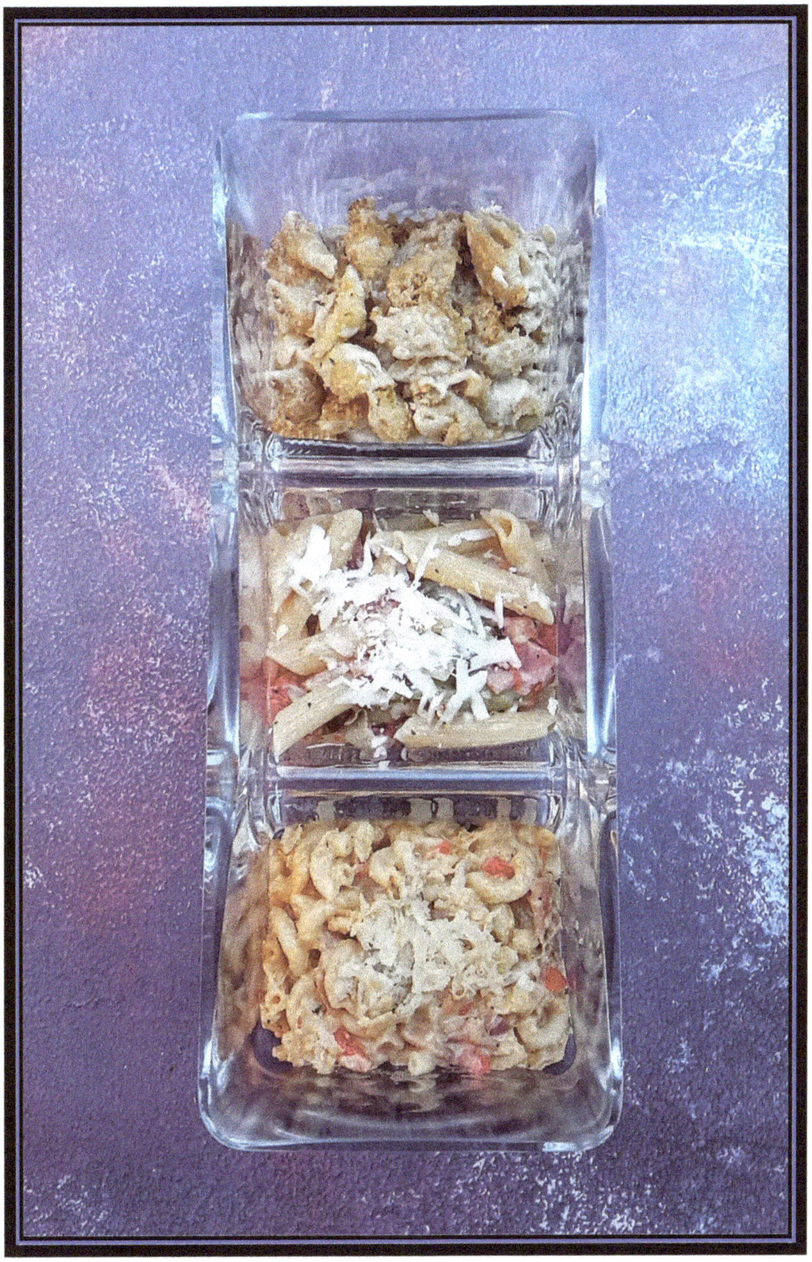

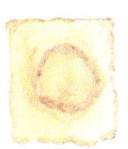
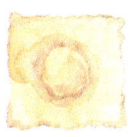
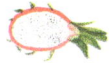

TOP TO BOTTOM:
Upscale Mac & Cheese, page 220
Vodka Penne, page 222
Hearty Bacony Mac & Cheese, page 223

Chapter Twelve: Pasta   221

Vodka Penne

START TO FINISH: ABOUT 40 MINUTES

Feel free to substitute some low-sodium chicken broth for the vodka if you like.

14.5-ounce can diced tomatoes
14-ounce can quartered artichoke hearts
8 ounces penne
2 tablespoons olive oil
½ cup onion, coarsely chopped
8 ounces cooked ham, coarsely chopped
½ cup plain vodka
¾ cup heavy cream
½ teaspoon dried basil
    (2–3 tablespoons fresh, minced)
½ teaspoon crushed red pepper flakes
½ teaspoon salt
½ teaspoon black pepper
3 ounces Parmesan and/or Romano cheese,
    finely shredded

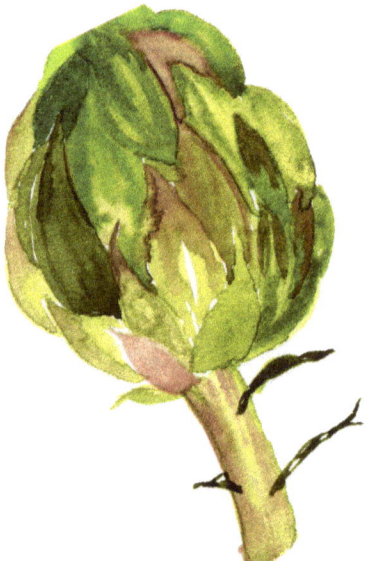

GARNISH: additional Parmesan and/or Romano cheese, finely shredded

DRAIN the tomatoes and artichoke hearts well, then set them aside in a medium bowl. Cook the pasta as directed on the package in a 4-quart saucepan. Reserve ¼ cup of the cooking liquid, then drain and set aside.

    MEANWHILE, sauté the oil, onion, and ham in a 5-quart deep skillet over rather high heat for 5 minutes. Add the vodka and boil for 2 minutes. Add the cream, the 4 seasonings, and the reserved tomatoes and artichoke hearts. Bring to a boil. Cook on a medium, gentle simmer, uncovered, 8 minutes. Stir a few times.

    ADD the cheese and raise the heat to medium. Cook another 2 minutes, mixing well. Add the pasta and combine well. Add any or all the reserved pasta cooking water only if it seems to need it. Season, as desired. Garnish with more cheese. Cover and refrigerate the leftovers. Makes 4–6 main-dish servings; 8–12 side-dish servings.

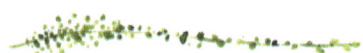

Hearty Bacony Mac & Cheese

Prep: about 44 minutes
Bake: 30 minutes
Stand: 5 minutes
Oven: 350°

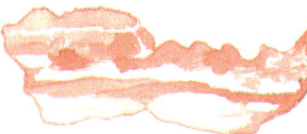

This is lovely with a green salad or vegetable on the side.

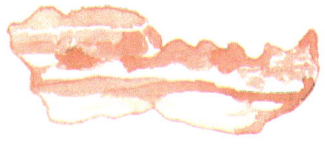

8 ounces elbow macaroni
4-ounce jar diced pimientos
2 tablespoons salted butter
½ cup red onion, coarsely chopped
1 tablespoon minced garlic
3 ounces precooked bacon, cut into ¼″ slices
2 tablespoons all-purpose flour
1 teaspoon smoked paprika
½ teaspoon black pepper
½ teaspoon salt
½ teaspoon crushed red pepper flakes
1 cup low-sodium chicken broth
12-ounce can evaporated milk (light and fat-free are okay)
8 ounces sharp cheddar cheese, shredded
2 tablespoons seasoned dry breadcrumbs
2 ounces Parmesan and/or Romano cheese, finely shredded

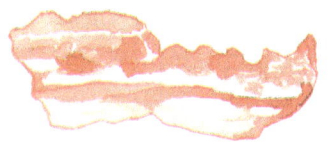

COOK the pasta as directed on the package in a 4-quart saucepan. Drain and let it stand. Pour the pimientos over the pasta and set aside. Reuse the pot.

    PREHEAT the oven to 350°. Coat a 2-quart casserole dish with cooking spray or grease lightly. Melt the butter in the saucepan and sauté the onion, garlic, and bacon over moderately high heat for 4 to 5 minutes, until the onions start to brown a bit. Add the flour and the 4 seasonings and whisk in. Add the broth and evaporated milk and cook over medium/high heat, whisking until thicker. Add the cheddar cheese and mix to melt. Add the pasta and pimientos and mix well. Pour into the prepared dish. Combine the breadcrumbs and Parmesan cheese in a small bowl. Sprinkle over the pasta evenly. Bake 30 minutes. Remove from the oven and let stand 5 minutes before serving. Cover and refrigerate the leftovers. Makes 4–6 main-dish servings; 8–12 side-dish servings.

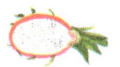

Santa Fe Fettuccine

START TO FINISH: ABOUT 40 MINUTES

Here is another dish loosely based on one of our favorites from our now-defunct noodle restaurant. The restaurant used to make this with curly-edged fettuccine, but this could be difficult to purchase. Nevertheless, any kind of long, rather wide pasta will work here. Half a pound of cooked protein can be added to the sauce; pretty much any variety will be fine, though chopped bacon gets my vote. Maybe chicken or shrimp. Chicken and bacon? YES. Don't like pine nuts? Substitute roasted and salted pumpkin seeds (pepitas).

⅔ cup pine nuts
¼ cup salted butter
1½ teaspoons salt, divided
1 teaspoon sugar
1 teaspoon black pepper
1 tablespoon minced garlic
2 cups onion, cut into ¼" slivers
12 ounces fettuccine
8 ounces roasted and chopped green chile, with juice
1¼ cups heavy cream
1 pound Roma tomatoes
4 ounces Parmesan and/or Romano cheese, finely shredded

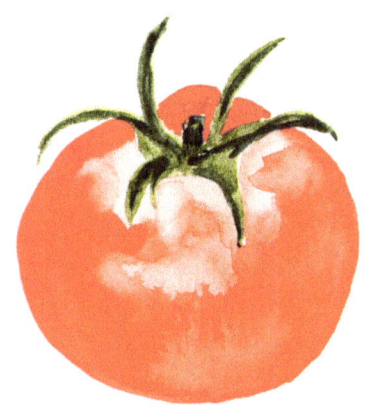

GARNISH: more finely grated fresh Parmesan and/or Romano cheese

PLACE nuts in a 5-quart deep skillet and toast them over rather high heat for 2–3 minutes, shaking the pan often. Pour into a small bowl and reuse the pan. Place the butter in the skillet and melt over rather high heat. Add 1 teaspoon salt, sugar, pepper, garlic, and onion and sauté over moderate heat 8 minutes, stirring often.

MEANWHILE, cook the fettuccine and ½ teaspoon salt in a 6-quart saucepan as directed on the package. Reserve ½ cup of the cooking liquid; drain and set aside.

ADD the chile and cream to the skillet and bring to a boil. Cook over low heat, uncovered, 15 minutes. Maintain a gentle, rolling simmer and stir a few times.

CUT the tomatoes into chunks, about ½" or so. Scoop them up with your hands and add them to the skillet, leaving most of any liquid on your cutting board. Raise the heat to medium/high and cook another minute. Add some (or all) of the reserved pasta cooking liquid only if it seems to need it. Add the drained pasta to the skillet and mix in well, cooking for another minute or so. Season, if desired. Sprinkle the cheese all over, then the nuts. Toss lightly, then garnish as you wish. Cover and refrigerate the leftovers. Makes 6–8 main-dish servings; 12–16 side-dish servings.

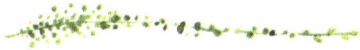

Creamy Dreamy Mac & Cheese

PREP: ABOUT 40 MINUTES
BAKE: 20 MINUTES
STAND: 5 MINUTES
OVEN: 350°

I'm normally not a fan of overly processed cheeses, but American adds the right touch to this dish. You can substitute yellow American and cheddar if the white varieties are unavailable, but I was trying to make this light and dreamy, like a cloud—a cheesy, buttery cloud coming out of your oven.

12 ounces elbow macaroni
4 tablespoons salted butter, divided
2 tablespoons all-purpose flour
¾ teaspoon salt
¾ teaspoon white pepper
1 cup 1% milk
1 cup half-and-half
¾ cup low-sodium chicken broth
4 ounces light cream cheese (Neufchâtel), softened
4 ounces white American cheese, coarsely chopped
4 ounces extra-sharp white cheddar cheese, shredded
¼ cup panko breadcrumbs
1 ounce Parmesan and/or Romano cheese, finely shredded

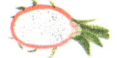

COOK pasta as directed on the package in a 6-quart saucepan. Drain and set aside. Reuse the pot.

PREHEAT the oven to 350°. Coat an 11″ by 7″ baking dish with cooking spray or grease lightly. Melt 2 tablespoons butter in the saucepan. Add the flour, salt, and pepper. Combine with a whisk over rather high heat until blended well. Slowly add the milk, half-and-half, and broth and whisk over medium heat until thicker and smooth. Add the 3 cheeses and whisk to melt. Add the pasta and mix in well. Season, if desired. Pour into the prepared dish. Place on a large baking sheet.

COMBINE the panko and Parmesan in a medium bowl. Sprinkle over the pasta evenly. Place the remaining butter in a small microwave-safe bowl. Microwave on HIGH for 20 seconds or so until completely melted, then drizzle over all. Bake 20 minutes. Remove from the oven and let stand 5 minutes before serving. Cover and refrigerate any leftovers. Makes 4–6 main-dish servings; 8–12 side-dish servings.

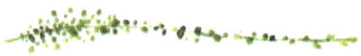

Frankenstein's Bowties

START TO FINISH: ABOUT 47 MINUTES

This recipe was originally based on leftovers from The Mile High Boil (page 138), but it sort of mutated and evolved into being a creature that had merit on its own; hence, it has its own spot in a separate chapter. And isn't that all the original Creature character wanted? Recognition? And vengeance. But mainly recognition. Any chunky, medium-sized pasta will work well here. Any sort of smoked sausage variety is also fine.

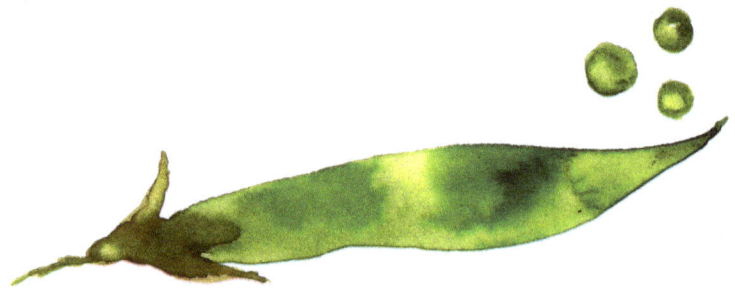

2 quarts water
1 teaspoon salt
8 ounces farfalle (bowtie pasta)
2 tablespoons salted butter
1 cup red onion, coarsely chopped
1 cup frozen peas
1 cup carrot, peeled and shredded
1 pound smoked sausage, cut into ¼" slices
½ cup heavy cream
2 tablespoons stone ground mustard
1 tablespoon packed light brown sugar
1 teaspoon Old Bay Seasoning
½ teaspoon crushed red pepper flakes
½ teaspoon prepared horseradish

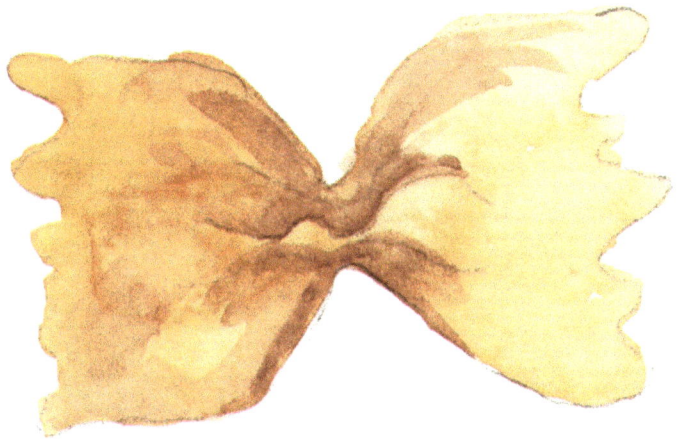

BRING the water and salt to a boil in a 6-quart saucepan. Add the pasta and cook as directed on the package. Reserve ½ cup of the cooking liquid in a 2-cup glass measuring cup and set aside. Drain the pasta and set aside. Reuse the pot.

COAT the saucepan with cooking spray. Melt the butter over rather high heat. Add the onion, peas, carrot, and sausage and sauté 5 minutes.

ADD the remaining ingredients to the reserved pasta water and whisk well. Add to the saucepan and bring to a boil. Cook on medium/low heat 5 minutes, uncovered. Stir a few times. Add the pasta and mix well. Cook another 3–4 minutes on rather high heat, stirring frequently until the pasta is completely coated with sauce. Season, as necessary. Cover and refrigerate the leftovers. Makes 4–6 main-dish servings; 8–12 side-dish servings.

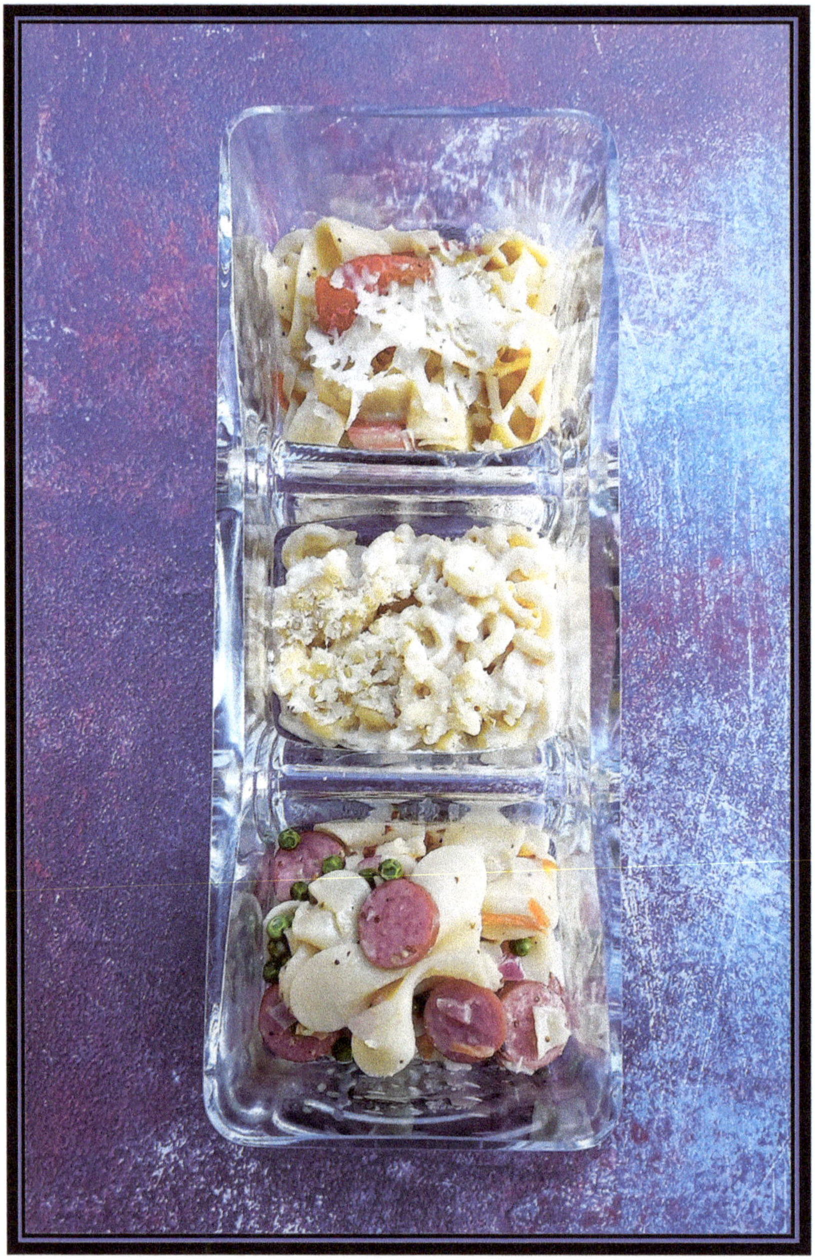

TOP TO BOTTOM:
Santa Fe Fettuccine, page 224
Creamy Dreamy Mac & Cheese, page 225
Frankenstein's Bowties, page 226

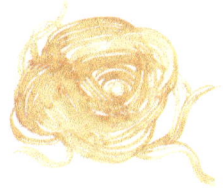

 228   Celebrating Comfy, Cozy Foods from North America: CH&M, Volume 3

Sheldon's Spaghetti

START TO FINISH: ABOUT 35 MINUTES

One day, we were watching *Young Sheldon,* and the beleaguered mom character put a giant bowl of spaghetti with hot dogs on the table. And (of course) my husband said that sounded really good. It is. You could go nuts and add a tablespoon of garlic powder to the sauce. I'm doubtful that Sheldon's mom, Mary, would do this (because garlic is Satan's seasoning), but you can. You could also substitute other varieties of hot dogs or items such as bratwurst. This is probably the easiest main-dish recipe in the whole cookbook. Bazinga!

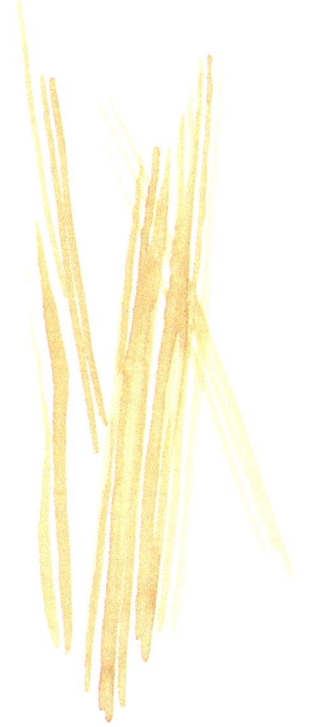

12 ounces spaghetti
24-ounce jar of prepared marinara sauce,
     any variety (3 cups)
2 tablespoons water
12-ounce package of good-quality beef hot dogs

GARNISH:

    Only dry Parmesan and/or Romano cheese will do here.

COOK the spaghetti as directed on the package in a 6-quart saucepan. Place the sauce and water in a 3-quart saucepan. Cut the hot dogs into ¼" slices and add to the sauce, along with any juices from the package. Cook on medium/low heat (a gentle simmer), covered, while the pasta cooks. Stir a few times.

    DRAIN the pasta; immediately place it back in the pot. Mix in the sauce. Season, if necessary. Garnish with lots of dry Parmesan cheese. Makes 6–8 main-dish servings; 12–16 side-dish servings.

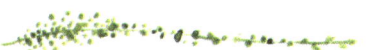

Tony's Tuna Casserole

PREP: ABOUT 38 MINUTES
BAKE: 30 MINUTES
STAND: 5 MINUTES
OVEN: 400°

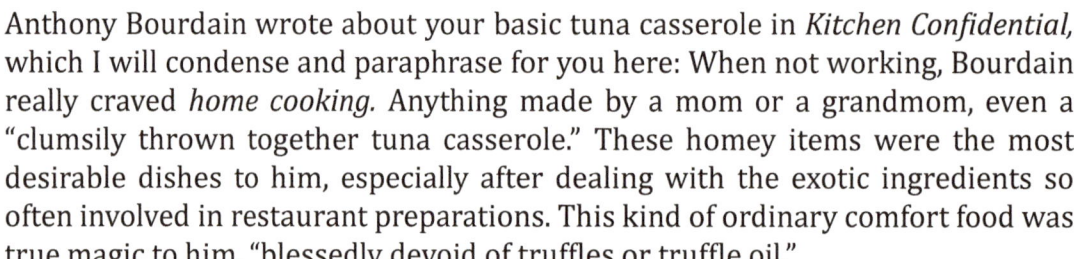

Anthony Bourdain wrote about your basic tuna casserole in *Kitchen Confidential,* which I will condense and paraphrase for you here: When not working, Bourdain really craved *home cooking.* Anything made by a mom or a grandmom, even a "clumsily thrown together tuna casserole." These homey items were the most desirable dishes to him, especially after dealing with the exotic ingredients so often involved in restaurant preparations. This kind of ordinary comfort food was true magic to him, "blessedly devoid of truffles or truffle oil."

    I always liked that down-to-earth quality he so easily conveyed. 2018 was a rough year in many ways; tragically, Bourdain committed suicide in June. I always thought someone like him would die in his late 70s, an incredibly tired victim of cholesterol, alcohol, drugs, and tobacco, his body simply worn out from all his travels and his indulgences. That would have been fitting. And this was before the COVID-19 pandemic started. It was a tumultuous time. Though what time isn't? I anticipate finishing this book in late 2023 sometime, but I'm fairly sure we will all still need comfort food.

    On a more personal note—Bob was always fond of his mother's version of tuna casserole and often talks about how he and his brother Bill would end up fighting over who would get the last of the casserole, especially the crispy topping. I have a feeling their dining room table sometimes became almost a battleground at mealtimes! This dish is based on my mom's recipe. My sister and I probably fought over the crispy topping when we were young, as well. Crispy toppings can be irresistible, don't you think?

    You may also substitute a one-pound bag of frozen peas and pearl onions if available. I often have trouble locating this product, so I just cut up an onion to go with the peas.

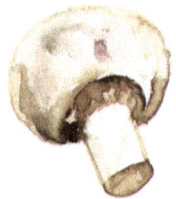
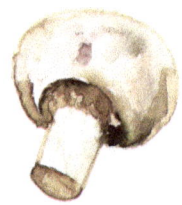

4-ounce jar diced pimientos
2 (7-ounce) cans water-packed albacore tuna
3 quarts water
8 ounces wide egg noodles (other medium-sized pasta will work well)
1 tablespoon dried parsley
1 teaspoon garlic salt
1 teaspoon celery salt
1 teaspoon onion salt
1 cup onion, coarsely chopped
1 cup frozen peas
10.5-ounce can cream of mushroom soup
10.5-ounce can cream of celery soup
½ teaspoon black pepper
½ cup 1% milk
¼ cup seasoned dry breadcrumbs
2 ounces Parmesan and/or Romano cheese, finely shredded

POUR the pimientos into a large colander. Break up the tuna into chunks and place on top of the pimientos to drain; let stand. Bring the water to a boil in a 6-quart saucepan. Add the noodles, parsley, and the 3 salts and boil for 5 minutes.

PREHEAT the oven to 400°. Coat an 11″ by 7″ baking dish with cooking spray or grease lightly; set aside. Add the onions and peas to the pasta and cook another 5–10 minutes, until the pasta is done. Pour over the tuna and let it stand. Reuse the pot.

PLACE the 2 soups, milk, and pepper in the pot and whisk well. Add the pasta to the pot and mix well. Season, as desired. Pour into the prepared dish. Combine the breadcrumbs and cheese in a small bowl. Sprinkle all over the pasta. Bake 30 minutes. Remove from the oven and let stand 5 minutes before serving. Cover and refrigerate the leftovers. Makes 4–6 main-dish servings; 8–12 side-dish servings.

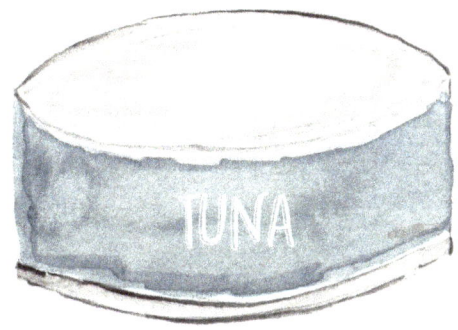

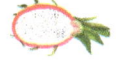

Halfling/Monster Mac & Cheese

START TO FINISH: 35–45 MINUTES, DEPENDING ON WHICH BATCH YOU MAKE

Let me carefully use a tiny quote from Anthony Bourdain's *Kitchen Confidential* again: "I have a fierce passion, when stoned, for unnaturally orange macaroni and cheese. Kraft. Velveeta."

My daughters certainly consumed their share of Kraft Mac & Cheese, with occasional detours to Annie's boxed varieties. But I really wanted to come up with something that would satisfy children and be REALLY homemade. I mean with actual cheese, not powder. Kids seem to think opening a box makes it homemade, which I suppose is technically true, since you are indeed making something at home. This recipe gets my grandchildren's approval. And it gets both of my daughters' approval, so you can definitely make it for adults who need comfy, cozy mac & cheese, stoned or not.

Your cheese choice can certainly be flexible. Generally, most of my cheese choices will be something like shredded colby/cheddar or a fiesta blend, plus something like a Gouda. If I have a couple of ounces of Gorgonzola hanging around, I can get away with throwing it in here and it adds a tangy bite. For the preschool variety, if I have an ounce of Swiss, an ounce of cream cheese, an ounce of fontina, and five ounces of cheddar, that will be fine. Some cheeses will end up producing a stickier sauce, which is yummy, of course, though it might make your pan harder to clean.

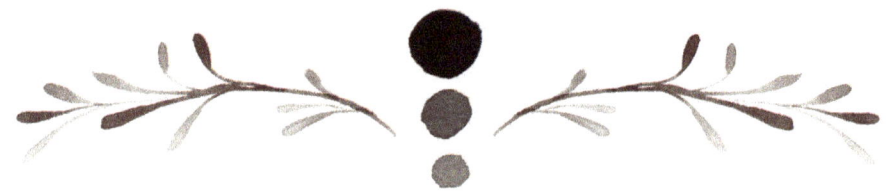

For your pasta, elbow macaroni is the classic choice, but you can certainly substitute whatever small or medium-sized pasta you like.

I'll supply you with three different quantities for this recipe, so you don't have to do the math. You've got your preschool quantity, then elementary, then secondary. Let's hope that by secondary school, your halflings/monsters might consider eating some vegetables or salad on the side. I'm dreading the day when I have to consider breaking out the 12- or 16-quart stockpot to make two pounds worth of mac & cheese to feed all of these darling little marauders…

Preschool (4-quart pot): **Elementary (6-quart):** **Secondary (8-quart):**

8 ounces elbow macaroni	12 ounces	1 pound
1 tablespoon salted butter	1½ tablespoons	2 tablespoons
1 tablespoon all-purpose flour	1½ tablespoons	2 tablespoons
½ teaspoon salt	¾ teaspoon	1 teaspoon
½ teaspoon black pepper	¾ teaspoon	1 teaspoon
1 cup 1% milk	1⅓ cups	1¾ cups
¼ cup heavy cream	½ cup	¾ cup
8 ounces (shredded) cheese	12 ounces	1 pound

cook the pasta in a 4-quart saucepan (or bigger; see above) as directed on the package until it has the desired tenderness. Drain and reuse the pot.

melt the butter over rather high heat. Whisk in the flour, salt, and pepper and cook over a rather high heat until combined. Add the milk and cream and cook until bubbly and a bit thicker. Add in the cheese and whisk until melted. Add a bit more milk if the cheese you have chosen makes the sauce extra thick. Add the pasta. Season, if you need to. If it seems too soupy, cover the pot and let it stand off the heat a minute or so (your choice of cheese might affect this since cheese can be unpredictable sometimes). Cover and refrigerate the leftovers. The preschool version makes 3–4 main-dish servings; 6–8 side-dish servings (the elementary serves 4–6 and the secondary serves 6–8, though these are all merely guidelines; they will serve more as side-dish portions).

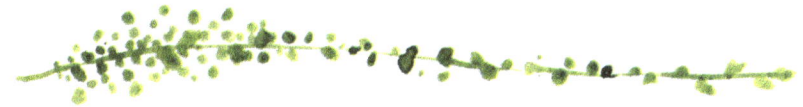

Chapter Twelve: Pasta   233

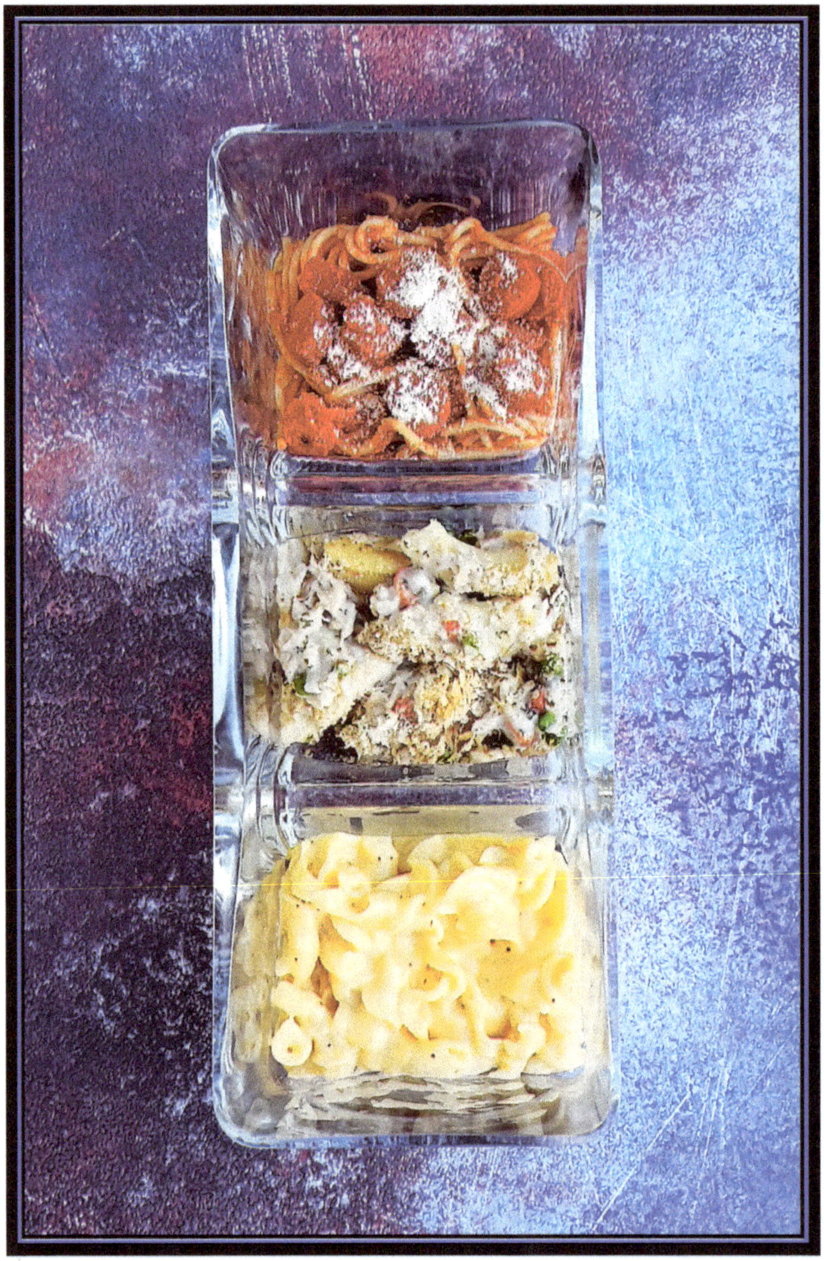

TOP TO BOTTOM:
Sheldon's Spaghetti, page 229
Tony's Tuna Casserole, page 230
Halfling/Monster Mac & Cheese, page 232

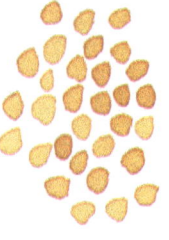

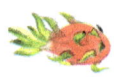 234   Celebrating Comfy, Cozy Foods from North America: CH&M, Volume 3

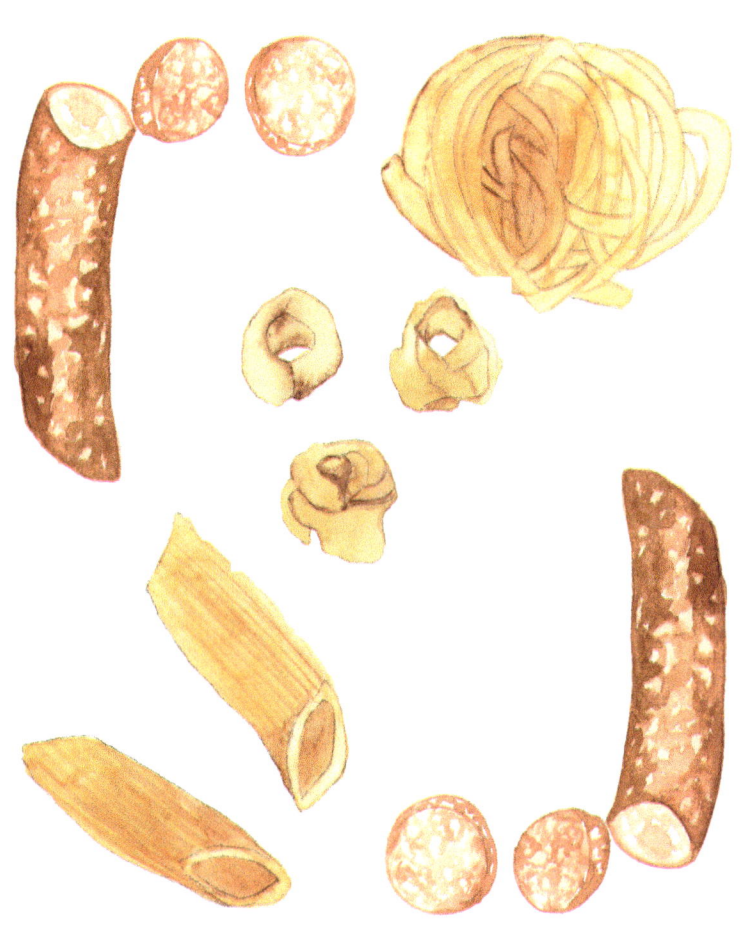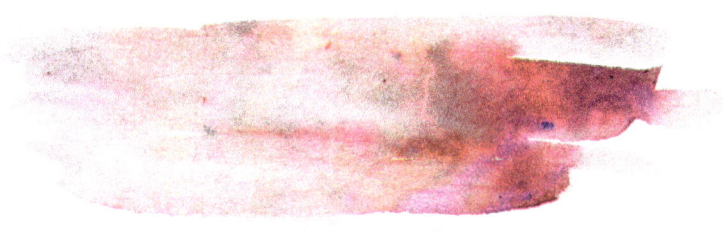

Chapter Thirteen

Bob's Birthday

Bob's Favorite Bowl

Mexican Flag Salad

Bob's Favorite Cake

Bob's Birthday

YES, I HAVE strangely set aside my husband's December birthday as a holiday. Why not? He is one of my favorite halflings/monsters.

Bob's Favorite Bowl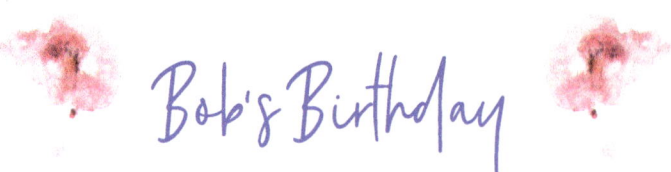

START TO FINISH: ABOUT 40 MINUTES

Beef. Potatoes. Beans. Chile. This is true New Mexican comfort in a bowl.

1½ pounds red potatoes, with peel; cut into ¾" chunks
1 quart water
¼ cup salted butter
1 teaspoon salt, divided
1 teaspoon black pepper, divided
1 pound ground beef sirloin
1 cup onion, coarsely chopped
1 tablespoon minced garlic
1 teaspoon dried oregano (2–3 tablespoons fresh, minced)
15.5-ounce can pinto beans, drained and rinsed (about 2 cups)
2 cups heated red chile sauce (purchased, or see the recipe on page xxviii)
2 cups sharp cheddar cheese, shredded

GARNISH:

> Besides the chile sauce and cheese, you could add anything you like from the **NICE NEW MEXICAN & MEXICAN GARNISHES** list. We usually don't, but you definitely could.

PLACE the potatoes in a large skillet with the water. Bring to a boil, then cook on a gentle boil 10 minutes. Drain and set aside; reuse the pan. Melt the butter in the skillet over very high heat. Add ½ teaspoon salt, ½ teaspoon pepper, and the potatoes and fry them until they are crispy golden brown, about 10–12 minutes. Shake the pan often.

MEANWHILE, coat a 3-quart deep skillet with cooking spray. Add the beef, onion, garlic, the remaining salt and pepper, and the oregano. Break up the meat and fry over very high heat until all the pink is gone, stirring often. Add the beans. Cook on a gentle simmer 5 minutes. Stir a few times.

TO SERVE: Season both items as desired, then place a portion of potatoes in a bowl. Top with beef, ladle the desired amount of chile all over, then sprinkle with cheese. Garnish, if desired. Cover and refrigerate the leftovers. Makes 3–4 servings.

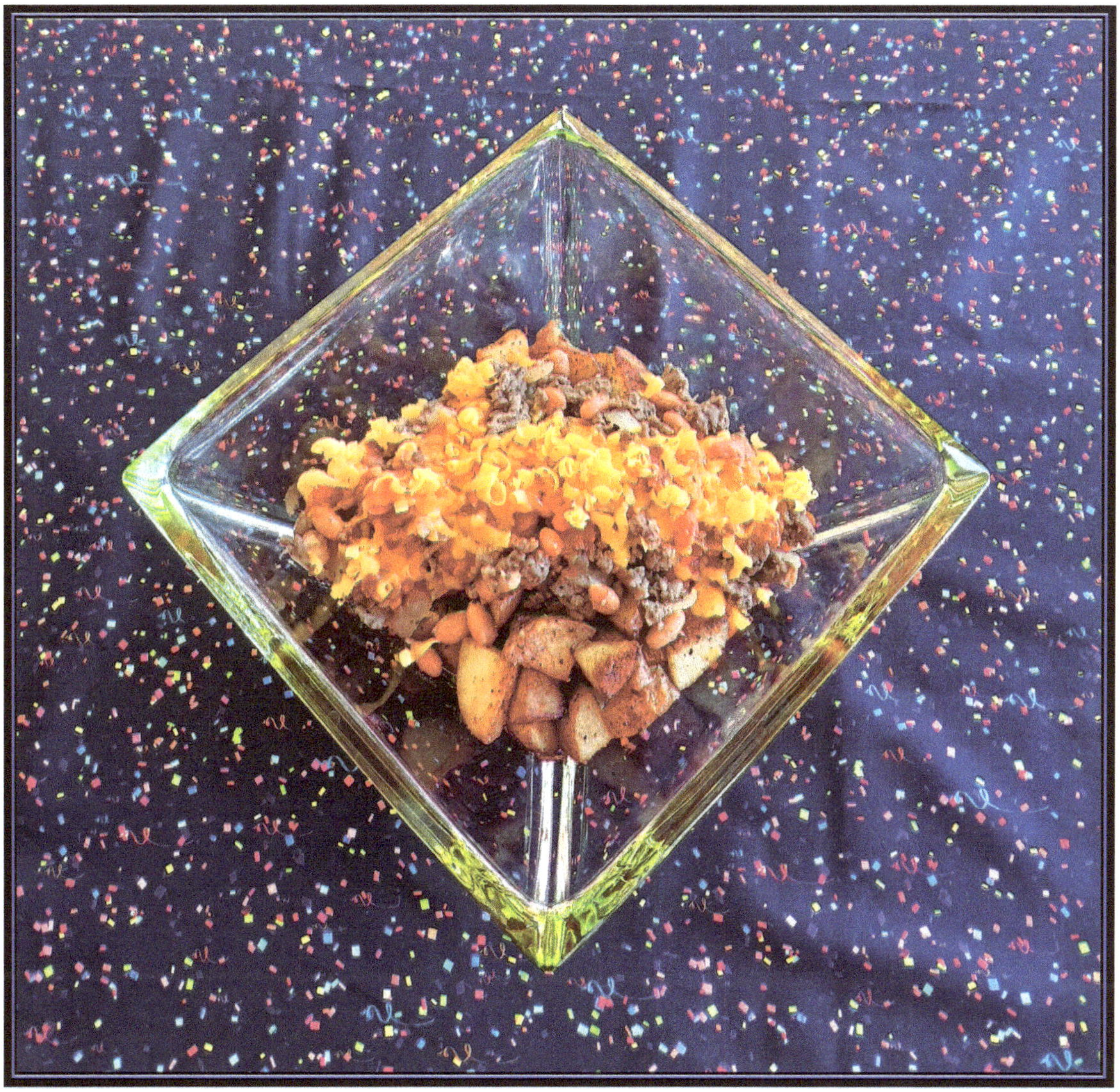

Chapter Thirteen: Bob's Birthday   239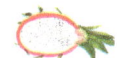

Mexican Flag Salad

PREP: ABOUT 22 MINUTES
CHILL: 1 HOUR

Here is a refreshing salad composed of the colors of the Mexican flag. If you have trouble locating jicama, you can always substitute the same quantity of other vegetables, such as radish, carrot, or celery, all sliced very thinly.

2 large limes
1 tablespoon sugar
2 tablespoons light agave syrup
1 tablespoon vegetable oil
1 tablespoon white wine vinegar
1 teaspoon crushed ginger
½ teaspoon salt
¼ teaspoon cayenne pepper
1½ cups red bell pepper, cored and chopped coarsely
1½ cups jicama, peeled and coarsely chopped
1½ cups seedless cucumber; partially peeled
  (cut off stems, cut lengthwise into quarters,
  then ¼" slices)

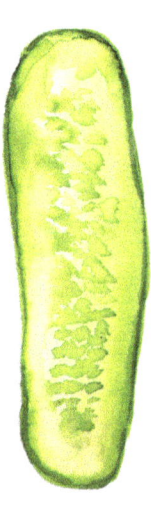
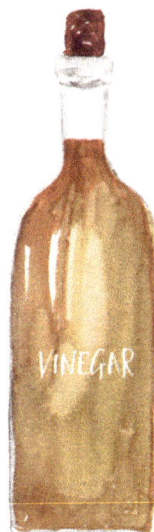

GARNISH:

  A sprinkling of Tajín seasoning would be yummy.

ZEST the limes and mince the zest; place in a large bowl. Juice the limes and add 2 tablespoons to the bowl (use any remaining juice for other purposes). Add the sugar, agave, oil, vinegar, ginger, salt, and cayenne; whisk well. Season, if desired. Add the vegetables. Combine well, cover, and refrigerate about 1 hour before serving; mix a couple of times. Serve with a slotted spoon. Cover and refrigerate the leftovers. Makes about 4½ cups.

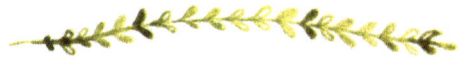

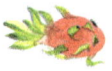

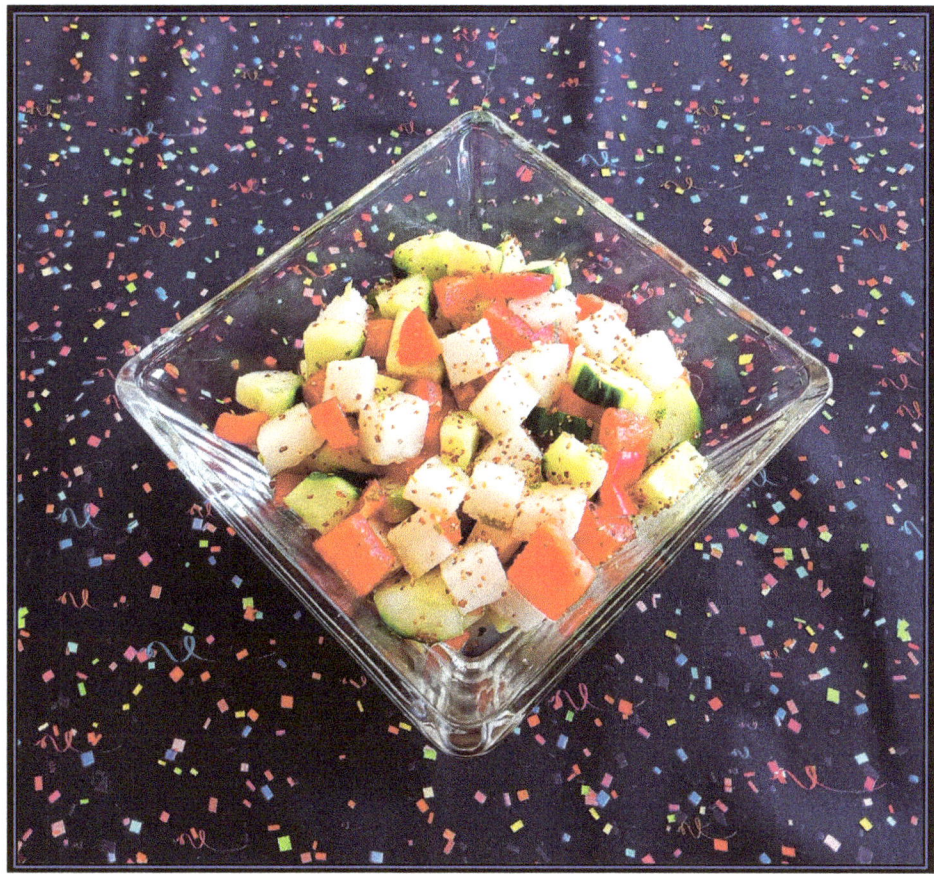

Bob's Favorite Cake

IN ADVANCE: TOASTING AND COOLING NUTS
ACTIVE PREP: ABOUT 38 MINUTES
BAKE: 28 MINUTES
COOL: 1 HOUR
CHILL: UP TO 45 MINUTES
OVEN: 350°

One of Bob's former bosses had never heard of putting white frosting on a chocolate cake. We both always thought that was strange. Regardless, this seems like a small cake, but it is rich and dense, definitely a Death by Chocolate experience. Top this cake with whatever brings you joy—coconut (toasted or not), sprinkles, etc.

Chapter Thirteen: Bob's Birthday

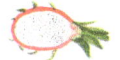

3 ounces sliced almonds, lightly toasted and cooled in advance
1¼ cups cake flour
⅓ cup unsweetened cocoa powder
½ teaspoon salt
½ teaspoon baking soda
All-purpose flour for dusting
¾ cup water, room temperature
4 teaspoons vanilla extract, divided
1 cup sugar
⅔ cup vegetable oil
2 large eggs, room temperature
8 ounces bittersweet chocolate chips (60–72% cacao)
4 ounces white chocolate, broken into smaller squares
3 cups powdered sugar
¼ cup very soft salted butter
3 tablespoons 1% milk

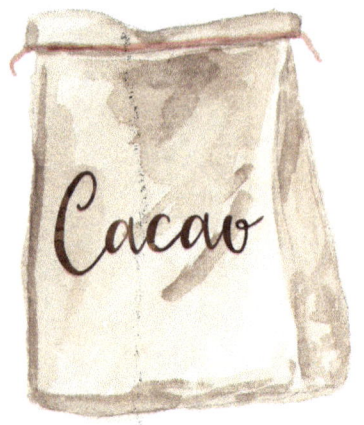

GRIND the cooled almonds in a small food processor, then place them in a medium bowl. Add the cake flour, cocoa powder, salt, and baking soda and combine well. Set aside.

PREHEAT the oven to 350°. Spritz a bit of cooking spray on the bottom of two 8" round baking pans. Cut some parchment paper to fit the bottom of the pans. Place the prepared paper in the pans, and coat the bottom and sides with cooking spray or grease lightly. Sprinkle some flour in the pans and shake to distribute lightly on the bottom and sides of each pan. Shake out the excess; set them aside.

COMBINE the water and 1 tablespoon vanilla in a 1-cup glass measuring cup and set aside. Place the sugar, oil, and eggs in a very large bowl and beat on medium speed 2 minutes. Add to the sugar mixture: ⅓ of the flour mixture, ½ of the water, ⅓ flour mixture, remaining water, and remaining flour. Mix well on medium after each addition and scrape down the sides as needed. Mix in the bittersweet chips and beat on medium another minute. Divide evenly between the prepared pans. Bake 28 minutes. Place on racks for 30 minutes. If needed, run a sharp knife along the edge to remove the cakes from the pans. Place the paper side down on the racks and cool 30 minutes.

PLACE the white chocolate in a small glass bowl and microwave on HIGH in 20-second intervals just until melted (this will take about 1 minute total). Let stand about 10 minutes. Place the powdered sugar, butter, remaining 1 teaspoon vanilla, milk, and white chocolate in a very large bowl and beat on low speed with a whisk attachment for 30 seconds. Scrape down the sides. Beat on medium speed about 2 minutes until fluffy and smooth.

REMOVE the paper from one cake layer and place on a plate. Spread about ½ cup frosting on top to the edge. Remove the paper from the other layer and place it on top. Spread a thin layer of frosting around the sides and refrigerate 15 minutes. Cover the remaining frosting with a towel and let it stand. Finish frosting the top and sides of the cake nicely. Refrigerate another 20–30 minutes or so to set the frosting before cutting. Cover and keep at room temperature (though you can keep it in the fridge, if the weather is warm; bring it out for an hour before serving again). Makes 10–12 servings.

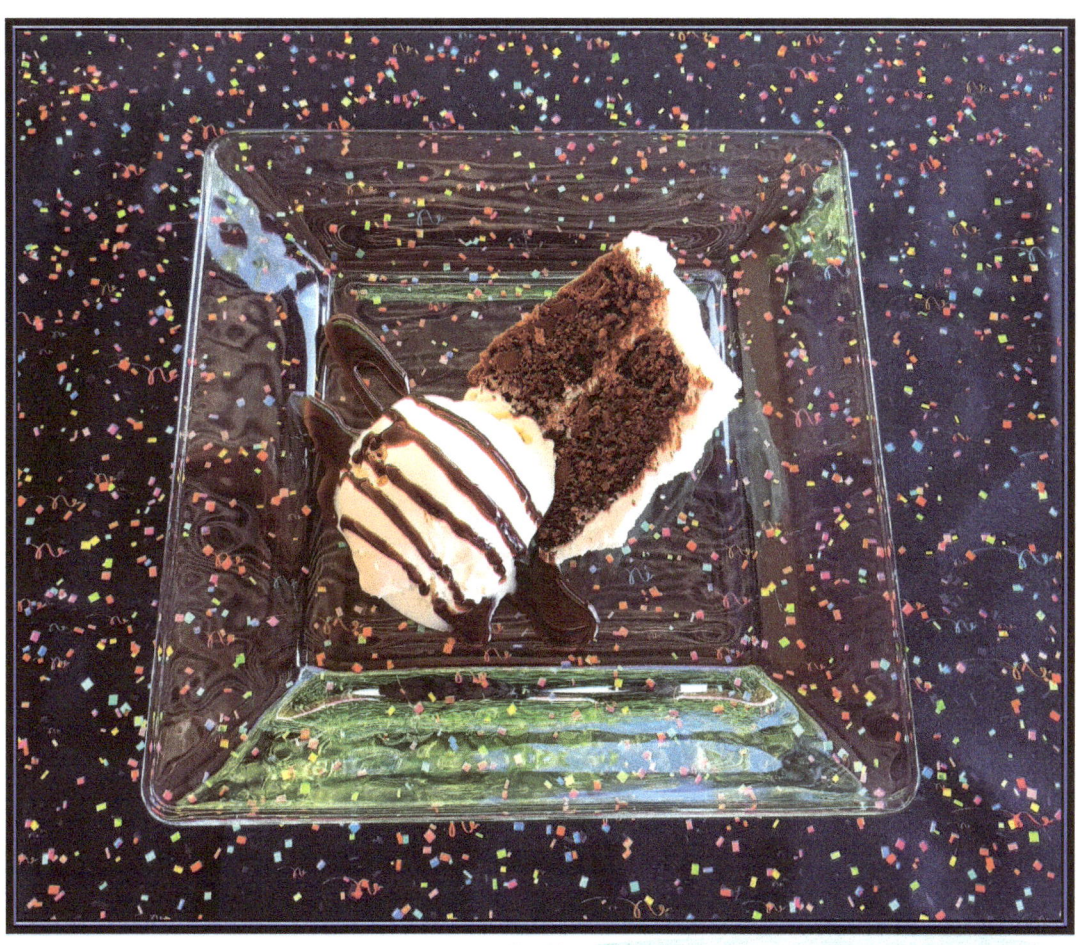

Chapter Fourteen

Sundry Sweeties

Skippy the Jedi Droid's Powerful Force Cookies

Chocolate Chip Cookies

Super Snickerdoodles

Perfect Polvorones

Amalgamation Cookies

Cherry Ginger Oatmeal Cookies

Jan's Moon Shadows

Blondie Rapture

Nirvana Newtons

Chocolate Chips in a Pan

P. D. G. Crisp

Joyful Almond Tart

Banana Muffincakes

Sundry Sweeties

ALTHOUGH SWEETS HAVE been scattered throughout this cookbook, here are a few more. Let me share my cookie philosophy in the following paragraphs. Use real butter, real extracts whenever possible, good quality ingredients, and definitely don't overbake them. When I took baking classes, my teacher said many people forget that when you let cookies cool on the baking sheet, they technically still bake for a couple of minutes. Remember, that pan is HOT!

I'm giving you a range of baking times. My time is always right in the middle. If you prefer your cookies to be a bit on the underbaked side, use the first measurement; if you prefer them to crisp up a bit more, use the second measurement. Remember, you can always bake your cookies for a minute more if they seem to need it, but if you bake them too long, you can't return from that. Cookies will stabilize while they rest on the hot pan, then become firmer after you place them on a rack to cool. Properly baked cookies should be rather fresh for a couple of days. On a third day, you could microwave a cookie for a few seconds to remind you of its original freshly baked quality.

Should you always toast your nuts before you make cookies (or any other dessert or other dish)? Maybe you should, but it's certainly not a requirement. If you do decide to toast nuts, toast them while they are whole, let them cool completely, then chop them. I often use a toaster oven to do this, but you might prefer to use your oven or heat them in a skillet on the stove. Just be sure not to burn them. Toasting times will depend on your method and the type of nut you are using.

For most of the following cookies, I'm suggesting a quantity of 24. This is a good-sized cookie—not too big, not too small. If you decide to make something like 36 cookies, the general rule of thumb is to bake them for two minutes less. If you decide to make 16 cookies, you will bake them for an additional two minutes. It's easy to fit 24 cookies on two large baking sheets and bake them at the same time, rotating the pans halfway through cooking. If you have a convection oven, you might not need to rotate your pans, but you might need to adjust your baking times.

I also like a cookie to look like a homemade cookie, so I don't use scoops. I want most cookies to have irregularities along the edges. To make 24 cookies, you need a scoop that measures out about an ounce of cookie dough. Then you have to fuss with the scoop and clean it. I like to take my dough and break off portions to place on the baking sheets. No muss. I might divide my dough into four portions, then each of those portions becomes six cookies. Sometimes, I just eyeball what I put on the sheet and add a little extra to those cookies that seem to need a bit more.

Don't get me wrong—there is certainly a place for perfectly formed crisp cookies. It is in your local bakery. It is also in the cookie aisle of your grocery store, and it is filled with Keebler and Pepperidge Farm products (and dozens of other brands, of course). There is nothing wrong with store-bought cookies. But when you choose to make some homemade cookies, that becomes a special occasion. Your house will smell good. If you have companions around, they will become excited about the prospect of eating freshly baked cookies. So, go do some baking right now!

Obviously, I have thought way too much about cookies.

Skippy the Jedi Droid's Powerful Force Cookies

IN ADVANCE: TOASTING NUTS, COOLING, AND CHOPPING
PREP: ABOUT 18 MINUTES
BAKE: 9–11 MINUTES
COOL: ABOUT 20 MINUTES
OVEN: 375°

A long time ago, in our neighborhood galaxy, my son-in-law (TOTAL *Star Wars* fan) and I were chatting about character names for future recipes. He is conversant in both canon and non-canon works, as well as all the films, books, and cartoons. He mentioned the strange story about a droid who happened to be strong in the Force. I said, "You must be kidding." He said, "I kid you not." Here is his story, according to non-canonical sources (a.k.a. Legends):

Chapter Fourteen: Sundry Sweeties 247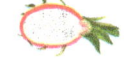

A long time ago in a galaxy far, far away... there was a little red droid named R5-D4, whom Luke Skywalker and his Uncle Owen purchased to work on their moisture farm, as seen in Episode IV of the *Star Wars* films, *A New Hope.* R5-D4 apparently once worked at Jabba the Hutt's palace serving drinks, just like R2-D2 does later on. One day, a drink nearly spilled, but R5, or Skippy, as he is more affectionately called, was able to prevent the glass from falling—by using the Force.

Later on, Skippy ended up on Tatooine in the same Jawa sandcrawler with R2-D2 and C-3PO. Skippy could sense the higher purpose of those storied droids. Apparently, Skippy used the Force to influence Luke Skywalker's Uncle Owen to choose him as his new droid. Skippy, however, was prone to visions. As he was walking along with his new owner, he began to sense that R2-D2 was truly the crucial droid in the scheme of these epic matters. He realized that he could do something heroic to further the cause of the Rebellion; if he didn't act quickly, all would be destroyed, the Empire would win, and Luke would never fulfill his destiny.

And so—he blew himself up. R2-D2 became the chosen droid. Skippy the Jedi Droid saved the day!

2 ounces roasted and salted peanuts, lightly toasted, cooled, and chopped coarsely in advance
½ cup soft salted butter
½ cup peanut butter (crunchy or smooth; use Skippy if you like! *He won't mind…*)
¾ cup packed light brown sugar
¼ cup sugar
1 large egg
1 tablespoon vanilla extract
1¼ cups all-purpose flour
½ cup old-fashioned oats
2 teaspoons ground cinnamon
½ teaspoon baking powder
½ teaspoon baking soda
¼ teaspoon salt
4 ounces sweetened coconut flakes

 248 Celebrating Comfy, Cozy Foods from North America: CH&M, Volume 3

PREHEAT the oven to 375°. Coat 2 large baking sheets with cooking spray or grease lightly; set aside. Cream together the butter, peanut butter, brown sugar, sugar, egg, and vanilla in a very large bowl on medium speed for a minute or two. Add the flour, oats, cinnamon, baking powder, baking soda, and salt. Mix well on low for 1 minute. Add the prepared peanuts and coconut and mix another minute or so on low, until well combined. Divide into 24 portions and place on the prepared pans. Bake 9–11 minutes. Let stand on the pans for 2 minutes. Rack carefully. Cover and store at room temperature. Makes 24.

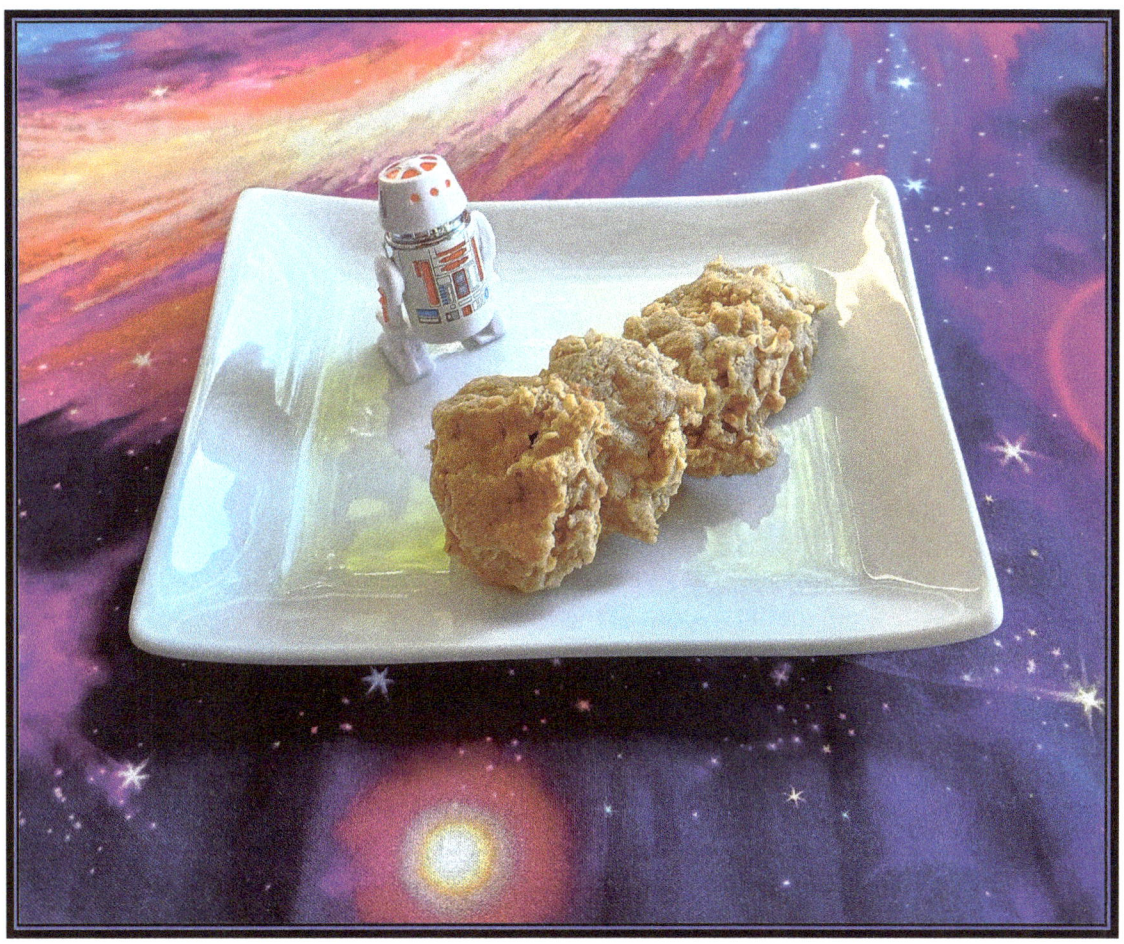

SKIPPY SAYS:

"You will eat these cookies…
these ARE the cookies you have been looking for…"

Chocolate Chip Cookies

IN ADVANCE: TOASTING NUTS, COOLING, AND CHOPPING
PREP: ABOUT 18 MINUTES
BAKE: 9–11 MINUTES
COOL: ABOUT 20 MINUTES
OVEN: 375°

No adjective needed; these are the bomb. That said, you can change out your chips and your nuts (try 4 ounces of white chocolate chips, 4 ounces of sweetened coconut flakes, and 4 ounces of chopped macadamia nuts, for a lovely variation). Maybe add cinnamon or other spices you might like, anywhere from a modest teaspoon to a bold tablespoon.

4 ounces pecans, lightly toasted, cooled, and chopped coarsely in advance
⅔ cup soft salted butter
½ cup sugar
½ cup packed light brown sugar
1 large egg
1 tablespoon vanilla extract
1¾ cups all-purpose flour
½ teaspoon salt
½ teaspoon baking soda
8 ounces semi-sweet chocolate chips

PREHEAT the oven to 375°. Coat 2 large baking sheets with cooking spray or grease lightly; set aside. Cream together the butter, sugar, brown sugar, egg, and vanilla in a very large bowl on medium speed for a minute or two. Add the flour, salt, and baking soda and mix well on low for 1 minute. Add the chips and the prepared pecans and mix another minute or so on low, until well combined. Divide into 24 portions and place on the prepared pans. Bake 9–11 minutes. Let stand on the pans for 2 minutes. Rack carefully. Cover and store at room temperature. Makes 24.

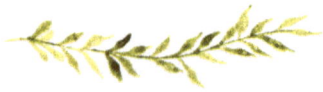

Super Snickerdoodles

PREP: ABOUT 18 MINUTES
BAKE: 10–12 MINUTES
COOL: ABOUT 20 MINUTES
OVEN: 375°

Add a teaspoon or two of chili powder to the cinnamon sugar for a fun Southwestern variation.

⅔ cup soft salted butter
1 cup plus 2 tablespoons sugar
1 large egg
1 teaspoon vanilla extract
2 cups all-purpose flour
¾ teaspoon cream of tartar
½ teaspoon baking soda
½ teaspoon salt
1 teaspoon ground cinnamon

PREHEAT the oven to 375°. Coat 2 large baking sheets with cooking spray or grease lightly; set aside. Cream together the butter, 1 cup sugar, egg, and vanilla in a very large bowl on medium speed for a minute or two. Add the flour, cream of tartar, baking soda, and salt and mix on low 1 minute or so, until well combined. Combine the 2 tablespoons sugar and cinnamon in a small bowl. Divide dough into 24 portions and shape into balls (about 1½″). Roll each in the prepared cinnamon sugar and place on the prepared pans (you can use any extra cinnamon sugar on other items). Bake 10–12 minutes. Let stand on the pans for 2 minutes. Rack carefully. Cover and store at room temperature. Makes 24.

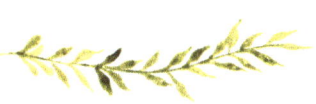

Perfect Polvorones

IN ADVANCE: TOASTING NUTS AND COOLING
ACTIVE PREP: 30 MINUTES
CHILL: 2 HOURS
BAKE: 12 MINUTES PER BATCH (TOTAL OF 24 MINUTES)
STAND: 20 MINUTES PER BATCH (TOTAL OF 40 MINUTES)
OVEN: 375°

A *polvorón* is a crumbly kind of shortbread cookie (from the word *polvo*, which is Spanish for "dust" or "powder"), often served around Christmastime or at weddings. I always think of them as wedding cookies. You might think some of the words used here (crumbly, dust, or powder) might indicate a rather blah cookie experience, but you would be mistaken. The main problem with good polvorones is preventing yourself from eating every single one of them.

For a fun flavor profile, try mixing about a half cup of finely ground strawberry powder with the powdered sugar used for rolling your cookies at the end.

6 ounces pecan halves, lightly toasted and cooled for about an hour
1¾ cups powdered sugar, divided
¼ teaspoon salt
2¼ cups all-purpose flour
1 cup soft salted butter
1 teaspoon vanilla extract
¼ cup warm tap water

PLACE the prepared pecans in a large food processor and process until they are ground. Add ½ cup powdered sugar, salt, and flour to the nuts and process well. Scrape sides and bottom and process again. Add butter, vanilla, and water and process thoroughly. Scrape sides down and process again. Scrape into a medium bowl, cover with a towel, and refrigerate 2 hours.

PREHEAT the oven to 375°. Coat 2 large baking sheets with cooking spray or grease lightly; set aside. Remove half of the dough from the bowl, cover, and refrigerate the other half. Divide the dough into 36 balls (about 1") and place 18 on each prepared pan. Bake 12 minutes. Let stand on the pans 20 minutes. Roll the remaining dough into another 36 balls while you wait, then you can use the bowl for the next step.

PLACE the remaining powdered sugar in the medium bowl. Using your hands, GENTLY roll 6 cookies at a time in the sugar, then place them on a rack. Repeat the rolling and baking process with the remaining dough; bake and roll them in sugar when they are ready. You may sprinkle any remaining sugar over all the cookies using a fine-mesh strainer. It's best to store these cookies covered at room temperature if possible, and preferably in a single layer. Makes 72.

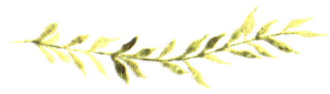

Amalgamation Cookies

IN ADVANCE: TOASTING NUTS, COOLING, AND CHOPPING
PREP: ABOUT 18 MINUTES
BAKE: 9–11 MINUTES
COOL: ABOUT 20 MINUTES
OVEN: 375°

This is my version of an "everything-but-the-kitchen-sink" cookie.

2 ounces pecans, lightly toasted, cooled, and chopped coarsely in advance
½ cup soft salted butter
½ cup sugar
½ cup packed light brown sugar
½ cup crunchy peanut butter
1 large egg
1 tablespoon vanilla extract
1 cup all-purpose flour
1 cup old-fashioned oats
1 teaspoon ground cinnamon
1 teaspoon baking powder
½ teaspoon salt
3 ounces raisins
2 ounces semi-sweet chocolate chips
2 ounces white chocolate chips
2 ounces sweetened coconut flakes

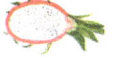

PREHEAT the oven to 375°. Coat 2 large baking sheets with cooking spray or grease lightly; set aside. Cream together the butter, sugar, brown sugar, peanut butter, egg, and vanilla in a very large bowl on medium speed for a minute or two. Add the flour, oats, cinnamon, baking powder, and salt. Mix well on low for 1 minute. Add the prepared pecans and the remaining ingredients and mix another minute or so on low, until well combined. Divide into 24 portions and place on the prepared pans. Bake 9–11 minutes. Let stand on the pans for 2 minutes. Rack carefully. Cover and store at room temperature. Makes 24.

Cherry Ginger Oatmeal Cookies

IN ADVANCE: TOASTING NUTS, COOLING, AND CHOPPING
PREP: ABOUT 18 MINUTES
BAKE: 9–11 MINUTES
COOL: ABOUT 20 MINUTES
OVEN: 375°

I would name these Halfling Alert Oatmeal Cookies, but I've probably used that phrase too much by now. But really, don't you think these would be devoured by hungry hobbits?

4 ounces walnuts, lightly toasted, cooled, and chopped coarsely in advance
⅔ cup soft salted butter
½ cup sugar
½ cup packed light brown sugar
1 large egg
1 tablespoon vanilla extract
1¼ cups all-purpose flour
1½ cups old-fashioned oats
1 teaspoon ground cinnamon
¾ teaspoon baking soda
½ teaspoon salt
½ teaspoon ground nutmeg
6 ounces dried cherries
2 ounces crystallized ginger, finely chopped

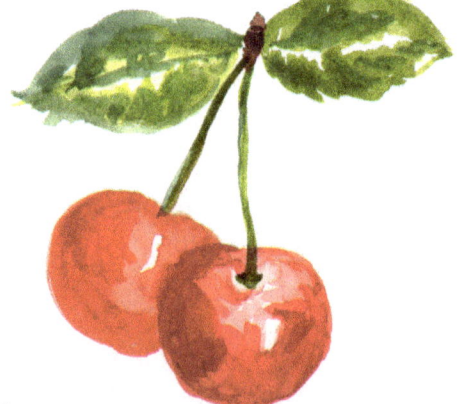

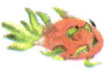

PREHEAT the oven to 375°. Coat 2 large baking sheets with cooking spray or grease lightly; set aside. Cream together the butter, sugar, brown sugar, egg, and vanilla in a very large bowl on medium speed for a minute or two. Add the flour, oats, cinnamon, baking soda, salt, and nutmeg and mix well on low for 1 minute. Add the prepared walnuts and the remaining ingredients and mix another minute or so on low, until well combined. Divide into 24 portions and place on the prepared pans. Bake 9–11 minutes. Let stand on the pans for 2 minutes. Rack carefully. Cover and store at room temperature. Makes 24.

Jan's Moon Shadows

IN ADVANCE: TOASTING NUTS, COOLING, AND CHOPPING
ACTIVE PREP: ABOUT 12 MINUTES
BAKE: 25 MINUTES
COOL: 1 HOUR
OVEN: 350°

This is based on a recipe from one of my college besties, Janis Ann Briggs, who died in 2008. Although she loved the songs of many musical artists, Cat Stevens held a special place in her heart.

3 ounces pecans, lightly toasted, cooled, and chopped coarsely in advance
½ cup salted butter
1 cup packed light brown sugar
2 large eggs, room temperature
1½ teaspoons vanilla extract
1 cup all-purpose flour
½ teaspoon baking powder
½ teaspoon salt
3 ounces semi-sweet chocolate chips
Powdered sugar

PREHEAT the oven to 350°. Coat an 8″ square baking dish with cooking spray or grease lightly; set aside. Melt the butter over moderate heat in a 3-quart saucepan. Add the brown sugar and whisk well. Let stand 5 minutes. Add the eggs and vanilla and whisk well. Add the flour, baking powder, and salt and whisk in well. Add the prepared nuts and mix well. Spread in the pan. Sprinkle the chocolate chips over all the dough. Bake 25 minutes. Cool 1 hour on a rack. Sprinkle with powdered sugar. Cover and keep at room temperature. Makes 16.

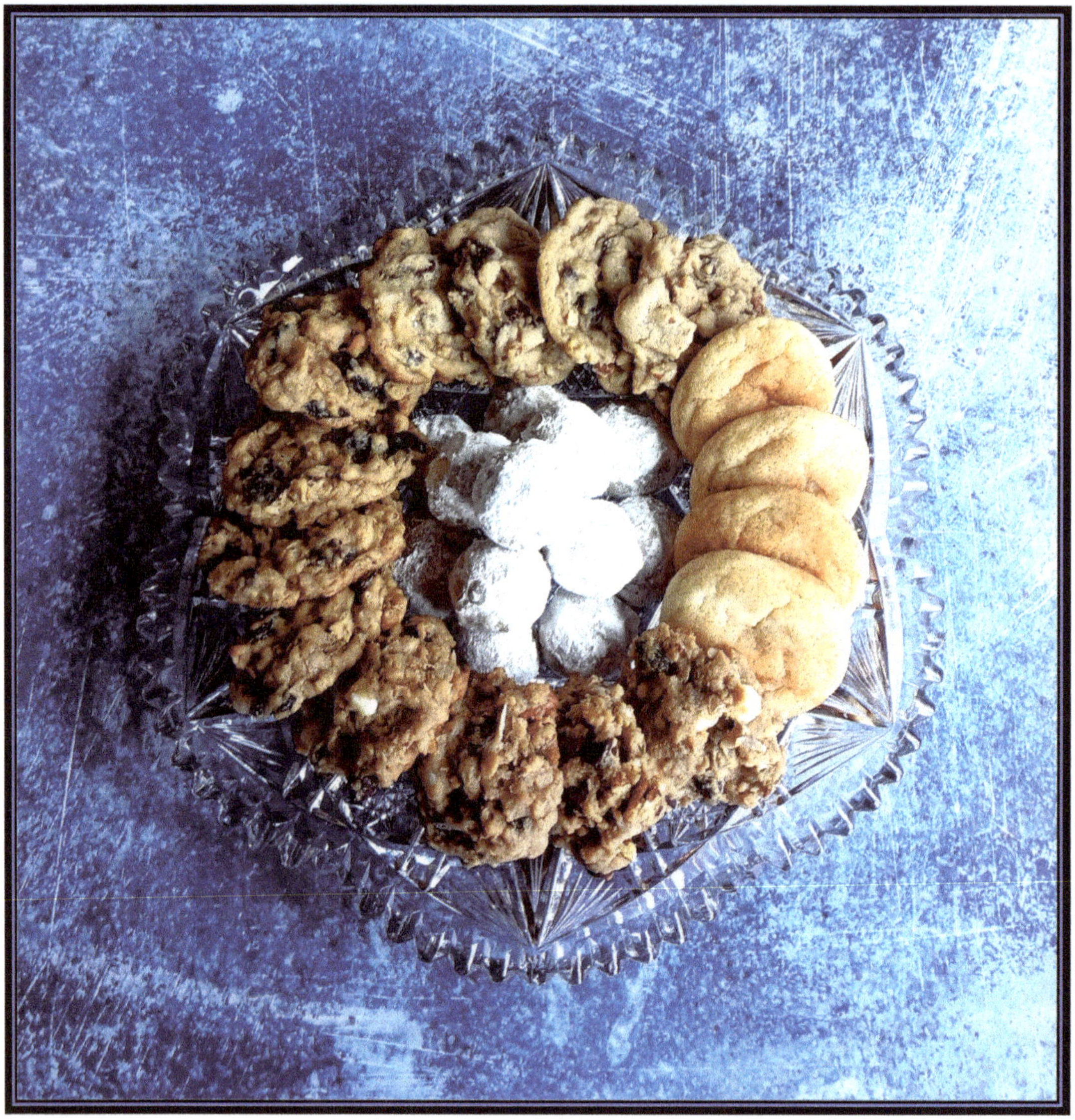

TOP, THEN CLOCKWISE:
Chocolate Chip Cookies, page 250
Super Snickerdoodles, page 251
Amalgamation Cookies, page 253
Cherry Ginger Oatmeal Cookies, page 254

CENTER:
Perfect Polvorones, page 252

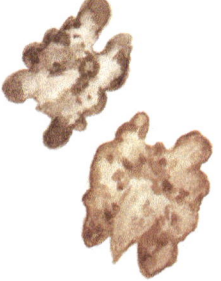

Blondie Rapture

IN ADVANCE: TOASTING NUTS AND COOLING
PREP: 18 MINUTES
BAKE: 47 MINUTES
COOL: 3 HOURS
OVEN: 325°

These are a delicious spin on brownies. I'm thinking of the Blondie song, in which the man from Mars is eating cars and guitars and bars, which couldn't possibly be healthy even for a space alien.

3 ounces sliced almonds, lightly toasted and cooled in advance
½ cup salted butter
12 ounces white chocolate, broken up (chips are okay)
1 cup sugar
4 large eggs, room temperature
1 tablespoon vanilla extract
2 cups all-purpose flour
1 teaspoon salt
½ teaspoon baking powder
8 ounces toffee chips (such as Heath, either plain toffee or chocolate toffee)

PREHEAT the oven to 325°. Place the butter and white chocolate in a very large glass bowl. Microwave on HIGH in 20-second intervals just until melted, about 90 seconds total. Whisk well. Let stand 5 minutes.

    MEANWHILE, coat a 13" by 9" baking dish with cooking spray or grease lightly; set aside. Whisk the sugar into the butter mixture well. Whisk in the eggs and vanilla. Add the flour, salt, and baking powder and whisk well. Add the toffee chips and the prepared almonds and mix in well. Pour into the prepared pan. Bake 47 minutes. Place on a rack to cool for 3 hours before cutting. Cover and keep at room temperature. Makes 24–32.

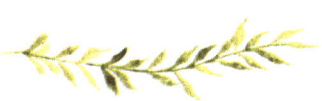

Nirvana Newtons

PREP: 20 MINUTES (PLUS FIG JAM PREP)
BAKE: 45 MINUTES
COOL: 2 HOURS
OVEN: 350°

Sometimes, it's fun to make up lyrics to songs where you can't understand what the vocalist is singing, especially in the car when you're driving around with teenagers. For the song "All Apologies" by Nirvana, I would always sing "Ah, the power of cheese." Now, I'll have to start doing that with my grandkids in the car so they can learn to appreciate some classic rock. When they're older, of course. It's hard to believe that song came out in 1993.

One of my least favorite cookies is your typical Fig Newton. These, however, will seem like Nirvana compared to a store-bought Newton. The fig jam is delicious on its own and can be used on any other bread product you like; it even freezes well.

Smells Like Yummy Fig Jam

PREP: ABOUT 15 MINUTES
STAND: ABOUT 1 HOUR

8 ounces dried figs, any variety
⅓ cup sugar
½ cup orange juice
1 teaspoon ground cinnamon
1 teaspoon dried orange peel
1 teaspoon vanilla extract

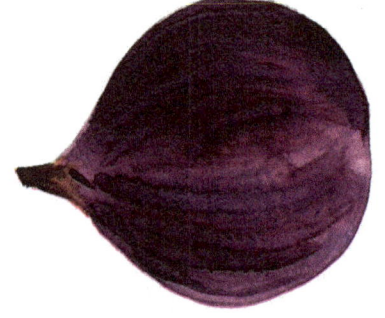

SNIP off all the stems of the figs. Place the figs and sugar in a large food processor and process until the figs are ground pretty finely (you will use this bowl again to finish the recipe below; no need to wash it). Place in a 1½-quart saucepan. Add the remaining ingredients and bring to a boil; stir to combine. Cook on medium/low heat 5 minutes, stirring frequently. Cover and let stand an hour or so (if you're just making this as a jam, store it covered in the refrigerator, or you can freeze it). Makes 1½ cups.

NIRVANA NEWTONS (PROPER)

A FULL RECIPE OF SMELLS LIKE YUMMY FIG JAM, PREPARED IN ADVANCE (SEE ABOVE)

1½ cups all-purpose flour
¼ cup cornstarch
½ cup old-fashioned oats, divided
⅓ cup sugar
½ teaspoon salt
¾ cup soft salted butter
2 tablespoons 1% milk
1 teaspoon vanilla extract
1 ounce pecans, finely chopped
2 tablespoons cinnamon sugar
2 tablespoons very soft salted butter

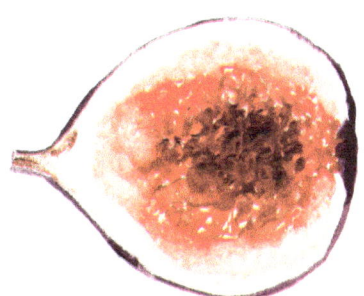

PREHEAT the oven to 350°. Line an 8″ square baking dish with foil, leaving a 2″ overhang on 2 sides. Coat the foil and pan well with cooking spray; set aside. Place the flour, cornstarch, ¼ cup oats, sugar, and salt in a large food processor and process well. Add the butter, milk, and vanilla and process well. Reserve ¾ cup of this mixture and set it aside in a medium bowl. Press the remainder evenly into the prepared pan.

SPREAD the prepared Yummy Fig Jam all over the dough. Add the remaining oats, pecans, cinnamon sugar, and very soft butter to the medium bowl and mix with your hands until crumbly. Sprinkle all over the jam in clumps. Bake 45 minutes. Place on a rack for 2 hours to cool. Using the foil overhang, lift the cookies out and place them on a cutting board to cut. Cover and keep at room temperature. Makes 16.

> Here are a couple of alternatives that are also delicious:
>
> You may substitute a 12-ounce jar of any sort of different jam for the fig jam. Mix it up to make it more spreadable. Or you may use a 13-ounce jar of Nutella. If your Nutella isn't completely spreadable, remove all the foil from the jar and microwave it on HIGH for 20–30 seconds.

Chapter Fourteen: Sundry Sweeties

Chocolate Chips in a Pan

IN ADVANCE: TOASTING NUTS, COOLING, AND CHOPPING
PREP: 16 MINUTES
BAKE: 19–21 MINUTES
COOL: 30 MINUTES
OVEN: 375°

Sometimes, you need your cookie to resemble a pizza. Baking a big cookie can be a challenge, so I prefer this to be a bit underdone in the middle; certainly not liquidy, but just a bit soft to the touch. It will stabilize when it stands for a while.

3 ounces pecans, lightly toasted, cooled, and chopped coarsely in advance
½ cup soft salted butter
⅓ cup sugar
⅓ cup packed light brown sugar
1 large egg
1 tablespoon vanilla extract
1¼ cups all-purpose flour
1 teaspoon ground cinnamon
½ teaspoon baking soda
½ teaspoon salt
4 ounces semi-sweet chocolate chips

GARNISH:

Ice cream would be a welcome addition to serve with this cookie.

PREHEAT the oven to 375°. Cut parchment paper to fit the bottom of an 8″ round pan and lay it in the pan. Coat the pan with cooking spray on the bottom and sides; set aside. Place the butter, sugar, brown sugar, egg, and vanilla in a very large bowl. Mix on medium speed with a stand or hand mixer for 2 minutes. Scrape down the sides. Add the flour, cinnamon, baking soda, and salt and mix well for another minute on low. Add the chips and the prepared pecans and mix on low just until combined. Spread in the prepared pan. Bake 19–21 minutes. Place on a rack to cool for 30 minutes. Run a knife around the edge, if necessary. Invert and remove the paper. Place this side down on a plate. Cut into wedges and serve warm. Cover and keep at room temperature. Makes 8 servings.

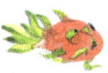

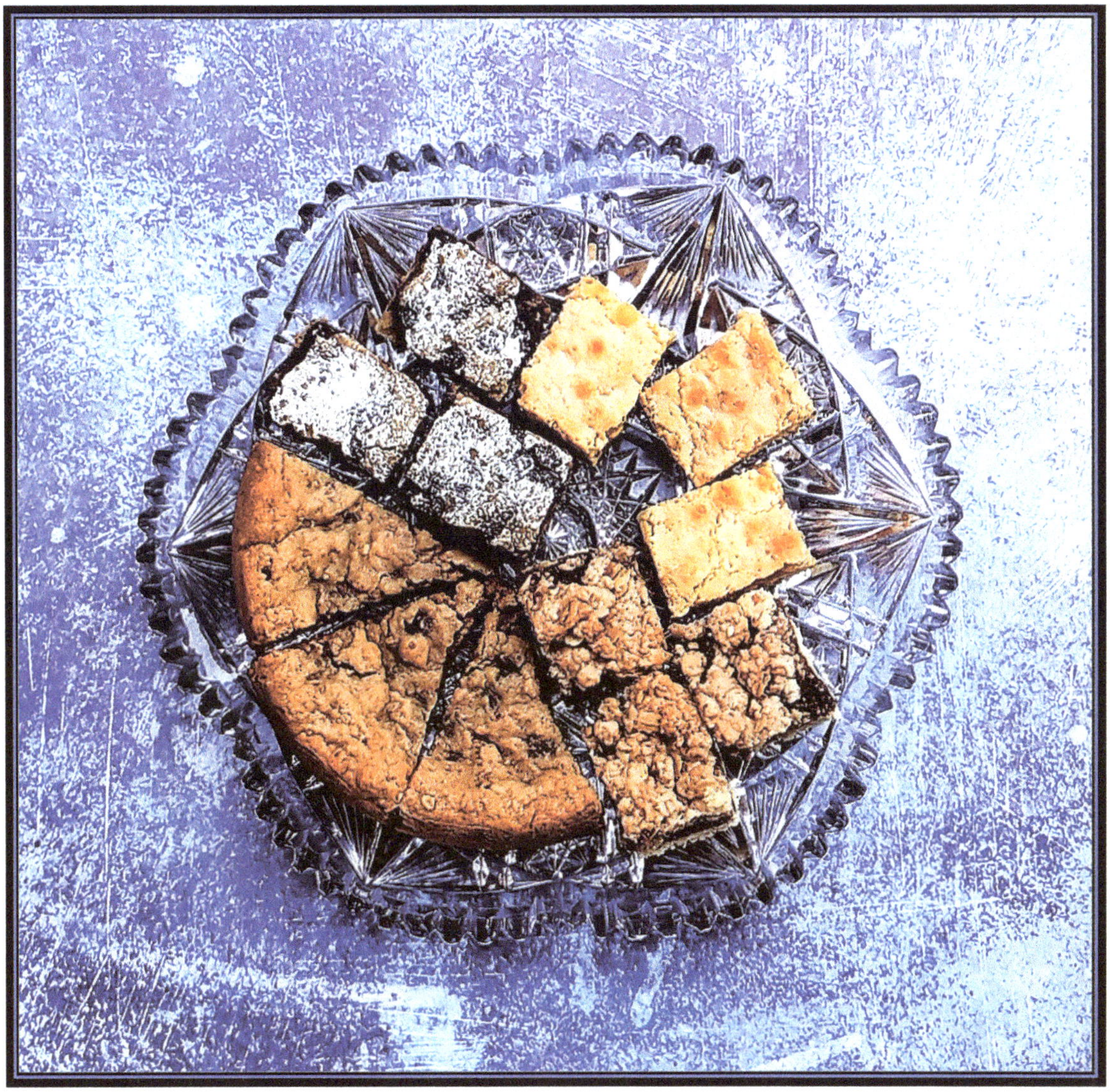

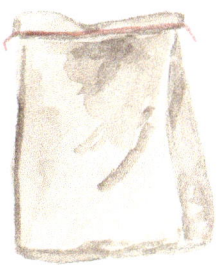

TOP LEFT, THEN CLOCKWISE:
Jan's Moon Shadows, page 255
Blondie Rapture, page 257
Nirvana Newtons, page 258
Chocolate Chips in a Pan, page 260

Chapter Fourteen: Sundry Sweeties 261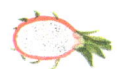

P. D. G. Crisp

IN ADVANCE: TOASTING NUTS, COOLING, AND CHOPPING
PREP: ABOUT 22 MINUTES
BAKE: 40 MINUTES
STAND: 30 MINUTES
OVEN: 375°

Bob christened this dessert a Pretty Damn Good Crisp, and it stuck. You may use yellow peaches, nectarines, or even apricots if you can't find white peaches.

2 ounces walnuts, lightly toasted, cooled, and chopped finely in advance
1½ pounds white peaches
6 ounces dried cherries
1 cup packed light brown sugar, divided
2 tablespoons minute tapioca
2 tablespoons lemon juice
¾ cup all-purpose flour
2 tablespoons cornmeal
2 tablespoons old-fashioned oats
1 teaspoon ground cinnamon
½ teaspoon salt
½ cup soft salted butter

GARNISH: vanilla ice cream or whipped cream

PREHEAT the oven to 375°. Coat a 2-quart baking or casserole dish with cooking spray or grease lightly; set aside. Wash the peaches, remove pits, then cut them into chunks around 1½". Place in a large bowl. Add the cherries, ½ cup brown sugar, tapioca, and lemon juice and combine well. Pour into the prepared dish. Rinse and dry the bowl to reuse.

COMBINE the flour, remaining brown sugar, cornmeal, oats, cinnamon, salt, and the prepared walnuts in the bowl. Add the butter and mix just until clumps form. Sprinkle all over the top of the fruit. Bake 40 minutes. Let stand 30 minutes before serving. Garnish, as desired. Cover and refrigerate any leftovers. You can microwave the leftovers, but as with all crisps, it's nicer to reheat them in a 350° oven for about 10 minutes or so. Makes 8–10 servings.

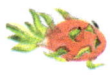

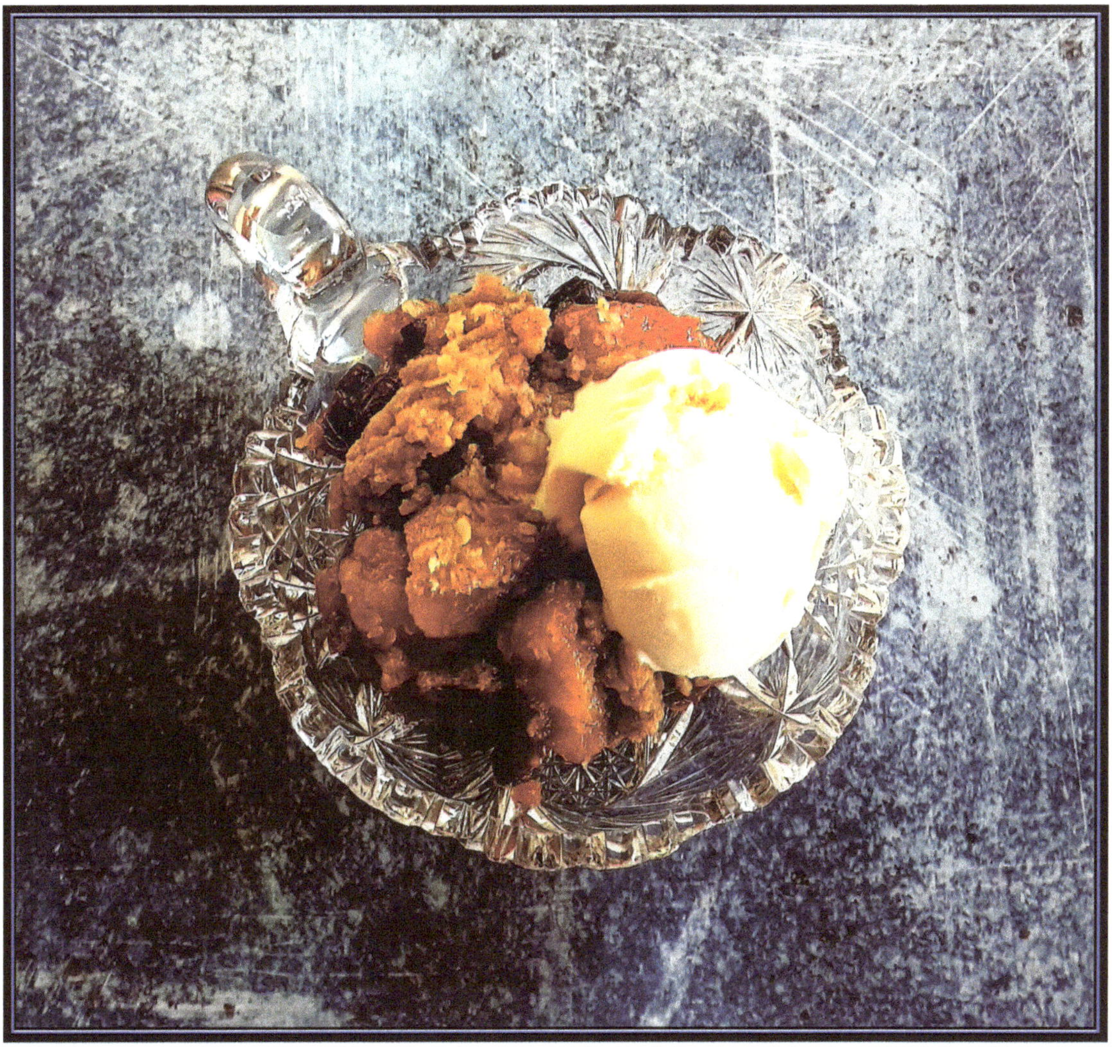

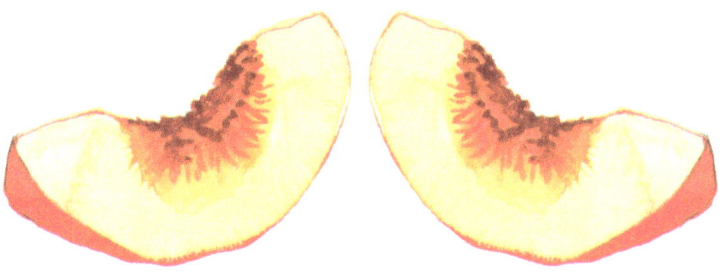

Chapter Fourteen: Sundry Sweeties 263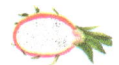

Joyful Almond Tart

ACTIVE PREP: 23 MINUTES
BAKE: 40 MINUTES
COOL: 30 MINUTES
CHILL: 2 HOURS
STAND: 1 HOUR
OVEN: 350°

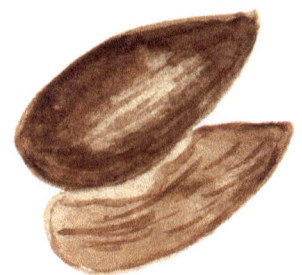

This is merely a giant, rather gooey version of the popular candy bar. If you don't happen to have the required pan, use a 9″ round, 1″ deep tart pan with removable sides and arrange your almonds in groups of three, in whatever fashion you like.

2 ounces sliced almonds
2 ounces graham crackers
¼ cup all-purpose flour
2 tablespoons sugar
½ teaspoon salt, divided
¼ cup salted butter, melted and cooled a bit
14-ounce can sweetened condensed milk (fat-free is okay)
4 ounces sweetened coconut flakes
1 large egg
½ teaspoon vanilla extract
½ teaspoon coconut extract
½ teaspoon almond extract
36 whole almonds
2 ounces milk chocolate chips
2 ounces semi-sweet chocolate chips
1 tablespoon vegetable oil

PLACE a sheet of foil in the oven which is large enough to fit under your baking pan with a couple of extra inches all around.

    PREHEAT the oven to 350°. Coat a 13½″ by 4½″ tart pan with removable sides with cooking spray well, especially on the sides. Combine the sliced almonds, graham crackers, flour, sugar, and ¼ teaspoon salt in a large food processor. Process thoroughly. Add the butter and process well. Pour into the prepared pan, pressing the mixture up the sides first, then the bottom evenly (don't wash the processor bowl; reuse). Bake 10 minutes.

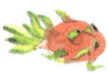

MEANWHILE, combine the sweetened condensed milk, coconut, egg, remaining salt, and the 3 extracts in the processor. Process thoroughly. Pour into the baked crust. Lay the 36 whole almonds on top of the coconut mixture, in 3 rows of 12 each. Bake 30 minutes. Place on a rack for 30 minutes.

IN a small glass bowl, combine all the chocolate chips and the oil. Microwave on HIGH in 20-second intervals to melt, which will take about a minute or so. Whisk to combine well. Pour over the tart; use a spoon or recessed spatula to spread the chocolate to the edge of the filling. Place the pan on the rack in the fridge for 2 hours to set. Remove and let it stand at room temperature for one hour. Use a sharp knife to carefully detach the sides. Carefully remove from the pan sides, then cut (press straight down to cut) into 12 pieces. Cover and refrigerate for longer storage; bring to room temperature 30–60 minutes for easier slicing. Makes 12 servings.

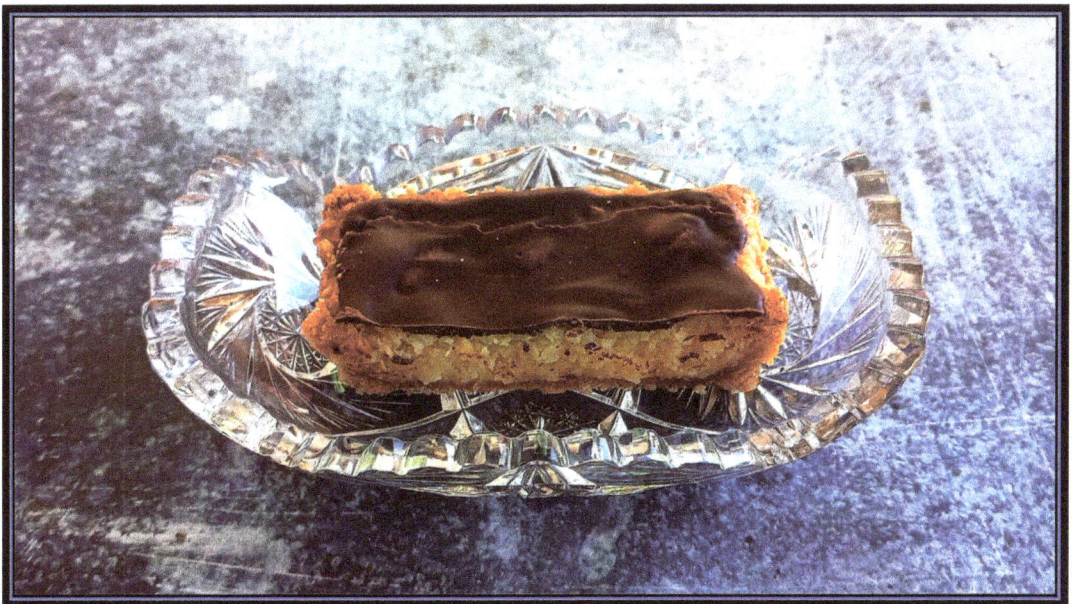

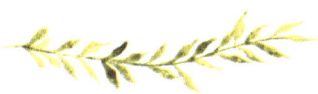

Banana Muffincakes

IN ADVANCE: TOASTING NUTS, COOLING, AND CHOPPING
ACTIVE PREP: ABOUT 55 MINUTES
BAKE: 28 MINUTES
COOL: 1 HOUR
OVEN: 400°

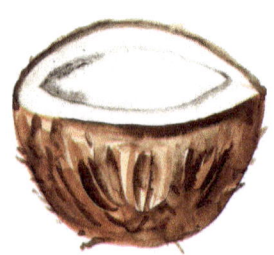

You can just make these as plain muffins or go all out and turn them into large cupcakes with the decadent frosting. Or you can make banana bread by placing the batter in a greased 8½" by 4½" loaf pan. Bake at 350° for an hour; place on a rack for 30 minutes. Turn the bread out of the pan and cool on the rack an additional 3–4 hours before cutting.

2 ounces pecans, lightly toasted, cooled, and chopped coarsely in advance
1¾ cups all-purpose flour
½ cup sugar
¼ cup packed light brown sugar
3–4 tablespoons orange zest, minced (1 tablespoon dried orange peel)
3–4 tablespoons lemon zest, minced (1 tablespoon dried lemon peel)
2 teaspoons baking powder
1 teaspoon baking soda
1 teaspoon ground cinnamon
1 teaspoon ground ginger
1 teaspoon ground nutmeg
1 teaspoon salt
½ cup vegetable oil
¼ cup plus 2 tablespoons orange juice
¼ cup buttermilk
½ cup sour cream (light is okay)
2 large eggs
1 cup mashed ripe bananas (about 3 medium)
1 tablespoon vanilla extract
9 ounces sweetened coconut flakes, divided
3 cups powdered sugar
¼ cup soft salted butter
2 tablespoons 1% milk

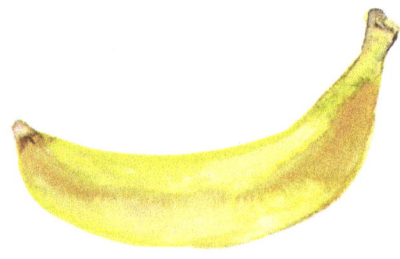

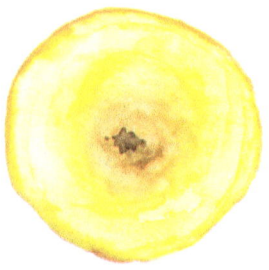

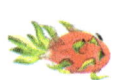

PREHEAT the oven to 400°. Coat 16 regular-size muffin cups with cooking spray or grease lightly. Combine the flour, sugar, brown sugar, orange and lemon zests, baking powder and soda, and the 4 seasonings in a very large bowl. In a 4-cup glass measuring cup, combine the oil, ¼ cup orange juice, buttermilk, sour cream, eggs, bananas, and vanilla well with a whisk. Add to the flour mixture. Whisk until well combined. Add the prepared pecans and 2 ounces of coconut and mix well. Divide between the prepared muffin cups. Bake 18–20 minutes. Place the pans on racks for 1 hour. Maintain oven temperature.

PLACE the remaining 7 ounces of coconut on a medium baking sheet and bake at 400° for 8–9 minutes. Stir at the 5-minute mark; shake the pan gently to distribute the coconut evenly. Stir again at 8 minutes and judge whether the coconut needs another minute. Be careful not to burn it! Remove from the oven and stir again. Let stand on the pan.

COMBINE the powdered sugar, butter, 2 tablespoons of orange juice, and milk in a very large bowl using a whisk attachment on your stand or hand mixer on low speed. Scrape the sides down, then mix on high speed a couple of minutes until the frosting is fluffy. Spread nicely on a muffin, then roll the top in the toasted coconut. Repeat with the remaining muffins. Cover and keep at room temperature (they freeze well). Extra toasted coconut is great for adding to pancake batter or topping ice cream sundaes. Makes 16.

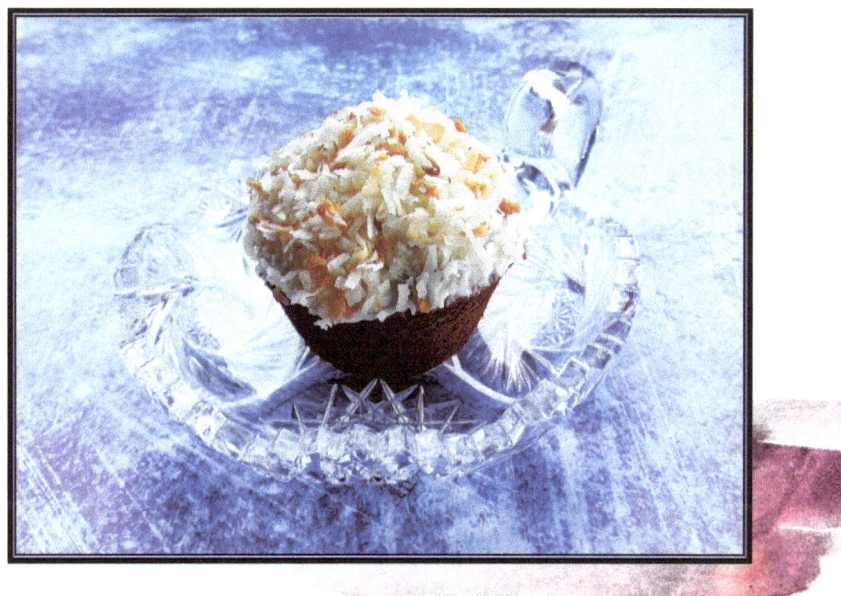

Chapter Fifteen

Monsters Scream for Ice Cream!

Silk Satin Sauce

Lobelia's Fudge Sauce

Peanut Butter Cup Sauce

White Chocolate Sauce

I Said Yeah, Yeah, Yeah Brown Sugar Sauce

German Chocolate Sauce

Mmm... Mocha Sauce

Nuts for You

Your Basic Vanilla Ice Cream

Apricot Ice Cream with Spicy Almond Crunch

Pretzel Nut Ice Cream

Tres Leches Ice Cream with Chili Pecans

Pucker Up, Buttercup!

Salty Goodness Caramel

Key Lime Pie Ice Cream

Monsters Scream for Ice Cream!

MY LATE MOTHER gave me a six-cup Cuisinart automatic ice cream maker a rather long while ago, so I worked on a few recipes. Any brand of machine can mix these up, as long as the capacity is at least six cups. No salt is required, as in the old-fashioned ice cream makers; plus, you don't have to do the mixing. I found that using a pasteurized liquid egg substitute creates an extra creaminess without the danger of curdling real eggs in your preparation. We'll start with a few sauces, which are probably best served on plainer flavors of ice creams such as vanilla. But these sauces are also great served over slices of pound cake or other types of desserts. Added bonus: once chilled, these sauces can be used as dips or spreads.

Silk Satin Sauce

PREP: 18 MINUTES
STAND: 30–45 MINUTES

Way back, when I was a dressmaker specializing in bridal garments, I occasionally was lucky enough to work with silk satin. I always thought if silk satin were a food, it would taste like this ice cream sauce.

2 ounces white chocolate chips
2 ounces bittersweet chocolate chips (60–72% cacao)
½ cup sugar
1 tablespoon salted butter
⅛ teaspoon salt
1 cup heavy cream
½ teaspoon vanilla extract

PLACE the chocolate chips, sugar, butter, salt, and cream in a 1½-quart saucepan. Cook over medium heat until bubbly and the chocolate has melted, whisking frequently. Turn heat to the lowest setting and cook, uncovered, 10 minutes. Whisk a couple of times. Turn off the heat and mix in the vanilla. Cover and let stand 30–45 minutes before serving. Stir and serve. Cover and refrigerate the leftovers; reheat slowly. Makes about 1¾ cups.

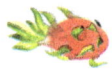

Lobelia's Fudge Sauce

PREP: 18 MINUTES
STAND: 30–45 MINUTES

This sauce was included in my first cookbook as a topping for some sort of pudding/pastry item named for Lobelia Sackville-Baggins, who is otherwise known as Bilbo Baggins's nemesis (although she turns out to be a rather sympathetic character at the end of her story). It involved using Pepperidge Farm puff pastry cups and a homemade pudding, topped with this sauce. After the Tolkien Estate got wind of my cookbook and I ended up rewriting the whole thing (I'm not bitter. Oh, maybe I am, a little…), that particular recipe was cut to make room for Turkish Delight, and I ended up salvaging only the sauce.

4 ounces semi-sweet chocolate chips
½ cup sugar
1 tablespoon salted butter
⅛ teaspoon salt
1 cup heavy cream
1 teaspoon vanilla extract
1 teaspoon almond extract

PLACE the chocolate chips, sugar, butter, salt, and cream in a 1½-quart saucepan. Cook over medium heat until bubbly and the chocolate has melted, whisking frequently. Turn heat to the lowest setting and cook, uncovered, 10 minutes. Whisk a couple of times. Turn off the heat and mix in the 2 extracts. Cover and let stand 30–45 minutes before serving. Stir and serve. Cover and refrigerate the leftovers; reheat slowly. Makes about 1¾ cups.

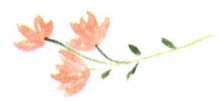

Chapter Fifteen: Monsters Scream for Ice Cream!

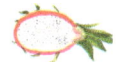

Peanut Butter Cup Sauce

PREP: 13 MINUTES
STAND: 30–45 MINUTES

This is rather reminiscent of the ubiquitous candy.

⅓ cup peanut butter (smooth or crunchy)
4 ounces semi-sweet chocolate chips
½ cup sugar
1 tablespoon salted butter
⅛ teaspoon salt
1 cup heavy cream
1 teaspoon vanilla extract

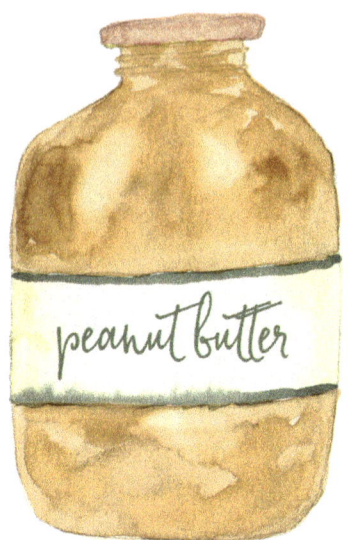

PLACE the peanut butter, chocolate chips, sugar, butter, salt, and cream in a 1½-quart saucepan. Cook over medium heat until bubbly and the chocolate has melted, whisking frequently. Turn heat to the lowest setting and cook, uncovered, 5 minutes. Whisk a couple of times. Turn off the heat and mix in the vanilla. Cover and let stand 30–45 minutes before serving. Stir and serve. Cover and refrigerate the leftovers; reheat slowly. Makes about 2 cups.

White Chocolate Sauce

PREP: 23 MINUTES
STAND: 30–45 MINUTES

A nice variation on this sauce is to add some orange flavor. Add a couple tablespoons of finely shredded orange zest and/or a tablespoon or two of any orange-flavored liqueur, either while it cooks or at the end, depending on if you want to retain the alcoholic content. This ends up being a thinner sauce than all the other chocolate-based sauces in this chapter. It's especially good on items like pound cake or other cakes. It's even good straight out of the refrigerator as a dip for items like cookies or strawberries.

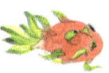

6 ounces white chocolate chips
1 tablespoon sugar
1 tablespoon salted butter
¼ teaspoon salt
¾ cup heavy cream
½ teaspoon vanilla extract

PLACE the chocolate chips, sugar, butter, salt, and cream in a 1½-quart saucepan. Cook over medium heat until bubbly and the chocolate has melted, whisking frequently. Turn heat to the lowest setting and cook, uncovered, 15 minutes. Whisk a couple of times. Turn off the heat and mix in the vanilla. Cover and let stand 30–45 minutes before serving. Stir and serve. Cover and refrigerate the leftovers; reheat very slowly, just for a few seconds in your microwave. Makes about 1½ cups.

I Said Yeah, Yeah, Yeah Brown Sugar Sauce

PREP: 18 MINUTES
STAND: 30–45 MINUTES

This is a rich, caramel-flavored sauce. If you have trouble locating cinnamon extract, you may substitute other flavors such as cake batter, rum, or caramel.

2 ounces white chocolate chips
1 ounce bittersweet chocolate chips (60–72% cacao)
½ cup packed light brown sugar
1 tablespoon salted butter
¼ teaspoon salt
1 cup heavy cream
1 teaspoon vanilla extract
1 teaspoon cinnamon extract

Chapter Fifteen: Monsters Scream for Ice Cream!

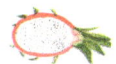

PLACE the chocolate chips, sugar, butter, salt, and cream in a 1½-quart saucepan. Cook over medium heat until bubbly and the chocolate has melted, whisking frequently. Turn heat to the lowest setting and cook, uncovered, 10 minutes. Whisk a couple of times. Turn off the heat and mix in the 2 extracts. Cover and let stand 30–45 minutes before serving. Stir and serve. Cover and refrigerate the leftovers; reheat slowly. Makes about 1½ cups.

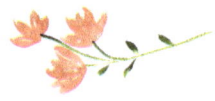

German Chocolate Sauce

IN ADVANCE: TOASTING NUTS, COOLING, AND CHOPPING
IN ADVANCE: TOASTING COCONUT
PREP: 18 MINUTES
STAND: 30–45 MINUTES

With this sauce, you won't need to add nuts to your deluxe ice cream sundae; they're already in the mix.

2 ounces pecans, lightly toasted, cooled, and chopped finely in advance
2 ounces sweetened coconut flakes, lightly toasted in advance
4 ounces German's sweet chocolate, broken into smaller squares
½ cup sugar
1 tablespoon salted butter
⅛ teaspoon salt
1⅓ cups heavy cream
1 teaspoon vanilla extract

PLACE the chocolate, sugar, butter, salt, and cream in a 1½-quart saucepan. Cook over medium heat until bubbly and the chocolate has melted, whisking frequently. Turn heat to the lowest setting and cook, uncovered, 10 minutes. Whisk a couple of times. Turn off the heat and mix in the vanilla and the prepared pecans and coconut. Cover and let stand 30–45 minutes before serving. Stir and serve. Cover and refrigerate the leftovers; reheat slowly. Makes about 2¼ cups.

Mmm... Mocha Sauce

PREP: 16 MINUTES
STAND: 30–45 MINUTES

Two tablespoons of espresso powder seemed to be the right amount for me and my family, but you can reduce or increase this amount according to how strong (or weak) you like your coffee flavor.

2 ounces unsweetened chocolate, broken into smaller squares
2 ounces semi-sweet chocolate chips
½ cup sugar
1 tablespoon salted butter
⅛ teaspoon salt
⅔ cup heavy cream
⅓ cup cold brewed coffee
2 tablespoons instant espresso powder
½ teaspoon vanilla extract

PLACE the 2 chocolates, sugar, butter, salt, and cream in a 1½-quart saucepan. Cook over medium heat until bubbly and the chocolate has melted, whisking frequently. Turn heat to the lowest setting and cook, uncovered, 3 minutes. Whisk a couple of times. Place the coffee, espresso powder, and vanilla in a 1-cup glass measuring cup. Microwave on HIGH for 1 minute. Stir this mixture, then add it to the saucepan. Raise the heat and cook on a gentle simmer 3 minutes, whisking frequently. Cover and let stand 30–45 minutes before serving. Stir and serve. Cover and refrigerate the leftovers; reheat slowly. Makes about 1½ cups.

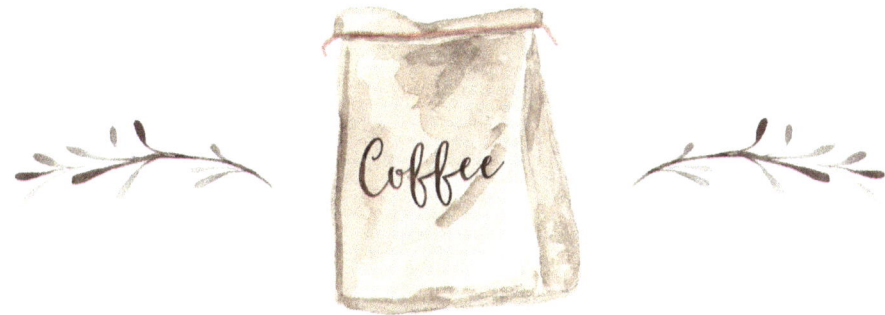

Chapter Fifteen: Monsters Scream for Ice Cream!

Nuts for You

ACTIVE PREP: ABOUT 15 MINUTES
BAKE: 12 MINUTES
COOL: ABOUT 1 HOUR
OVEN: 350°

It's nice to have a ready-to-use assortment of chopped nuts around the house for when those sundae-making urges hit you. This is my favorite combination below, but you can use pretty much any nut you like. Be sure to use two roasted and salted nuts (for example, macadamias and pistachios) with three plain nuts (such as hazelnuts, Brazils, or slivered almonds). When you get to the end of these nuts, you'll have a bunch of dust that is perfect to add to your next batch of pancakes or any other baked goods you might like. I know it takes more time, but it's better to chop the nuts by hand; a food processor will merely pulverize them all. Don't have time to toast your nuts? They will still be fine.

- 2 ounces pecan halves
- 2 ounces walnut halves
- 2 ounces sliced almonds
- 2 ounces roasted, salted peanuts
- 2 ounces roasted, salted cashews

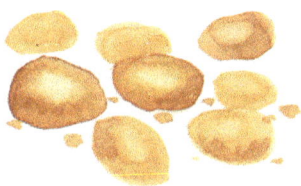

PREHEAT the oven to 350°. Place all the nuts in an 8" square baking dish. Bake 12 minutes. Stir halfway through. Cool in the pan for an hour or so. Chop all the nuts rather finely. Place in a 3-cup covered container. Store them tightly covered at room temperature, or you may store them in the refrigerator or freezer. Makes about 2½ cups.

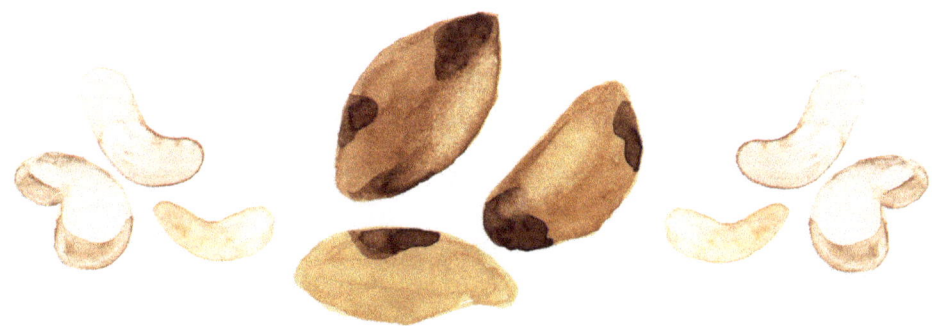

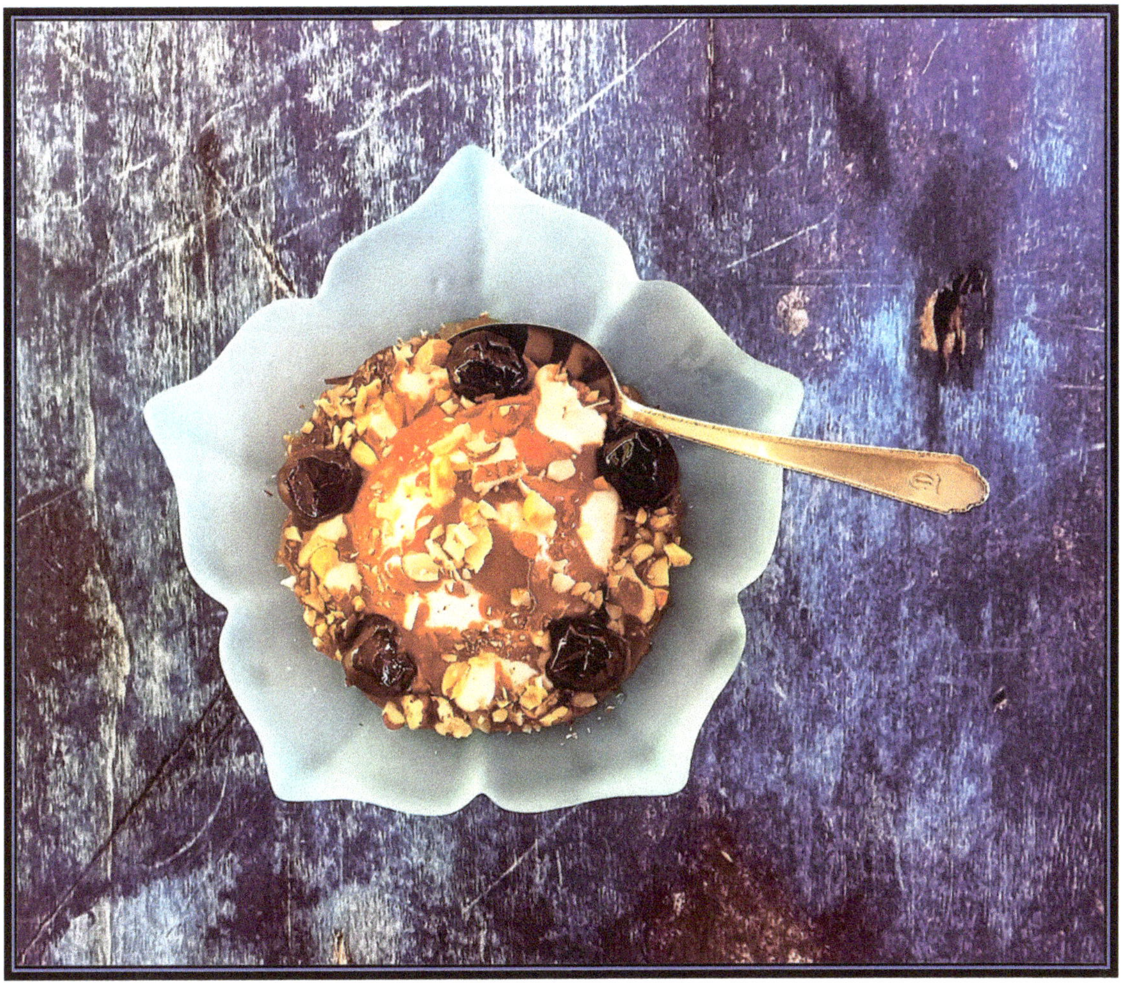

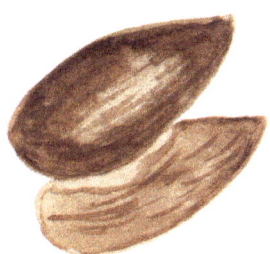

Your Basic Vanilla Ice Cream, page 278
Silk Satin Sauce, page 270
Nuts for You, page 276
Garnished with Luxardo Maraschino Cherries

Chapter Fifteen: Monsters Scream for Ice Cream!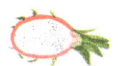

Your Basic Vanilla Ice Cream

ACTIVE PREP: 8 MINUTES
MIX: 30 MINUTES
FREEZE: 3–4 HOURS

This is the soft building block of any sundae. You can flavor this with real vanilla extract or use the seeds out of a very fresh pod; carefully cut the pod lengthwise with a small, very sharp knife, then scrape the seeds out with the tip of the knife. To jazz this up, add a cup or so of chopped (toasted) nuts or various fruits. Add a quarter to a half cup of your favorite liqueur for an alcoholic version (this will probably keep the ice cream somewhat softer).

As with all ice creams, both homemade and purchased, take all the following products out of your freezer 10–15 minutes before serving, once they have been frozen over six hours or so. All the following recipes can be served after freezing anywhere from three to four hours and will already be rather soft.

One more note: I also discovered that using milk substitutes, such as oat or soy, will keep your ice cream a bit on the softer side. You can keep the half-and-half and cream as stated in the recipe but switch to a milk substitute with good results.

1¼ cups heavy cream
¾ cup 1% milk
½ cup liquid egg substitute
¾ cup sugar
¼ teaspoon salt
1 tablespoon real vanilla extract (or the seeds from a large, fresh pod)

PLACE all the ingredients in a 4-cup glass measuring cup. Whisk well until the sugar has dissolved. Place in a 6-cup automatic ice cream maker and mix for 30 minutes. Place in a 6-cup container; cover and freeze at least 3–4 hours. Stir a couple of times. Cover and freeze any leftover ice cream; let it stand at room temperature for 10–15 minutes once it has fully frozen. Makes about 5 cups.

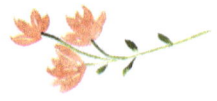

Apricot Ice Cream with Spicy Almond Crunch

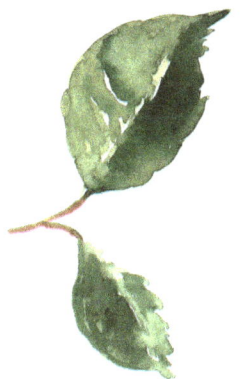

ACTIVE PREP: ABOUT 17 MINUTES
MIX: 35 MINUTES
FREEZE: 3–4 HOURS

If you have trouble locating canned apricots, canned mangos or peaches will also work out fine.

15-ounce can light apricot halves, with juice
1 tablespoon lemon juice
½ cup heavy cream
½ cup 1% milk
½ cup liquid egg substitute
¾ cup plus 2 tablespoons sugar
½ teaspoon salt, divided
½ teaspoon vanilla extract
3 tablespoons salted butter
½ teaspoon ground cinnamon
¼ teaspoon cayenne pepper
3 ounces sliced almonds

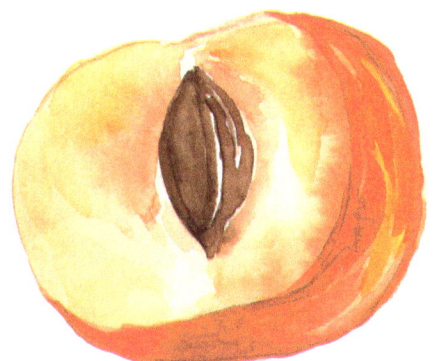

PLACE the apricots with juice, lemon juice, cream, milk, egg substitute, ¾ cup sugar, ¼ teaspoon salt, and vanilla in a blender and puree well. Pour into a 6-cup automatic ice cream maker and mix 30 minutes.

MEANWHILE, place the butter in a medium skillet and melt over very high heat. Add the 2 tablespoons sugar, ¼ teaspoon salt, cinnamon, and cayenne and mix. Add the almonds and sauté 1 minute, stirring constantly. Let stand in the pan. When the ice cream has been mixed for 30 minutes, carefully break up the nuts into smallish chunks and add to the mixer. Mix another 5 minutes. Pour into a 6-cup container. Cover and freeze 3–4 hours; stir a few times. Cover and freeze any leftover ice cream; let it stand at room temperature for 10–15 minutes once it has fully frozen. Makes about 6 cups.

Pretzel Nut Ice Cream

ACTIVE PREP: ABOUT 18 MINUTES
CHILL: ABOUT 1 HOUR
MIX: 35 MINUTES
FREEZE: 3–4 HOURS

If you omit the pretzel nut treatment, this is a lovely plain chocolate ice cream. You could also use caramel or butterscotch syrup instead of chocolate syrup for a subtle caramel flavor. Add an extra half a teaspoon of salt for more of a salted caramel option.

Deconstruct this recipe even further by simply making the candy. Double or triple the first three ingredients, spread the mixture on a larger baking sheet and refrigerate for a couple of hours. Break it all up and enjoy it as a candy-bark treat.

4 ounces white chocolate chips
2 ounces dry roasted and salted peanuts
1 ounce very thin, salted pretzel sticks, broken into approximately ½" bits
1 cup 1% milk
½ cup heavy cream
½ cup liquid egg substitute
½ cup chocolate syrup (such as Hershey's)
¼ cup sugar
½ teaspoon vanilla extract
¼ teaspoon salt

PLACE a piece of wax paper on a medium baking sheet; set aside. Place the white chocolate in a medium glass bowl and microwave on HIGH in 20-second intervals just until melted. Mix in the nuts and pretzel bits. Pour this onto the wax paper and spread it around to make a rather thin layer. Refrigerate until firm, about 1 hour.

MEANWHILE, place the remaining ingredients in a 4-cup glass measuring cup and whisk well to combine. Place in a 6-cup automatic ice cream maker and mix 30 minutes. Chop the prepared nut mixture coarsely and add to the mixer (break it up by hand if you would prefer larger chunks). Mix another 5 minutes. Pour into a 6-cup container. Cover and freeze 3–4 hours; stir a few times. Cover and freeze any leftover ice cream; let it stand at room temperature for 10–15 minutes once it has fully frozen. Makes about 6 cups.

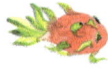

Tres Leches Ice Cream with Chili Pecans

ACTIVE PREP: ABOUT 17 MINUTES
MIX: 35 MINUTES
FREEZE: 3–4 HOURS

Tres leches simply means "three milks," which you see represented in this recipe.

¾ cup 1% milk
¾ cup half-and-half
½ cup heavy cream
½ cup liquid egg substitute
1 tablespoon Mexican vanilla blend extract (regular vanilla extract is also fine)
½ cup sugar
½ cup packed light brown sugar, divided
1 teaspoon ground cinnamon, divided
¾ teaspoon salt, divided
3 tablespoons salted butter
¾ teaspoon chili powder
4 ounces pecans, coarsely chopped

COMBINE the milk, half-and-half, cream, egg substitute, Mexican vanilla, sugar, ¼ cup brown sugar, ½ teaspoon cinnamon, and ¼ teaspoon salt in a 4-cup glass measuring cup and whisk well to combine. Pour into a 6-cup automatic ice cream maker and mix 30 minutes.

MEANWHILE, place the butter in a medium skillet and melt over very high heat. Add the remaining brown sugar, ½ teaspoon salt, ½ teaspoon cinnamon, and the chili powder and mix. Add the pecans and sauté 1 minute, stirring constantly. Let stand in the pan. When the ice cream has been mixed for 30 minutes, carefully break up the nuts into smallish chunks and add to the mixer. Mix another 5 minutes. Pour into a 6-cup container. Cover and freeze 3–4 hours; stir a few times. Cover and freeze any leftover ice cream; let it stand at room temperature for 10–15 minutes once it has fully frozen. Makes about 6 cups.

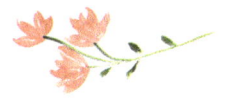

Chapter Fifteen: Monsters Scream for Ice Cream! 281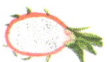

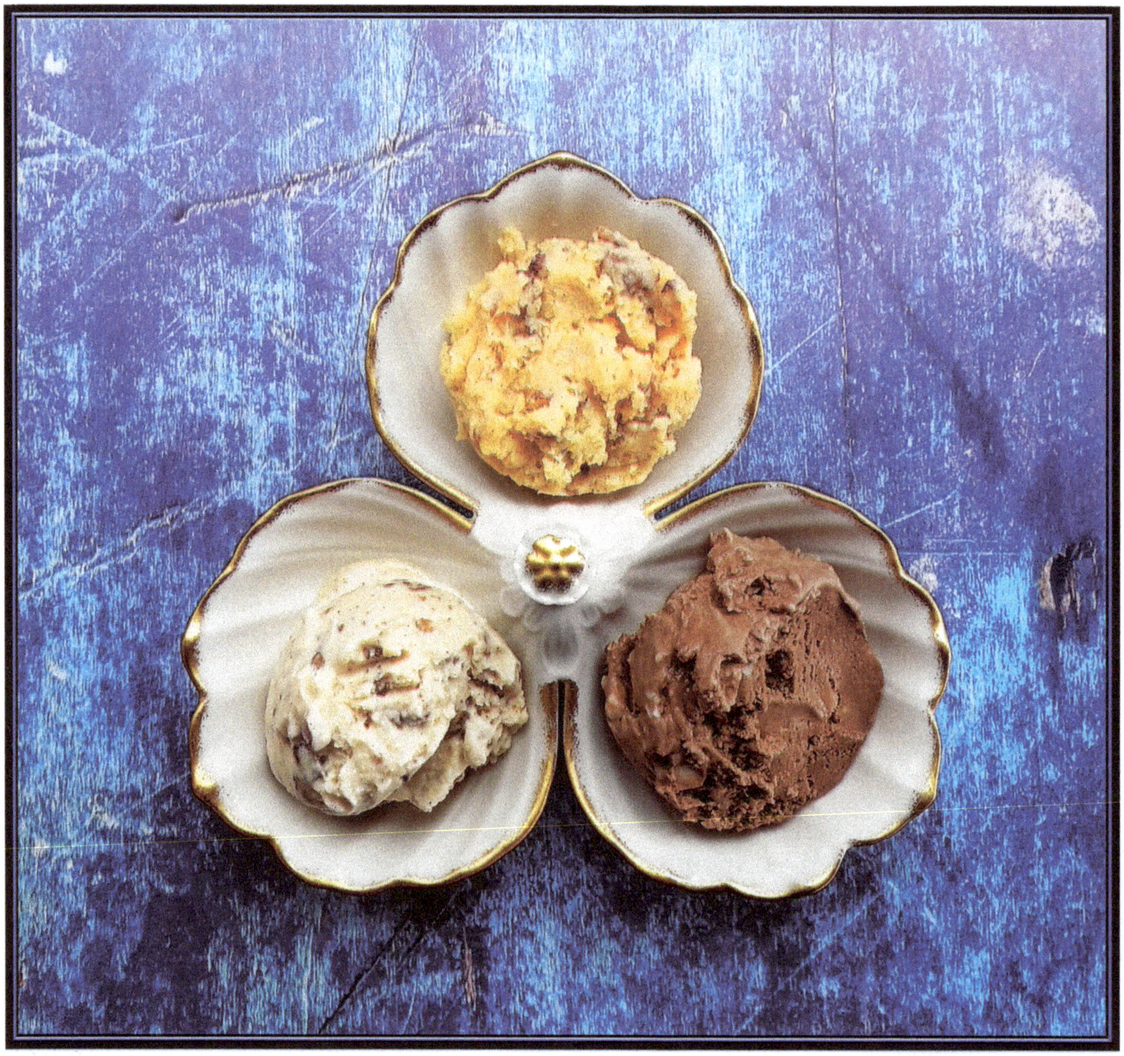

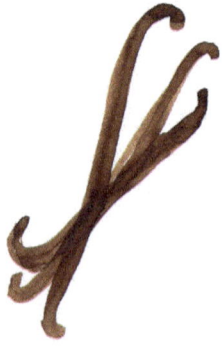

Clockwise, from top:
Apricot Ice Cream with Spicy Almond Crunch, page 279
Pretzel Nut Ice Cream, page 280
Tres Leches Ice Cream with Chili Pecans, page 281

 Celebrating Comfy, Cozy Foods from North America: CH&M, Volume 3

Pucker Up, Buttercup!

ACTIVE PREP: ABOUT 27 MINUTES
MIX: 35 MINUTES
FREEZE: 3–4 HOURS

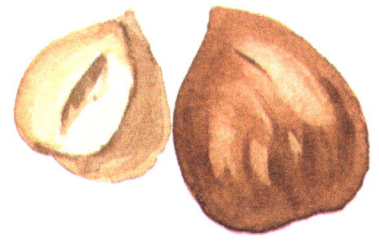

This will knock your socks off. Limes are just as good as lemons, or you might try combining both. Try oranges as well for a much milder version. This might remind you of the candy Lemon Heads.

1 cup chilled ginger ale (diet or regular)
4 good-sized lemons
½ cup liquid egg substitute
¼ cup heavy cream
1 cup lemon yogurt
1 cup sugar
1 teaspoon ground cardamom
½ teaspoon salt, divided
2 tablespoons salted butter
2 tablespoons raw sugar (turbinado)
4 ounces hazelnuts, coarsely chopped

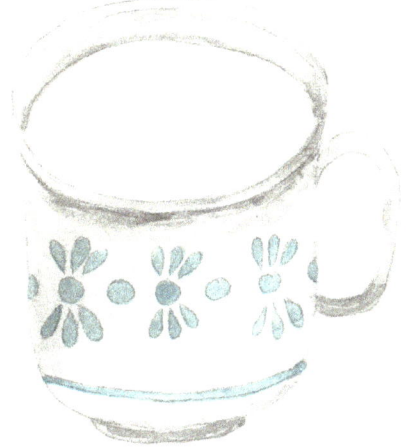

POUR the ginger ale into a 4-cup glass measuring cup and let it settle. Place a fine mesh strainer on top of the cup. Zest the lemons well and chop the zest finely; set aside. Cut lemons in half and juice them. Strain enough juice into the cup to measure 1½ cups total. Add the egg substitute, cream, yogurt, sugar, cardamom, ¼ teaspoon salt, and the reserved zest. Combine well with a whisk. Pour into a 6-cup ice cream maker and mix 30 minutes.

MEANWHILE, melt the butter in a medium skillet. Add the raw sugar and the remaining salt and cook until the sugar dissolves. Add the nuts and sauté over rather high heat 1 minute; stirring frequently. Let stand in the pan. When the ice cream has been mixed for 30 minutes, carefully break up the nuts into smallish chunks and add to the mixer. Mix another 5 minutes. Pour into a 6-cup container. Cover and freeze 3–4 hours; stir a few times. Cover and freeze any leftover ice cream; let it stand at room temperature for 10–15 minutes once it has fully frozen. Makes about 6 cups.

Salty Goodness Caramel

ACTIVE PREP: 7 MINUTES
MIX: 30 MINUTES
FREEZE: 3–4 HOURS

Just because salty and sweet are fantastic to eat.

1 cup 1% milk
1 cup heavy cream
½ cup liquid egg substitute
1 cup packed brown sugar (light or dark)
1 teaspoon coarse kosher salt
1 teaspoon vanilla extract

PLACE all the ingredients in a 4-cup glass measuring cup. Whisk well until the sugar has dissolved. Place in a 6-cup automatic ice cream maker and mix for 30 minutes. Place in a 6-cup container; cover and freeze at least 3–4 hours. Stir a couple of times. Cover and freeze any leftover ice cream; let it stand at room temperature for 10–15 minutes once it has fully frozen. Makes about 5 cups.

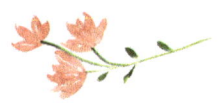

Key Lime Pie Ice Cream

ACTIVE PREP: ABOUT 18 MINUTES
BAKE: 5 MINUTES
STAND: 15 MINUTES
MIX: 35 MINUTES
FREEZE: 3–4 HOURS
OVEN: 425°

This final ice cream will remind you of a slice of mellow key lime pie. Increase the key lime juice up to half a cup if you need a bigger jolt.

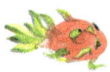

3 ounces graham crackers
3 tablespoons salted butter, softened
⅓ cup packed light brown sugar (raw sugar will also work)
1 cup 1% milk
½ cup heavy cream
½ cup liquid egg substitute
¼ cup key lime juice
¼ teaspoon salt
1 cup sugar

PREHEAT the oven to 425°. Spread the butter evenly on all the graham crackers. Place on a medium baking sheet. Sprinkle evenly with the brown sugar. Bake 5 minutes. Let stand on the pan at least 15 minutes. Place on a cutting board and chop coarsely. Set aside on the pan.

PLACE the remaining ingredients in a 4-cup glass measuring cup. Whisk well until the sugar has dissolved. Place in a 6-cup automatic ice cream maker and mix for 30 minutes. When the ice cream has been mixed for 30 minutes, add the prepared graham cracker mixture and mix another 5 minutes. Pour into a 6-cup container. Cover and freeze 3–4 hours; stir a few times. Cover and freeze any leftover ice cream; let it stand at room temperature for 10–15 minutes once it has fully frozen. Makes about 5 cups.

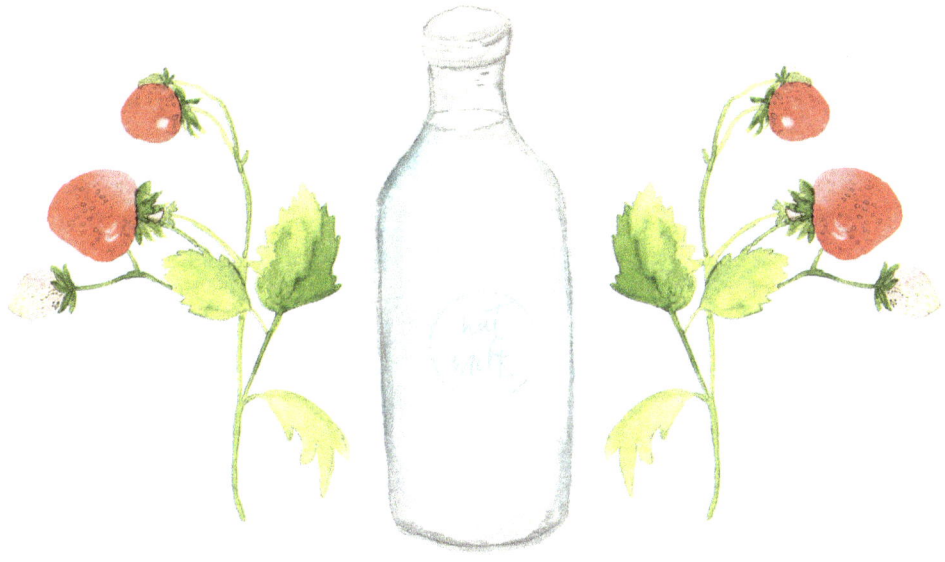

Chapter Fifteen: Monsters Scream for Ice Cream!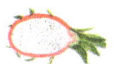

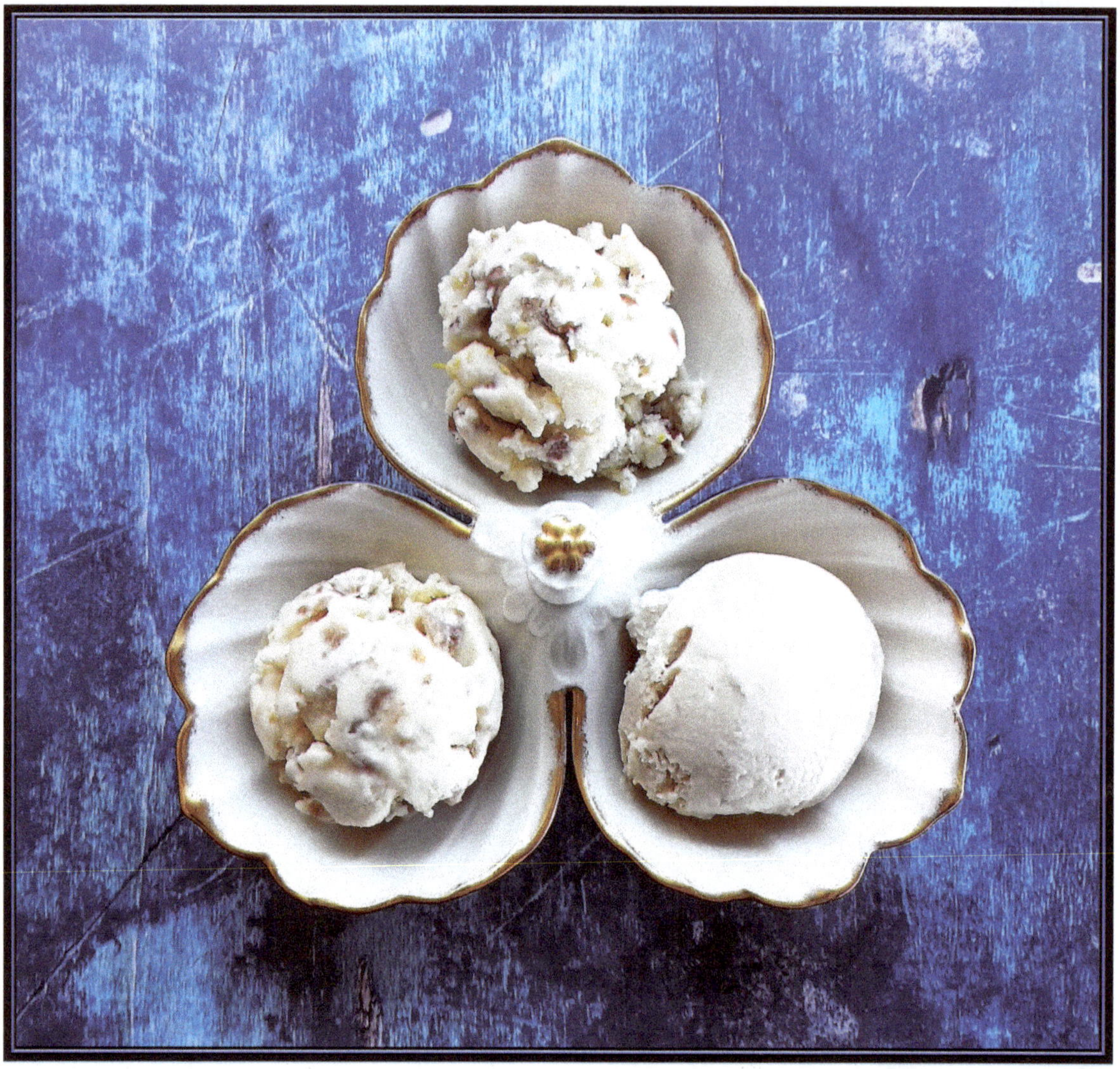

CLOCKWISE, FROM TOP:
Pucker Up, Buttercup!, page 283
Salty Goodness Caramel, page 284
Key Lime Pie Ice Cream, page 284

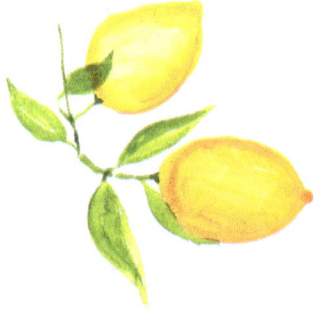

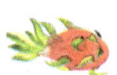 286   Celebrating Comfy, Cozy Foods from North America: CH&M, Volume 3

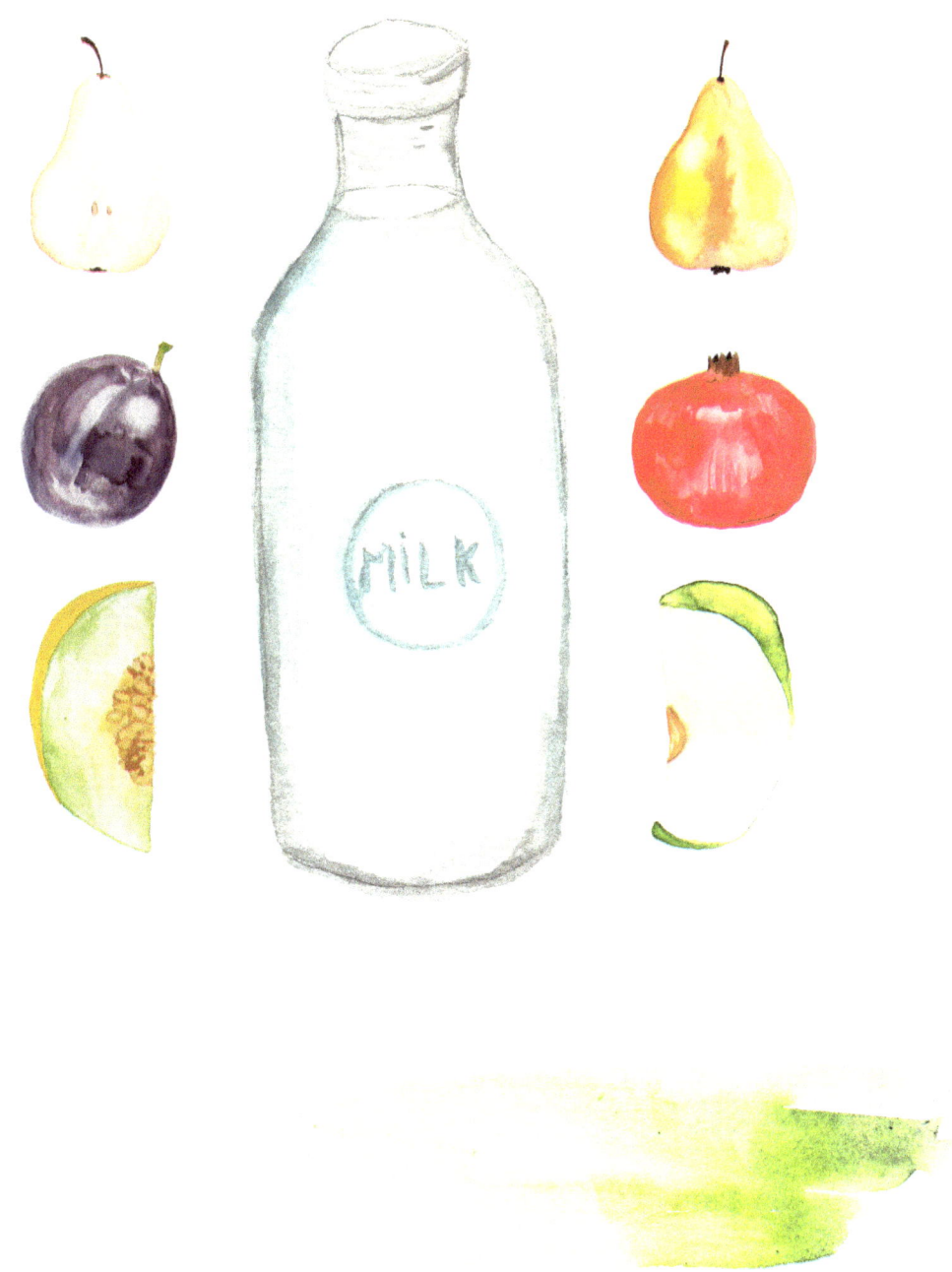

conclusion

I'M GOING TO carefully channel my favorite hobbit, Frodo Baggins, and his friend Gandalf here, and paraphrase some of their musings. You know that proverb "May you live in interesting times?" It is usually attributed to the Chinese language as a relatively mild curse for an enemy, but English has probably degraded and simplified the nuance of any original phrasing here. Meaning, sure, interesting times can be just that: *interesting*; and they are stressful and frightening. And even though we may wish that various events need not have happened in our time, all we can do is decide what we will do during these times. The times were pretty damn interesting while I wrote this cookbook. A global pandemic. A domestic insurrection. Ukraine. The Middle East. AI. Climate change… And so many other *interesting* happenings, that I can't even begin to enumerate them.

Two things I always choose to do during these *interesting* times are cooking and baking, as if these activities might impart some sort of magical healing powers, like Julieta's gift does in Disney's *Encanto* (which I think I have now seen with my granddaughter maybe 15 times—so far). But don't you usually feel a little bit better after preparing something delicious and sharing it with some loved ones or even just yourself? Give it a try more often. Make the enchiladas. Adopt a sourdough starter. Pour that homemade fudge sauce freely.

I hope you will find some new favorites within this quirky cookbook. And I also hope this world is blessed with a few absolutely boring times for a few years so we can recover.

List of Kitchen Utensils

MOST OF THESE items are fairly common and you probably already have them in a well-stocked kitchen. Saucepan sizing sometimes changes slightly, like fashion trends, but these capacities still seem popular. If I list a brand name, it's just because that's what I happen to have around; I'm not making a product endorsement. Cooking and baking times might need to be adjusted if you are using metal, glass, ceramic, or other types of cookware.

Cooking Utensils & Miscellaneous Items

- Measuring cups for dry ingredients (⅛, ¼, ⅓, ½, ⅔, ¾, and 1-cup)
- Glass measuring cups for liquid ingredients (1, 2, and 4-cup)
- Measuring spoons (⅛, ¼, ½, ¾, and 1 teaspoon, ½ tablespoon and 1 tablespoon)
- Kitchen scale (with a minimum capacity of 1 pound—I have a digital 30-pound capacity, which I love)
- Knife set (a few good, sharp knives, including a serrated one; I also use a cleaver)
- Storage containers with lids (various sizes; plastic and glass)
- Assorted mixing bowls, both glass and stainless steel (various sizes, from small to very large)
- Vegetable peeler / spatula / wooden spoon / cutting boards
- Towels / cloth napkins / potholders / box grater / pastry blender
- Whisks—various sizes / strainers and colanders—assorted sizes
- Dinner plates / forks, knives, and spoons / ice cube trays
- Rolling pin / timer / spray bottle for water / pastry brush / bent (or recessed) spatula
- Zester / tongs / slotted serving spoon / potato masher
- 16-ounce shaker jar for salad dressings
- Aluminum foil, both light and heavy-duty / parchment paper
- Medium-sized punchbowl / cocktail picks / meat thermometer
- Jigger / cocktail shaker with strainer / metal straw or cocktail stirrer
- Glassware for the bar:
	coupe 5–8 ounces / lowball 6–10 ounces
	highball 10–14 ounces / pint glass 16 ounces

List of Kitchen Utensils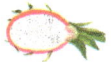

Small & Large Appliances

- Gas stove with conventional oven / microwave
- Panini press
- Hand mixer
- Blender (You need at least a 6-cup capacity; my newest one accommodates 8 cups. But you can always blend in stages if you need to.)
- Small food processor (Cuisinart "Mini-Prep"—4-cup variety; a 3-cup is also fine)
- Large food processor (Cuisinart—12-cup variety, with standard accessories)
- 5–5½-quart stand mixer (KitchenAid—with the standard beater, whisk, and dough hook)
- A slow cooker or Crock-Pot (minimum capacity 5 quarts)
- An automatic ice cream maker (or attachment) with at least a 6-cup capacity (1½ quarts)

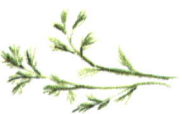

Pots & Pans

- Saucepans (pots) with lids (1, 1½, 2, 3, 4, 6, and 8-quart)
- Small skillet, 8" / medium skillet, 10" / large skillet, 12"
- 3-quart deep skillet, with cover
- 5-quart (5½-quart) deep skillet, with cover
- 10" cast iron skillet
- Griddle

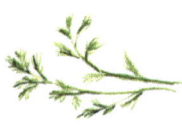

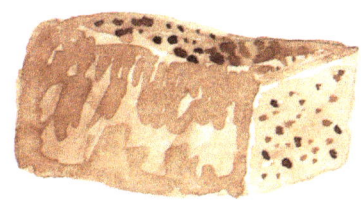

Baking Essentials

- Two 1-cup ramekins
- Two ¾-cup ramekins
- Quarter sheet (medium) baking pan (13″ by 9″—heavy aluminum, with 1″ rim)
- Two half sheet (large) baking pans (18″ by 13″—heavy aluminum, with 1″ rim)
- Small baking sheet pan (I use the 10″ square one from my toaster oven)
- Two pizza pans or stones
- Cooling racks
- 9″ springform pan (2″ sides)
- 11″ by 7″ baking dish (glass, metal, or ceramic are fine)
- 13″ by 9″ baking dish
- 8″ square baking dish
- 9″ square baking dish
- Two 8″ round baking pans
- Two 9″ by 5″ loaf pans
- 9½″ (glass) pie dish (metal or ceramic are fine)
- 2-quart baking or casserole dish with cover (round, square, oval, or rectangular will work)
- Two muffin pans—regular size (to make 24) / miniature muffin pans (enough to make 48)
- 13½″ by 4½″ tart pan with removable bottom (1″ deep; a 9″ round tart pan will substitute)

CONVERSION CHARTS

Here are some basic measurement conversion charts. All equivalents are approximate.

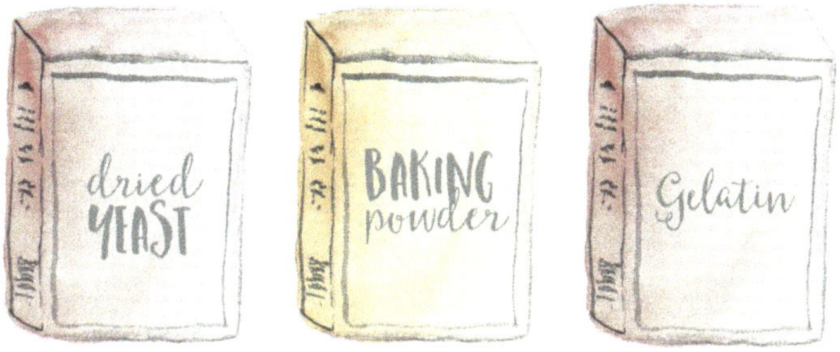

Dry Ingredients by Weight

Multiply the number of ounces by 28 to convert to grams.

⅛ teaspoon	a pinch			
3 teaspoons	1 tablespoon			
⅛ cup	2 tablespoons	1 ounce		28 grams
¼ cup	4 tablespoons	2 ounces	⅛ pound	56 grams
⅓ cup	5 tablespoons plus 1 teaspoon	3 ounces		84 grams
½ cup	8 tablespoons	4 ounces	¼ pound	112 grams
⅔ cup	10 tablespoons plus 2 teaspoons	5⅓ ounces	⅓ pound	144 grams
¾ cup	12 tablespoons	6 ounces		170 grams
1 cup	16 tablespoons	8 ounces	½ pound	230 grams
1¼ cups		10⅔ ounces	⅔ pound	300 grams
1½ cups		12 ounces	¾ pound	340 grams
2 cups		16 ounces	1 pound	450 grams
4 cups		32 ounces	2 pounds	900 grams
			2.2 pounds	1 kilogram

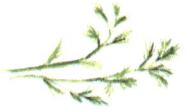

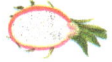

Liquid Ingredients by Volume

The column with parenthetical measurements on the right is for rounding up, if you don't need very precise conversions. Multiply the number of ounces by 30 to convert to milliliters.

¼ teaspoon				
½ teaspoon				
1 teaspoon			5 milliliters	
1 tablespoon	3 teaspoons	½ ounce	15 milliliters	
1 fluid ounce	2 tablespoons	⅛ cup	30 milliliters	
2 ounces	¼ cup		60 milliliters	
3 ounces	⅓ cup		90 milliliters	
4 ounces	½ cup		120 milliliters	
5⅓ ounces	⅔ cup		160 milliliters	
6 ounces	¾ cup		180 milliliters	
8 ounces	1 cup	half a pint	240 milliliters	(250 milliliters)
12 ounces	1½ cups		355 milliliters	
16 ounces	2 cups	1 pint	475 milliliters	(500 milliliters)
24 ounces	3 cups		700 milliliters	(750 milliliters)
32 ounces	4 cups	1 quart	950 milliliters	(1 liter)
128 ounces	16 cups	1 gallon	3.8 liters	(4 liters)

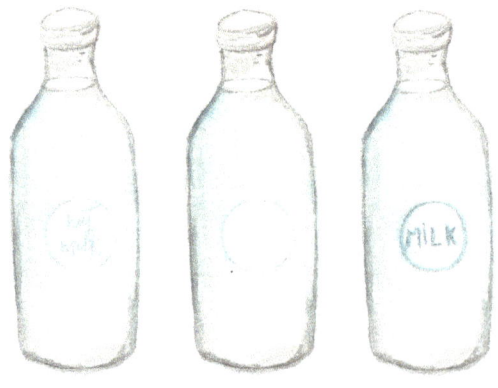

Lengths & Widths

Multiply number of inches by 2.5 to convert to centimeters.

1 inch			2.5 centimeters	
6 inches	½ foot		15 centimeters	
12 inches	1 foot		30 centimeters	
36 inches	3 feet	1 yard	90 centimeters	
40 inches			100 centimeters	1 meter

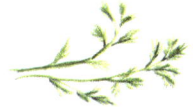

Temperatures

Fahrenheit	Celsius	Gas Mark
32°	0°	(freezes water)
212°	100°	(boils water)
225°	110°	¼
250°	130°	½
275°	140°	1
300°	150°	2
325°	160°	3
350°	180°	4
375°	190°	5
400°	200°	6
425°	220°	7
450°	230°	8
475°	240°	9

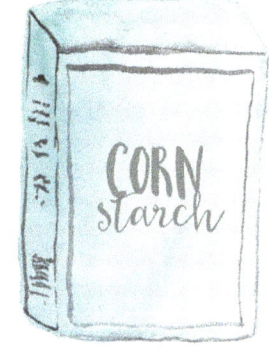
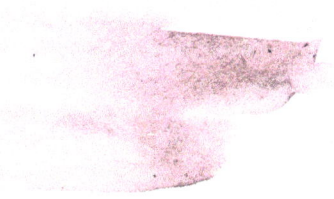

Acknowledgments

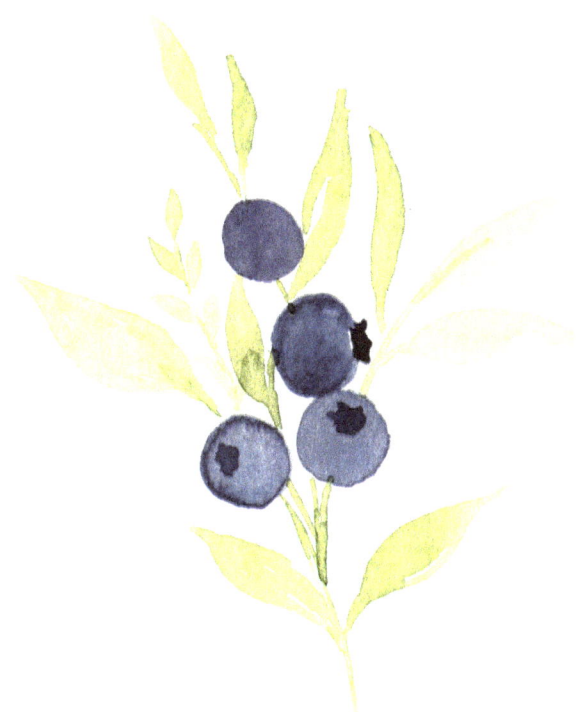

A FEW OF the *Star Wars* figurines and bobbleheads belong to my meager collection, but the majority belong to my son-in-law. I am forever grateful that he trusted me to use his beloved collectibles in my photographs! *Teeha*, Walter (this word is Ewok for thank you ✺).

Many thanks to my wonderful family members who were first readers. Some of them have missed their callings as editors and/or proofreaders. I am honored to share life's journey with all of you.

Thanks so much to my excellent and eagle-eyed editorial staff for their thoughtful suggestions: the delightful Dawn Catanach, the awesome Ann Tinkham, the terrific Tina Ramsey, and the zesty, yet zen, Zach Hively (and Casa Urraca Press, Ltd.). If any of them had seen this particular paragraph, they might have advised me to avoid all of this alliteration. Oh, well.

The Fellowship of the Recipe Testers

Thank You!

THANKS A MILLION to the committed squadron of Recipe Testers I recruited for this cookbook, who went above and beyond to help these recipes be the best they can be! Although recipes are always rather subjective, aren't they? I left plenty of white space within this cookbook, so you can make all the notes you need to in the margins.

ARASIZ
DAWN BENSE
ELVISH BLACK
DUSTY BROOKS
GENIE BULLARD (VAUGHN'S MUM)
SHARON CIRAULO
MICHELLE CROWDER
SUZAN DENTRY
CELIA GARLAND
MARCIA GLENN
JOHN HARSTINE
KATE JERACKI
THE RAMSEY FAMILY: TINA, YVONNE, AND MICHELLE
MARK & ELLEN STURMER
VAUGHN SVOBODA
LINDA VELWEST
ERIC WAGONER
THE WINEGAR-VALDEZ FAMILY

Works Cited -&- Sourced

30 Rock. Television series, created by Tina Fey. Perf. Tina Fey et al. United States: NBCUniversal Television Distribution, 2006–2013. Season 2, episode 6, "Somebody to Love." Dir. Beth McCarthy-Miller, aired on November 15, 2007.

And Just Like That… Television series, created by Darren Star. Perf. Sarah Jessica Parker et al. United States: Warner Bros. Discovery Global Streaming & Interactive Entertainment, 2021–unknown. Season 1, episode 5, "Tragically Hip." Dir. Gillian Robespierre, aired on December 30, 2021.

Blondie. "Rapture." *Autoamerican.* Songwriters Debbie Harry and Chris Stein. Producer Mike Chapman. Chrysalis, 1981.

Bourdain, Anthony. *Kitchen Confidential* (Updated Edition). New York: Ecco Books, an imprint of HarperCollins Publishers, 2000 and 2007.

Christmas with Southern Living 2005. Ed. Rebecca Brennan. Alabama: Oxmoor House, Inc., 2005.

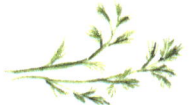

Encanto. Dir. Jared Bush and Byron Howard. Screenplay by Charise Castro Smith and Jared Bush. Perf. Stephanie Beatriz et al. United States: Walt Disney Studios Motion Pictures, 2021.

Gabriel, Peter. "Steam." *Us.* Songwriter Peter Gabriel. Producers Daniel Lanois and Peter Gabriel. Geffen, 1993.

How I Met Your Mother. Television series, created by Carter Bays and Craig Thomas. Perf. Josh Radnor et al. United States: 20th Century Fox Television, 2005–2014. Season 8, episode 20, "The Time Travelers." Dir. Pamela Fryman, aired on March 25, 2013.

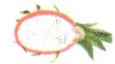

The Late Show with Stephen Colbert. Television series, created by David Letterman. Perf. Stephen Colbert. United States: CBS Media Ventures, 2015–unknown. Episode 865, guests Patrick Stewart and Dick Cavett, aired on January 21, 2020.

—. Episode 880, guests Sam Heughan et al., aired on February 13, 2020.

—. Episode 1347, guests Andy Cohen and Anderson Cooper, aired on December 15, 2022.

—. Episode 1351, guests Tom Hanks et al., aired on January 9, 2023.

—. Episode 1355, guests Hugh Jackman et al., aired on January 16, 2023.

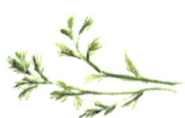

Nirvana. "All Apologies." *In Utero.* Songwriter Kurt Cobain. Producer Steve Albini. DGC, 1993.

Quiz RPG: The World of Mystic Wiz. Video game, developed by Colopl and Core Edge (PC Version). Platforms: iOS, Android, Windows, 2013.

Scrubs. Television series, created by Bill Lawrence. Perf. Zach Braff et al. United States: Disney—ABC Domestic Television, 2001–2010. Season 8, episode 2, "My Last Words." Dir. Bill Lawrence, aired on January 6, 2009.

Star Trek: The Next Generation. Television series, created by Gene Roddenberry. Perf. Patrick Stewart et al. United States: Paramount Domestic Television, 1987–1994. Season 7, Episode 24, "Preemptive Strike." Dir. Patrick Stewart, aired on May 16, 1994.

Star Wars: Episode V—The Empire Strikes Back. Dir. Irvin Kershner. Screenplay by Leigh Brackett and Lawrence Kasdan. Perf. Mark Hamill et al. United States: 20th Century Fox, 1980.

Star Wars: Episode VII—The Force Awakens. Dir. J. J. Abrams. Screenplay by Lawrence Kasdan et al. Perf. Harrison Ford et al. United States: Walt Disney Studios Motion Pictures, 2015.

Star Wars: Episode IV—A New Hope. Dir. George Lucas. Screenplay by George Lucas. Perf. Mark Hamill et al. United States: 20th Century Fox, 1977.

Star Wars: Episode I—The Phantom Menace. Dir. George Lucas. Screenplay by George Lucas. Perf. Liam Neeson et al. United States: 20th Century Fox, 1999.

Tucci, Stanley. *Stanley Tucci shows how to make a perfect Negroni cocktail at home. YouTube,* uploaded by Good Morning America. 21 April 2020, https://www.youtube.com/watch?v=L7yV_ctYOVs.

Whitaker, Holly. *Quit Like a Woman.* New York: The Dial Press, 2019.

Young Sheldon. Television series, created by Chuck Lorre and Steven Molaro. Perf. Iain Armitage et al. United States: CBS, 2017–2024. Multiple episodes.

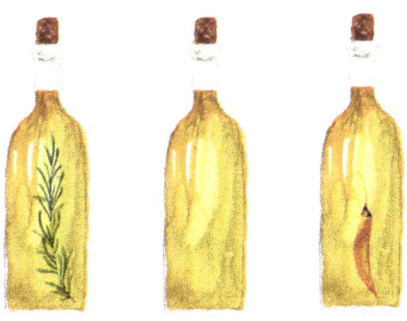

shopping sources

THERE IS ALWAYS Amazon for various ingredients you might have trouble finding, but here are a few smaller companies that you might prefer to use. Lots of fun can be had looking at King Arthur Baking Company. Here is where I purchased my beloved yeast measuring spoon, and I also treated myself to precut parchment paper rounds in both the eight- and nine-inch sizes. Worth it! www.kingarthurbaking.com

For many spices and spice mixes, try Spices, Inc. I like to order the glass jars with half a cup of spice, though they can also accommodate your larger needs. Their prices are competitive, and their selection is massive. www.spicesinc.com

Here are popular options for prepared chile sauces and salsas, still in business as of October 2024:

505 Southwestern	www.505southwestern.com
Bueno Foods	www.buenofoods.com
Cervantes Salsa	www.cervantessalsa.com
Chile Traditions	www.chiletraditions.com
El Pinto	www.elpinto.com
Hatch Chile Store	www.hatch-green-chile.com
La Salita	www.lasalita.com
Monroe's	www.monroeschile.com
Sadie's	www.sadiesofnewmexico.com

INDEX

WITH ONLY A few exceptions, recipes are assigned to a maximum of five groups: the title, the overall type of recipe, and no more than three dominant ingredients. Various ingredients have been grouped together, such as fruit.

A

Agave Shrimp, 102

ALCOHOL
Aperol Spritzie, 24
The Black-eyed Susan, 40
Carrie's Crazy Cosmo, 35
The Cavett, 25
Chocolate Chip Cookie, 32
Cinnamon Bun, 34
The Colbert, 26
Cupid Cocktail, 76
Fruity Martuity, 36
Hot Tamale, 42
Jackie D's Nancy Drew, 27
J.D.'s Awesome Appletini, 38
Just Another Tequila Sunrise, 42
Kickin' Moscow Mule, 28
Lemon Cake, 32
Manhattan Madness, 36
Marvelous Margarita, 40
The More Mature Scherbatsky, 38
Negroni Spritzie, 24
Old-Fogey-Fashioned, 37
Ooooo-ti-ni!, 30
Screaming Orgasm, 34
Sloe Your Roll Fizz, 28
Steaks with Benefits, 72
Tequila Peppers, 85
Tickin' Time Bomb, 29
Vodka Penne, 222
The Watergate, 43
XOXO, 78

All Hail the Caesar Salad, 66
Amalgamation Cookies, 253
Aperol Spritzie, 24

APPETIZERS
Mom's Spicy Meatballs, 2
Tauntaun Wontons, 128

Apricot Ice Cream with Spicy Almond Crunch, 279

ASPARAGUS
The Evening-After Salad, 79

AVOCADO
Guacamole, 5
Tomatillo Salsa, 48

B

BACON
Bacon Mac Salad, 63
Hearty Bacony Mac & Cheese, 223
Valentine's Day Taters, 73

Bacon Mac Salad, 63
Banana Muffincakes, 266

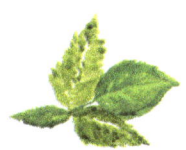

BEANS
Black Bean Salad, 58
Bob's Favorite Bowl, 238
Búho Beans, 92
Callista's Birthday Pizza, 177
Marcella's Flat Enchiladas, 167
NMNYBEP, 9
NMNYBEP Soup, 11
Three Bean Salad, 62
Ultimate Nachos, 46
The Whole Enchilada, 170

BEEF
Beefy Enchiladas, 152
Bob's Favorite Bowl, 238
Bodacious Brisket, 160
Burqueño Beef, 134
Callista's Birthday Pizza, 177
Chile Joes, 131
The Evening-After Salad, 79
Hidden Treasure Meatloaf, 156
Marcella's Flat Enchiladas, 167
Roast Beef & Gorgonzola
    Sandwich, 126
Sheldon's Spaghetti, 229
Spaghetti Western, 216
Steaks with Benefits, 72
Super Savory Salad, 64
Taco Rice Casserole, 164
Taco Tuesday Tacos, 171
Ultimate Nachos, 46

Beefy Enchiladas, 152

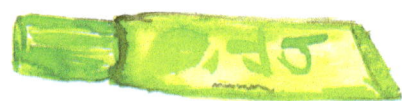

BEETS
Lobo Beets & Greens, 90

BELL PEPPERS
Cajun-Style Fettuccine, 219
Mexican Flag Salad, 240
Mom's Bell Pepper, 133
Puebla Coleslaw, 105
Tequila Peppers, 85
Three Bean Salad, 62
Truth or Consequences Stuffed
    Peppers, 165

BEVERAGES
Aperol Spritzie, 24
The Black-eyed Susan, 40
Carrie's Crazy Cosmo, 35
The Cavett, 25
Chocolate Chip Cookie, 32
Cinnamon Bun, 34
The Colbert, 26
Cupid Cocktail, 76
Fruity Martuity, 36
Hot Tamale, 42
Jackie D's Nancy Drew, 27
J.D.'s Awesome Appletini, 38
Just Another Tequila Sunrise, 42
Kickin' Moscow Mule, 28
Lemon Cake, 32
Manhattan Madness, 36
Marvelous Margarita, 40
The More Mature Scherbatsky, 38
Negroni Spritzie, 24
Old-Fogey-Fashioned, 37
Ooooo-ti-ni!, 30
Screaming Orgasm, 34
Sloe Your Roll Fizz, 28
Tickin' Time Bomb, 29

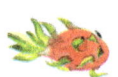

Uncle Donny's Tropical Apple Cider Punch, 145
The Watergate, 43

Biscochitos, 107
Black Bean Salad, 58
The Black-eyed Susan, 40
Blondie Rapture, 257
Bob's Favorite Bowl, 238
Bob's Favorite Cake, 241
Bodacious Brisket, 160
Boil Bonus Soup, 142

BREAD & CEREAL
All Hail the Caesar Salad, 66
Chloë's Grits Dressing, 190
English Muffins, xxi
Pumpkin Pancakes, 210
Sandia Spoon Bread, 86

BROCCOLI
Roasted Tiny Trees, 87

BRUSSELS SPROUTS
Caulisprouts, 186

Búho Beans, 92
Burque Turkey, 133
Burqueño Beef, 134

C

CABBAGE
Puebla Coleslaw, 105

Cajun Mix, xv
Cajun-Style Fettuccine, 219

CAKES
Banana Muffincakes, 266
Bob's Favorite Cake, 241
Cranberry Cheesecake, 195
The Half-Pound Cake, 198
Warren's Pumpkin Cheesecake, 202

Calabacitas, 104
Callista's Birthday Pizza, 177
Carrie's Crazy Cosmo, 35

CARROT
Roasted Baby Carrots, 184

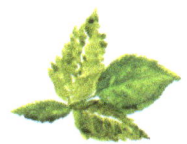

CAULIFLOWER
Caulisprouts, 186

Caulisprouts, 186
The Cavett, 25

CELERY
Chloë's Grits Dressing, 190

CHEESE (ONLY SAVORY ITEMS)
All Hail the Caesar Salad, 66
Bacon Mac Salad, 63
Beefy Enchiladas, 152
Black Bean Salad, 58
Burque Turkey, 133
Burqueño Beef, 134
Callista's Birthday Pizza, 177
Chile con Queso, 6
Chile Joes, 131
Creamy Dreamy Mac & Cheese, 225

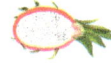

Giant Funky Ham Sandwich, 122
Halfling/Monster Mac & Cheese, 232
Hasperat, 120
Hearty Bacony Mac & Cheese, 223
It's My Pie; Nacho Pie, 50
Jakkubano, 124
Mom's Bell Pepper, 133
The One-Bowl Thanksgiving Leftover Casserole, 192
Roast Beef & Gorgonzola Sandwich, 126
Saucy Soupy Mac & Cheese, 218
Savory Seasoning Pork Chops, 162
Spaghetti Western, 216
Spinach au Gratin, 188
Super Savory Salad, 64
Taco Rice Casserole, 164
Taco Tuesday Tacos, 171
Tauntaun Wontons, 128
Thank Goodness for Enchilada Casseroles, 194
Ultimate Nachos, 46
Upscale Mac & Cheese, 220
Vader's Killer Taters, 174
Valentine's Day Taters, 73
The Whole Enchilada, 170
Zaragoza's Lasagna, 100

Cherry Ginger Oatmeal Cookies, 254

CHICKEN & POULTRY
Burque Turkey, 133
Chicken Salad, 116
Hidden Treasure Meatloaf, 156
The One-Bowl Thanksgiving Leftover Casserole, 192
"Perhaps This Chicken Needs Paprika?", 154
Post-Watergate Chicken Salad, 56
Thank Goodness for Enchilada Casseroles, 194
Truth or Consequences Stuffed Peppers, 165
The Whole Enchilada, 170

Chicken Salad, 116
Chile con Queso, 6
Chile Joes, 131

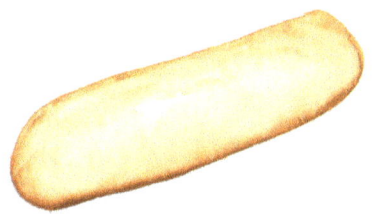

CHILE PEPPERS (ALL VARIETIES; RED, GREEN, OR CHRISTMAS—WHICH MEANS BOTH AT THE SAME TIME)
Beefy Enchiladas, 152
Búho Beans, 92
Burque Turkey, 133
Burqueño Beef, 134
Calabacitas, 104
Chile con Queso, 6
Chile Joes, 131
Green Chile Dip, 3
Guacamole, 5
It's My Pie; Nacho Pie, 50
Marcella's Flat Enchiladas, 167
NMNYBEP, 9
"Perhaps This Chicken Needs Paprika?", 154
Perky Pico de Gallo, xxix
Red Chile Sauce, xxviii
Roasted Green Chile: A Big Bunch of Chiles, xxvi

Roasted Green Chile: Just a Few Chiles, xxvi
Sandia Spoon Bread, 86
Santa Fe Fettuccine, 224
Taco Rice Casserole, 164
Thank Goodness for Enchilada Casseroles, 194
Tomatillo Salsa, 48

Chipotle Mayo, 115
Chloë's Grits Dressing, 190

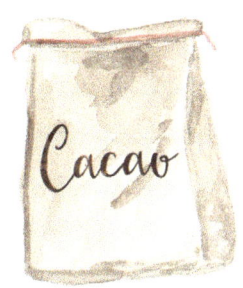

CHOCOLATE (ALL VARIETIES)
Amalgamation Cookies, 253
Blondie Rapture, 257
Bob's Favorite Cake, 241
Chocolate Chip Cookies, 250
Chocolate Chips in a Pan, 260
Fudge Bomb Brownies, 52
German Chocolate Sauce, 274
I Said Yeah, Yeah, Yeah Brown Sugar Sauce, 273
Jan's Moon Shadows, 255
Joyful Almond Tart, 264
Lobelia's Fudge Sauce, 271
Mmm… Mocha Sauce, 275
Peanut Butter Cup Sauce, 272
Pecan Pie, 12
Pretzel Nut Ice Cream, 280
Pumpkin Pancakes, 210

Silk Satin Sauce, 270
Snickers Salad, 147
White Chocolate Sauce, 272
XOXO, 78

Chocolate Chip Cookie, 32
Chocolate Chip Cookies, 250
Chocolate Chips in a Pan, 260
Cinnamon Bun, 34
The Colbert, 26

COLD SALADS
Agave Shrimp, 102
All Hail the Caesar Salad, 66
Bacon Mac Salad, 63
Black Bean Salad, 58
Chicken Salad, 116
Cranberry Spinach Salad, 143
Egg Salad, 117
The Evening-After Salad, 79
Ham Salad, 117
Mexican Flag Salad, 240
Mom's Bell Pepper, 133
Naked Ambrosia, 68
Post-Watergate Chicken Salad, 56
Puebla Coleslaw, 105
Super Savory Salad, 64
Three Bean Salad, 62
Tuna Salad, 118
You Can't Name Everything After Bob Potato Salad, 59

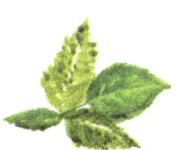

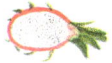

Index   313

COOKIES (DROP OR BAR)
- Amalgamation Cookies, 253
- Biscochitos, 107
- Blondie Rapture, 257
- Cherry Ginger Oatmeal Cookies, 254
- Chocolate Chip Cookies, 250
- Chocolate Chips in a Pan, 260
- Fudge Bomb Brownies, 52
- Jan's Moon Shadows, 255
- Nirvana Newtons, 258
- Perfect Polvorones, 252
- Skippy the Jedi Droid's Powerful Force Cookies, 247
- Super Snickerdoodles, 251

CORN
- Puebla Coleslaw, 105
- Sandia Spoon Bread, 86

Corn Sauce, 140
Cran-Apple Streusel Pie, 199
Cranberry Cheesecake, 195
Cranberry Spinach Salad, 143

CREAMY
- Cajun-Style Fettuccine, 219
- Creamy Dreamy Mac & Cheese, 225
- Frankenstein's Bowties, 226
- Green Chile Dip, 3
- Sam's Fairly Large Crowd Po—ta—toes, 183
- Santa Fe Fettuccine, 224
- Snickers Salad, 147

Creamy Dreamy Mac & Cheese, 225

CUCUMBERS
- Jakkubano, 124
- Mexican Flag Salad, 240

Cupid Cocktail, 76
Cyrus's No-Bake Pumpkin Tarts, 203

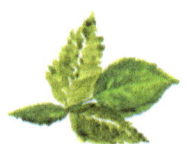

D

DESSERTS
- Amalgamation Cookies, 253
- Apricot Ice Cream with Spicy Almond Crunch, 279
- Banana Muffincakes, 266
- Biscochitos, 107
- Blondie Rapture, 257
- Bob's Favorite Cake, 241
- Cherry Ginger Oatmeal Cookies, 254
- Chocolate Chip Cookies, 250
- Chocolate Chips in a Pan, 260
- Cran-Apple Streusel Pie, 199
- Cranberry Cheesecake, 195
- Cyrus's No-Bake Pumpkin Tarts, 203
- Fudge Bomb Brownies, 52
- The Half-Pound Cake, 198
- Isabella's Pumpkin Pie Ice Cream, 208
- Jan's Moon Shadows, 255
- Joyful Almond Tart, 264
- Key Lime Pie Ice Cream, 284
- Nirvana Newtons, 258
- P. D. G. Crisp, 262
- Perfect Polvorones, 252
- Pretzel Nut Ice Cream, 280
- Pucker Up, Buttercup!, 283
- Pumpkin Sparkle Pie, 204
- R2-DChews, 7
- Salty Goodness Caramel, 284

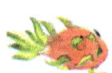

Skippy the Jedi Droid's
    Powerful Force Cookies, 247
Snickers Salad, 147
Super Snickerdoodles, 251
Tres Leches Ice Cream with
    Chili Pecans, 281
Warren's Pumpkin Cheesecake, 202
William's Chili Pumpkin Bread
    with Pepitas Honey Butter, 207
XOXO, 78
Your Basic Vanilla Ice Cream, 278

**DRY SEASONING MIXES
    (SWEET & SAVORY)**
Cajun Mix, xv
Easy Herbes de Provence, xii
Just the Basics, xiv
Mexican Mix, xiv
New England Mix, xv
Pumpkin Pie Spice, xvi
Savory Seasoning, xi
Simple Cinnamon Sugar, xvi

E

Easy Herbes de Provence, xii
Egg Salad, 117

EGGS
Egg Salad, 117
It's My Pie; Nacho Pie, 50
You Can't Name Everything After
    Bob Potato Salad, 59

English Muffins, xxi
Evening-After Dressing, 79
The Evening-After Salad, 79

F

FISH & SEAFOOD
Agave Shrimp, 102
All Hail the Caesar Salad, 66
Boil Bonus Soup, 142
The Mile High Boil, 138
Partial to Panko Fish, 158
Tony's Tuna Casserole, 230
Tuna Salad, 118

Frankenstein's Bowties, 226

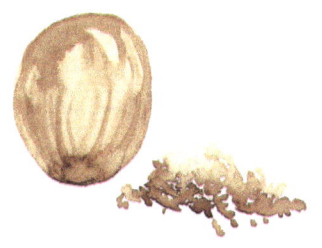

FRUIT (IN ANY FORM)
Amalgamation Cookies, 253
Apricot Ice Cream with Spicy
    Almond Crunch, 279
Banana Muffincakes, 266
Cherry Ginger Oatmeal Cookies, 254
Cran-Apple Streusel Pie, 199
Cranberry Cheesecake, 195
Cranberry Spinach Salad, 143
German Chocolate Sauce, 274
The Half-Pound Cake, 198
Joyful Almond Tart, 264
Key Lime Pie Ice Cream, 284
Naked Ambrosia, 68
Nirvana Newtons, 258

Index   315
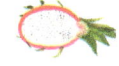

P. D. G. Crisp, 262
Post-Watergate Chicken Salad, 56
Pucker Up, Buttercup!, 283
Pumpkin Sparkle Pie, 204
R2-DChews, 7
Skippy the Jedi Droid's
    Powerful Force Cookies, 247
Smells Like Yummy Fig Jam, 258
Snickers Salad. 147
Uncle Donny's Tropical Apple
    Cider Punch, 145
Walter's Favorite Cranberry
    Relish, 192

Fruity Martuity, 36
Fudge Bomb Brownies, 52

G

German Chocolate Sauce, 274
Giant Funky Ham Sandwich, 122
Green Chile Dip, 3
Guacamole, 5

H

Hail Caesar Dressing, 66
Halfling Alert Pie Crust, xix
Halfling Alert Taters, 89
Halfling/Monster Mac & Cheese, 232
The Half-Pound Cake, 198
Ham Salad, 117
Hasperat, 120
Hearty Bacony Mac & Cheese, 223
Hidden Treasure Meatloaf, 156
Honey Mustard Sauce, 113
Horsey Mayo, 114

HOT SIDES
Búho Beans, 92
Calabacitas, 104
Caulisprouts, 186
Halfling Alert Taters, 89
Lobo Beets & Greens, 90
Mellow Mexican Rice, 84
Roasted Baby Carrots, 184
Roasted Tiny Trees, 87
Sam's Fairly Large Crowd
    Po—ta—toes, 183
Sandia Spoon Bread, 86
Spinach au Gratin, 188
Tequila Peppers, 85
Valentine's Day Taters, 73
Very Versatile Vegetables, 96

Hot Tamale, 42

I

ICE CREAM
Apricot Ice Cream with Spicy
    Almond Crunch, 279
Isabella's Pumpkin Pie Ice
    Cream, 208
Key Lime Pie Ice Cream, 284
Pretzel Nut Ice Cream, 280
Pucker Up, Buttercup!, 283
Salty Goodness Caramel, 284
Tres Leches Ice Cream with
    Chili Pecans, 281
Your Basic Vanilla Ice Cream, 278

Isabella's Pumpkin Pie Ice Cream, 208
I Said Yeah, Yeah, Yeah Brown
    Sugar Sauce, 273
It's My Pie; Nacho Pie, 50

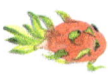

J

Jackie D's Nancy Drew, 27
Jakkubano, 124
Jan's Moon Shadows, 255
J.D.'s Awesome Appletini, 38

JICAMA
Mexican Flag Salad, 240

Joyful Almond Tart, 264
Just Another Tequila Sunrise, 42
Just the Basics, xiv

K

Key Lime Pie Ice Cream, 284
Kickin' Moscow Mule, 28

L

Lemon Cake, 32
Lobelia's Fudge Sauce, 271
Lobo Beets & Greens, 90

M

Magical Mythical Garlic: Elephant Roast, xviii
Magical Mythical Garlic: Regular Roast, xvii

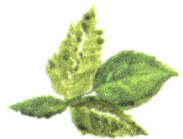

MAIN DISHES
Beefy Enchiladas, 152
Bob's Favorite Bowl, 238
Bodacious Brisket, 160
Callista's Birthday Pizza, 177
Hidden Treasure Meatloaf, 156
It's My Pie; Nacho Pie, 50
Marcella's Flat Enchiladas, 167
The Mile High Boil, 138
NMNYBEP, 9
The One-Bowl Thanksgiving Leftover Casserole, 192
Partial to Panko Fish, 158
"Perhaps This Chicken Needs Paprika?", 154
Savory Seasoning Pork Chops, 162
Steaks with Benefits, 72
Taco Rice Casserole, 164
Taco Tuesday Tacos, 171
Thank Goodness for Enchilada Casseroles, 194
Truth or Consequences Stuffed Peppers, 165
Ultimate Nachos, 46
Vader's Killer Taters, 174
The Whole Enchilada, 170
Zaragoza's Lasagna, 100

Manhattan Madness, 36
Marcella's Flat Enchiladas, 167
Marvelous Margarita, 40
Mellow Mexican Rice, 84
Mexican Flag Salad, 240
Mexican Mix, xiv
The Mile High Boil, 138

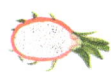

Index 317

MISCELLANEOUS
   Halfling Alert Pie Crust, xix
   Magical Mythical Garlic:
      Elephant Roast, xviii
   Magical Mythical Garlic:
      Regular Roast, xvii
   Nuts for You, 276
   Pepitas Honey Butter, 208
   Rich Simple Syrup, 22
   Roasted Green Chile: A Big
      Bunch of Chiles, xxvi
   Roasted Green Chile: Just a
      Few Chiles, xxvi
   Smells Like Yummy Fig Jam, 258

Mmm... Mocha Sauce, 275
Mom's Bell Pepper, 133
Mom's Spicy Meatballs, 2
The More Mature Scherbatsky, 38

N

Naked Ambrosia, 68
Negroni Spritzie, 24
New England Mix, xv
Nirvana Newtons, 258
NMNYBEP, 9
NMNYBEP Soup, 11

NUTS
   Apricot Ice Cream with Spicy
      Almond Crunch, 279
   Banana Muffincakes, 266
   Blondie Rapture, 257
   Bob's Favorite Cake, 241
   Cherry Ginger Oatmeal Cookies, 254
   Chocolate Chip Cookies, 250
   Chocolate Chips in a Pan, 260
   Cran-Apple Streusel Pie, 199
   Cranberry Spinach Salad, 143
   The Evening-After Salad, 79
   Fudge Bomb Brownies, 52
   German Chocolate Sauce, 274
   Isabella's Pumpkin Pie Ice
      Cream, 208
   Jan's Moon Shadows, 255
   Joyful Almond Tart, 264
   Naked Ambrosia, 68
   Nirvana Newtons, 258
   Nuts for You, 276
   P. D. G. Crisp, 262
   Peanut Butter Cup Sauce, 272
   Pecan Pie, 12
   Perfect Polvorones, 252
   Post-Watergate Chicken Salad, 56
   Pretzel Nut Ice Cream, 280
   Pucker Up, Buttercup!, 283
   Pumpkin Pancakes, 210
   Pumpkin Sparkle Pie, 204
   Roasted Tiny Trees, 87
   Skippy the Jedi Droid's
      Powerful Force Cookies, 247
   Tres Leches Ice Cream with
      Chili Pecans, 281
   Truth or Consequences Stuffed
      Peppers, 165
   Walter's Favorite Cranberry
      Relish, 192
   Warren's Pumpkin Cheesecake, 202
   William's Chili Pumpkin Bread
      with Pepitas Honey Butter, 207

Nuts for You, 276

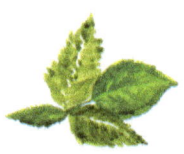

O

Old-Fogey-Fashioned, 37
The One-Bowl Thanksgiving
    Leftover Casserole, 192

ONION (ALL VARIETIES, BUT ONLY IF THEY ARE RATHER PROMINENT IN A DISH)
    Agave Shrimp, 102
    Cajun-Style Fettuccine, 219
    Caulisprouts, 186
    Chloë's Grits Dressing, 190
    Lobo Beets & Greens, 90
    Roast Beef & Gorgonzola
        Sandwich, 126
    Tauntaun Wontons, 128
    Three Bean Salad, 62
    Upscale Mac & Cheese, 220

Ooooo-ti-ni!, 30

P

Partial to Panko Fish, 158

PASTA
    Bacon Mac Salad, 63
    Cajun-Style Fettuccine, 219
    Creamy Dreamy Mac & Cheese, 225
    Frankenstein's Bowties, 226
    Halfling/Monster Mac & Cheese, 232
    Hearty Bacony Mac & Cheese, 223
    Santa Fe Fettuccine, 224
    Saucy Soupy Mac & Cheese, 218
    Sheldon's Spaghetti, 229
    Spaghetti Western, 216
    Tony's Tuna Casserole, 230
    Upscale Mac & Cheese, 220
    Vodka Penne, 222
    Zaragoza's Lasagna, 100

P. D. G. Crisp, 262
Peanut Butter Cup Sauce, 272

PEAS
    Frankenstein's Bowties, 226
    Tony's Tuna Casserole, 230

Pecan Pie, 12
Pepitas Honey Butter, 208
Perfect Polvorones, 252
"Perhaps This Chicken Needs
    Paprika?", 154
Perky Pico de Gallo, xxix
Pesto Mayo, 114

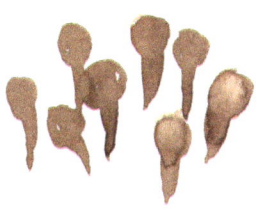

PICKLES (HOMEMADE OR PURCHASED)
    Giant Funky Ham Sandwich, 122
    Ham Salad, 117
    Hasperat, 120
    Tuna Salad, 118
    You Can't Name Everything After
        Bob Potato Salad, 59

PIES (ONLY SWEET)
    Cran-Apple Streusel Pie, 199
    Cyrus's No-Bake Pumpkin Tarts, 203
    Pecan Pie, 12
    Pumpkin Sparkle Pie, 204

Index 319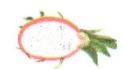

PIMIENTOS
    Hearty Bacony Mac & Cheese, 223
    Tony's Tuna Casserole, 230

PORK & HAM
    Boil Bonus Soup, 142
    Chloë's Grits Dressing, 190
    Frankenstein's Bowties, 226
    Giant Funky Ham Sandwich, 122
    Ham Salad, 117
    Hidden Treasure Meatloaf, 156
    Jakkubano, 124
    The Mile High Boil, 138
    Mom's Spicy Meatballs, 2
    NMNYBEP, 9
    NMNYBEP Soup, 11
    "Perhaps This Chicken Needs
        Paprika?", 154
    Savory Seasoning Pork Chops, 162
    Tauntaun Wontons, 128
    Vader's Killer Taters, 174
    Vodka Penne, 222
    Zaragoza's Lasagna, 100

Post-Watergate Chicken Salad, 56

POTATOES (ALL VARIETIES)
    Bob's Favorite Bowl, 238
    Boil Bonus Soup, 142
    Halfling Alert Taters, 89
    The Mile High Boil, 138
    The One-Bowl Thanksgiving
        Leftover Casserole, 192
    Sam's Fairly Large Crowd
        Po—ta—toes, 183
    Vader's Killer Taters, 174
    Valentine's Day Taters, 73
    You Can't Name Everything After
        Bob Potato Salad, 59

Potato Sauce, 141
Pretzel Nut Ice Cream, 280
Pucker Up, Buttercup!, 283
Puebla Coleslaw, 105

PUMPKIN
    Cyrus's No-Bake Pumpkin Tarts, 203
    Isabella's Pumpkin Pie Ice
        Cream, 208
    Pumpkin Pancakes, 210
    Pumpkin Sparkle Pie, 204
    Warren's Pumpkin Cheesecake, 202
    William's Chili Pumpkin Bread
        with Pepitas Honey Butter, 207

Pumpkin Pancakes, 210
Pumpkin Pie Spice, xvi
Pumpkin Sparkle Pie, 204

R2-DChews, 7
Red Chile Sauce, xxviii

RICE
    Mellow Mexican Rice, 84

Rich Simple Syrup, 22
Roast Beef & Gorgonzola Sandwich, 126
Roasted Baby Carrots, 184
Roasted Green Chile: A Big
    Bunch of Chiles, xxvi
Roasted Green Chile: Just a
    Few Chiles, xxvi
Roasted Tiny Trees, 87

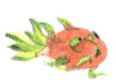

S

SALAD DRESSINGS
Evening-After Dressing, 79
Hail Caesar Dressing, 66
Savory Seasoning Ranch Dressing, 65

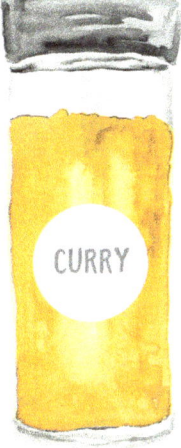

Salty Goodness Caramel, 284
Sam's Fairly Large Crowd Po—ta—toes, 183
Sandia Spoon Bread, 86

SANDWICHES
Burque Turkey, 133
Burqueño Beef, 134
Chile Joes, 131
Giant Funky Ham Sandwich, 122
Hasperat, 120
Jakkubano, 124
Roast Beef & Gorgonzola Sandwich, 126

Santa Fe Fettuccine, 224

SAUCES, RELISHES, AND DIPS (ONLY SAVORY)
Chile con Queso, 6
Chipotle Mayo, 115
Corn Sauce, 140
Green Chile Dip, 3
Guacamole, 5
Honey Mustard Sauce, 113
Horsey Mayo, 114
Perky Pico de Gallo, xxix
Pesto Mayo, 114
Potato Sauce, 141
Red Chile Sauce, xxviii
Sausage Sauce, 140
Shrimp Sauce, 140
Smoky BBQ Sauce, 113
Sriracha Mayo, 114
Tomatillo Salsa, 48
Tomato Mayo, 115

SAUCES, RELISHES, AND DIPS (ONLY SWEET)
German Chocolate Sauce, 274
I Said Yeah, Yeah, Yeah Brown Sugar Sauce, 273
Lobelia's Fudge Sauce, 271
Mmm... Mocha Sauce, 275
Peanut Butter Cup Sauce, 272
Silk Satin Sauce, 270
Walter's Favorite Cranberry Relish, 192
White Chocolate Sauce, 272

Saucy Soupy Mac & Cheese, 218
Sausage Sauce, 140
Savory Seasoning, xi
Savory Seasoning Pork Chops, 162
Savory Seasoning Ranch Dressing, 65
Screaming Orgasm, 34

Index 321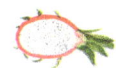

Sheldon's Spaghetti, 229
Shrimp Sauce, 140
Silk Satin Sauce, 270
Simple Cinnamon Sugar, xvi
Skippy the Jedi Droid's
   Powerful Force Cookies, 247
Sloe Your Roll Fizz, 28
Smells Like Yummy Fig Jam, 258
Smoky BBQ Sauce, 113
Snickers Salad, 147

SOUP
   Boil Bonus Soup, 142
   NMNYBEP Soup, 11

Spaghetti Western, 216

SPINACH
   Cranberry Spinach Salad, 143
   Spinach au Gratin, 188
   Super Savory Salad, 64

Spinach au Gratin, 188

SQUASH (ALL VARIETIES)
   Calabacitas, 104

Sriracha Mayo, 114
Steaks with Benefits, 72
Super Savory Salad, 64
Super Snickerdoodles, 251

T

Taco Rice Casserole, 164
Taco Tuesday Tacos, 171
Tauntaun Wontons, 128
Tequila Peppers, 85

Thank Goodness for Enchilada
   Casseroles, 194
Three Bean Salad, 62
Tickin' Time Bomb, 29
Tomatillo Salsa, 48
Tomato Mayo, 115

TOMATOES
   Black Bean Salad, 58
   Calabacitas, 104
   Chile con Queso, 6
   Guacamole, 5
   Mellow Mexican Rice, 84
   Perky Pico de Gallo, xxix
   Santa Fe Fettuccine, 224
   Sheldon's Spaghetti, 229
   Spaghetti Western, 216
   Vodka Penne, 222

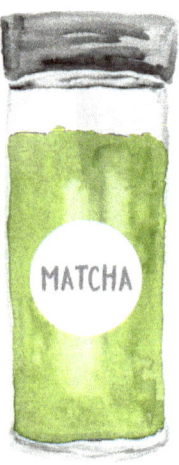

Tony's Tuna Casserole, 230
Tres Leches Ice Cream with
   Chili Pecans, 281
Truth or Consequences Stuffed
   Peppers, 165
Tuna Salad, 118

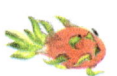

U

Ultimate Nachos, 46
Uncle Donny's Tropical Apple
    Cider Punch, 145
Upscale Mac & Cheese, 220

V

Vader's Killer Taters, 174
Valentine's Day Taters, 73
Very Versatile Vegetables, 96
Vodka Penne, 222

W

Walter's Favorite Cranberry Relish, 192
Warren's Pumpkin Cheesecake, 202
The Watergate, 43
White Chocolate Sauce, 272
The Whole Enchilada, 170
William's Chili Pumpkin Bread
    with Pepitas Honey Butter, 207

X

XOXO, 78

Y

You Can't Name Everything After
    Bob Potato Salad, 59
Your Basic Vanilla Ice Cream, 278

Z

Zaragoza's Lasagna, 100

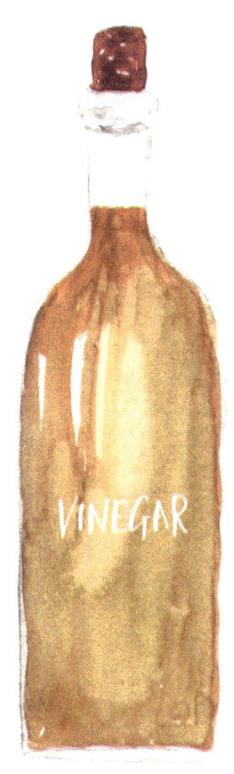
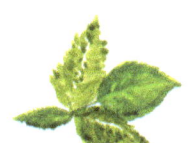

Author's Biography

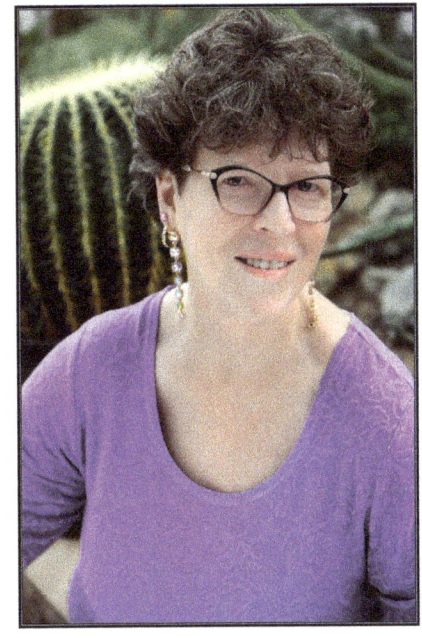

ASTRID TUTTLE WINEGAR is the author of the *Cooking for Halflings & Monsters* series. She is a nerd and a geek, but only in the most positive senses of the words. She loves Star things, both Trek and Wars. She loves J. R. R. Tolkien. She cooks and bakes too much, reads too much, watches television shows and movies way too much, then she writes about all of these activities in comfy, cozy cookbooks. She lives in Albuquerque, New Mexico, which is otherwise known as the Land of Enchantment.

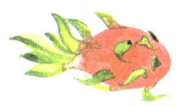

Her first book, *Cooking for Halflings & Monsters: 111 Comfy, Cozy Recipes for Fantasy-Loving Souls,* was a finalist in the 2018 New Mexico/Arizona Book Awards. Her second book, *Cooking for Halflings & Monsters, Volume 2: A Year of Comfy, Cozy Soups, Stews, and Chilis,* was a finalist in the 2020 New Mexico Press Women's Communications Contest and the 2020 New Mexico/Arizona Book Awards. She holds bachelor's and master's degrees from the University of New Mexico. For more information, go to astridwinegar.com.

ETSY SHOP: Elegant Sufficiencies
FACEBOOK: Astrid Tuttle Winegar
INSTAGRAM: a111tw

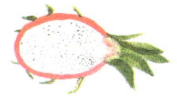

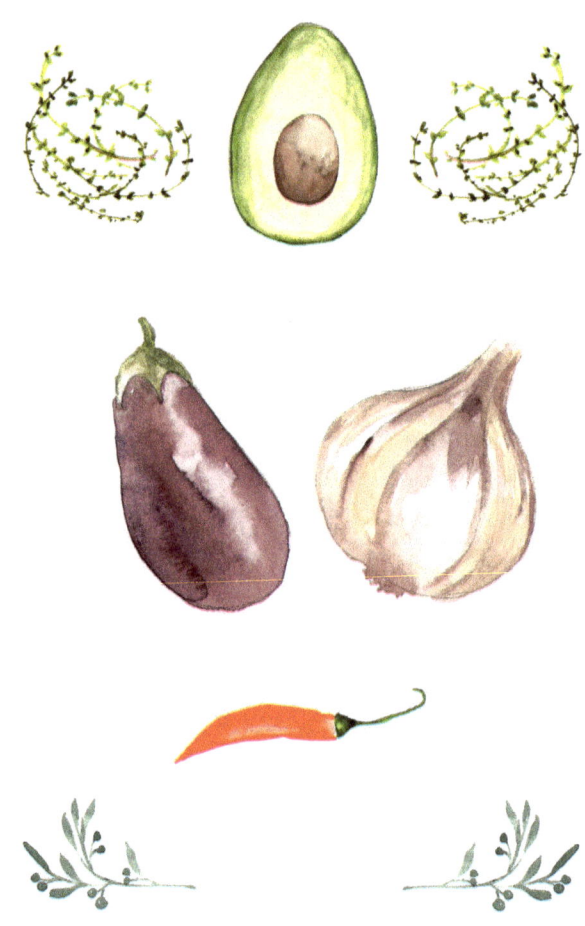

www.ingramcontent.com/pod-product-compliance
Lightning Source LLC
Chambersburg PA
CBHW061152010526
44118CB00027B/2946